COUNSELS ON HEALTH

Counsels on Health

and Instruction to
Medical Missionary
Workers

by

ELLEN G. WHITE

A compilation from the published writings of Mrs. White as found in her books, leaflets, and periodical articles covering a period of over fifty years.

"Incline thine ear unto My sayings."
"For they are life unto those that find them, and health to all their flesh."
Proverbs 4:20, 22.

PACIFIC PRESS® PUBLISHING ASSOCIATION
Nampa, Idaho
Oshawa, Ontario, Canada

Cover design by Willie Duke
Cover illustration by Lee Christiansen

ISBN 13: 978-0-8163-1926-8
ISBN 10: 0-8163-1926-X

08 09 10 11 12 • 6 5 4 3 2

PREFACE

In the lobby of the White Memorial Hospital, which was founded in memory of the writer of the "Counsels" which compose this book, is a bronze tablet bearing the inscription:

"This hospital is dedicated to the memory of Ellen Gould White, whose long life was unselfishly devoted to the alleviation of the woes and sorrows of the sick, the suffering, and the needy; and to inspiring young men and women to consecrate their lives to the work of Him who said, 'Heal the sick.'"

To those who knew Mrs. White these words are freighted with tender memories of almost countless incidents in the life of that most kindly soul. Of the women who have lived in modern days, no other, in all probability, has exercised so deep and lasting an influence upon the lives of her fellows as Ellen G. White. In no realm were her teachings more far-reaching and thorough than in that relating to the care of the body—the temple of the Holy Spirit.

From many and varied sources, during the last half century, a flood of light has been thrown upon this important theme. From out the mind of the renowned Pasteur came shafts of light of brilliant and penetrating power on matters relating to health and disease. From him the world received its knowledge of bacteria, the causative factors of so many diseases. From Louis Pasteur came the cure that conquered anthrax, that devastating sickness afflicting both man and beast. He it was whose unremitting toil culminated in the discovery of a cure for hydrophobia, one of the most dread diseases of all the ages.

Lord Lister, by applying the principles of Pasteur to the operating room, made surgery safe for mankind. His genius transformed hospitals from being shambles of horror and gangrene to places of comfort and cure. He demonstrated that pus in surgical wounds is unnecessary, and reduced surgical mortality to a relatively insignificant figure.

Then there was Semmelweiss, the obstetrician, to whom Kugelmann wrote: "With few exceptions the world has crucified and burned its benefactors. I hope you will not grow weary in the honorable fight which still remains before you." It was this Semmelweiss who wrestled with the dread monster of puerperal fever, and through whose brain there throbbed the queries: "Why do these mothers die? What is childbirth fever?" His efforts cost his life, but he conquered the fearful malady.

And I might continue to tell of the blessings the world has received at the hands of many others, from Koch, Ehrlich, Nicolaier, Kitasato, Von Behring, Flexner, Ronald Ross, and many another. But to Ellen G. White a different role was given. While her lifework and teaching were in harmony with truly scientific medicine, it was in the realm of the spiritual side of the healing art that she shone with a brilliance of holy luster. In the matter of appealing to men and women to regard their bodies as a sacred trust from the Highest One, and to obey the laws of nature and of nature's God, she stands without a peer. She it was who exalted the sacredness of the body and the necessity of bringing all the appetites and passions under the control of an enlightened conscience. Others emphasized science in health; to her it was left to impress the spiritual in the treatment of the temple of the body.

No other one of modern day has entered this field of spiritual endeavor to anything like the extent she did. Her efforts were tireless from the days of her young womanhood to the hour of her death at a very advanced age. In books, in magazine articles, in papers, in tracts and pamphlets, she constantly and unswervingly called men and women, old and young, in clarion tones, to a more rational, a higher, purer plane of spiritual living. From the platform in churches and lecture halls, at convocations and conferences, her voice was continually heard urging the need of consecrated, Christian living in things relating to the body and its care. Others brought to light scientific facts concerning disease, its cause, and its cure; Ellen G White drove home those facts on the spiritual side to the innermost citadel of the souls of men and women.

It is fitting, therefore, that though she sleeps in her quiet grave, her tired hands folded across the sainted breast, her works should follow her. It is meet that in this volume her "Counsels" should live, to bless, to fortify, and to direct the lives of those who seek to point their fellow beings to that blest One who alone has healing in His wings.

It was the apostle Paul who wrote in his second letter to the youthful Timothy:

"In a great house there are not only vessels of gold and of silver, but also of wood and of earth; and some to honor, and some to dishonor. If a man therefore purge himself from these, he shall be a vessel unto honor, sanctified, and meet for the Master's use, and prepared unto every good work."

Paul wrote especially concerning the members of the Lord's church. But how wonderfully applicable also are the words to the human stones which form the structure of the great house of the healing art on earth today! In it there are doctors and nurses of gold, and doctors and nurses of silver, doctors and nurses of wood and of earth, and some to honor and some to dishonor. To purify the great house of healing, to help to mold it after the similitude of the Mighty Healer, is the object of "Counsels."

In this sordid day, when everything that was once sacred is being commercialized, when the golden calf is being worshiped on every hand, there are and ever will be some men and women wistfully longing for the highest ideals that properly belong with a profession second in sacredness only to the ministry of the word of God. In the hope and with the simple prayer that this volume may contribute to the purest and most unselfish profession of medicine, it is now launched upon its mission.

PERCY T. MAGAN.

Preface to the Second Edition

The Trustees are pleased to bring forth the second edition of *Counsels on Health.* Issued first in 1923, this compilation of E. G. White writings on the subject of health proved to be an indispensable reference work, and the first edition in its several printings far exceeded expectations for its distribution. The text of the book is unchanged, and the original paging has been maintained. A new feature which will be much appreciated by the careful student is the inclusion of the date of writing or of first publication which appears in connection with source reference to each article. That this volume in its reissued form may continue to fill an important place in keeping before the church and its ministerial and medical workers the significant place of our health message is the sincere wish of the publishers and—

THE TRUSTEES OF THE
ELLEN G. WHITE PUBLICATIONS.

Washington, D.C.
January 29, 1957.

CONTENTS

SECTION III. DIET AND HEALTH

SECTION IV. OUTDOOR LIFE AND PHYSICAL ACTIVITY

SECTION V. SANITARIUMS—THEIR OBJECTS AND AIMS

SECTION VI. SUCCESSFUL INSTITUTIONAL WORK

Section VII. THE CHRISTIAN PHYSICIAN

Section VIII. NURSES AND HELPERS

Section IX. TEACHING HEALTH PRINCIPLES

SECTION XII. ENSAMPLES TO THE FLOCK

SECTION XIII. HOLINESS OF LIFE

THE WORLD'S NEED

Multitudes in Distress

When Christ saw the multitudes that gathered about Him, "He was moved with compassion on them, because they fainted, and were scattered abroad, as sheep having no shepherd." Christ saw the sickness, the sorrow, the want and degradation of the multitudes that thronged His steps. To Him were presented the needs and woes of humanity throughout the world. Among the high and the low, the most honored and the most degraded, He beheld souls who were longing for the very blessing He had come to bring; souls who needed only a knowledge of His grace, to become subjects of His kingdom. "Then saith He unto His disciples, The harvest truly is plenteous, but the laborers are few; pray ye therefore the Lord of the harvest, that He will send forth laborers into His harvest." Matthew 9:36-38.

Today the same needs exist. The world is in need of workers who will labor as Christ did for the suffering and the sinful. There is indeed a multitude to be reached. The world is full of sickness, suffering, distress, and sin. It is full of those who need to be ministered unto—the weak, the helpless, the ignorant, the degraded.

In the Path of Destruction

Many of the youth of this generation, in the midst of churches, religious institutions, and professedly Christian

Testimonies for the Church, vol. 6, pp. 254-258 (1900).

homes, are choosing the path to destruction. Through intemperate habits they bring upon themselves disease, and through greed to obtain money for sinful indulgences they fall into dishonest practices. Health and character are ruined. Aliens from God, and outcasts from society, these poor souls feel that they are without hope either for this life or for the life to come. The hearts of parents are broken. Men speak of these erring ones as hopeless; but God looks upon them with pitying tenderness. He understands all the circumstances that have led them to fall under temptation. This is a class that demands labor.

Poverty and Sin Abound

Nigh and afar off are souls, not only the youth but those of all ages, who are in poverty and distress, sunken in sin, and weighed down with a sense of guilt. It is the work of God's servants to seek for these souls, to pray with them and for them, and lead them step by step to the Saviour.

But those who do not recognize the claims of God are not the only ones who are in distress and in need of help. In the world today, where selfishness, greed, and oppression rule, many of the Lord's true children are in need and affliction. In lowly, miserable places, surrounded with poverty, disease, and guilt, many are patiently bearing their own burden of suffering, and trying to comfort the hopeless and sin-stricken about them. Many of them are almost unknown to the churches or to the ministers; but they are the Lord's lights, shining amid the darkness. For these the Lord has a special care, and He calls upon His people to be His helping hand in relieving their wants. Wherever there is a church, special attention should be given to searching out this class and ministering to them.

Needs of the Rich

And while working for the poor, we should give attention also to the rich, whose souls are equally precious in the sight of God. Christ worked for all who would hear His word. He sought not only the publican and the outcast, but the rich and cultured Pharisee, the Jewish nobleman, and the Roman ruler. The wealthy man needs to be labored for in the love and fear of God. Too often he trusts in his riches, and feels not his danger. The worldly possessions which the Lord has entrusted to men are often a source of great temptation. Thousands are thus led into sinful indulgences that confirm them in habits of intemperance and vice.

Among the wretched victims of want and sin are found many who were once in possession of wealth. Men of different vocations and different stations in life have been overcome by the pollutions of the world, by the use of strong drink, by indulgence in the lusts of the flesh, and have fallen under temptation. While these fallen ones excite our pity and demand our help, should not some attention be given also to those who have not yet descended to these depths, but who are setting their feet in the same path? There are thousands occupying positions of honor and usefulness who are indulging habits that mean ruin to soul and body. Should not the most earnest effort be made to enlighten them?

Ministers of the gospel, statesmen, authors, men of wealth and talent, men of vast business capacity and power for usefulness, are in deadly peril because they do not see the necessity of strict temperance in all things.

They need to have their attention called to the principles of temperance, not in a narrow or arbitrary way, but in the light of God's great purpose for humanity. Could the principles of true temperance be thus brought before them, there are very many of the higher classes who would recognize their value and give them a hearty acceptance.

Durable Riches for Earthly Treasure

There is another danger to which the wealthy classes are especially exposed, and here also is a field for the work of the medical missionary. Multitudes who are prosperous in the world and who never stoop to the common forms of vice are yet brought to destruction through the love of riches. Absorbed in their worldly treasures, they are insensible to the claims of God and the needs of their fellow men. Instead of regarding their wealth as a talent to be used for the glory of God and the uplifting of humanity, they look upon it as a means of indulging and glorifying themselves. They add house to house and land to land, they fill their homes with luxuries, while want stalks the streets and all about them are human beings in misery and crime, in disease and death. Those who thus give their lives to self-serving are developing in themselves, not the attributes of God, but the attributes of Satan.

These men are in need of the gospel. They need to have their eyes turned from the vanity of material things to behold the preciousness of the enduring riches. They need to learn the joy of giving, the blessedness of being co-workers with God.

Persons of this class are often the most difficult of access, but Christ will open ways whereby they may be reached. Let the wisest, the most trustful, the most hopeful laborers seek for these souls. With the wisdom and tact born of divine love, with the refinement and courtesy that result alone from the presence of Christ in the soul, let them work for those who, dazzled by the glitter of earthly riches, see not the glory of the heavenly treasure. Let the workers study the Bible with them, pressing sacred truth home to their hearts. Read to them the words of God: "But of Him are ye in Christ Jesus, who of God is made unto us wisdom, and righteousness, and sanctification, and redemption." "Thus saith the Lord, Let not the wise man glory in his wisdom, neither let the mighty man glory in his might, let not the rich man glory in his riches: but let him that glorieth glory in this, that he understandeth and knoweth Me, that I am the Lord which exercise loving-kindness, judgment, and righteousness, in the earth: for in these things I delight, saith the Lord." "In whom we have redemption through His blood, the forgiveness of sins, according to the riches of His grace." "But my God shall supply all your need according to His riches in glory by Christ Jesus." 1 Corinthians 1:30; Jeremiah 9:23, 24; Ephesians 1:7; Philippians 4:19.

Such an appeal, made in the spirit of Christ, will not be thought impertinent. It will impress the minds of many in the higher classes.

By efforts put forth in wisdom and love, many a rich man may be awakened to a sense of his responsibility and his accountability to God. When it is made plain that the Lord expects them as His representatives to relieve suffering humanity, many will respond, and will give of their means and their sympathy for the benefit of the poor. When their minds are thus drawn away from their own selfish interests, many will be led to surrender themselves to Christ. With their talents of influence and means they will gladly unite in the work of beneficence with the humble missionary who was God's agent in their conversion. By a right use of their earthly treasure they will lay up "a treasure in the heavens that faileth not, where no thief approacheth, neither moth corrupteth." They will secure for themselves the treasure that wisdom offers, even "durable riches and righteousness."

A Degenerate Race

The present enfeebled condition of the human family was presented before me. Every generation has been growing weaker, and disease of every form afflicts the race. Thousands of poor mortals with deformed, sickly bodies, shattered nerves, and gloomy minds are dragging out a miserable existence. Satan's power upon the human family increases. If the Lord should not soon come and destroy his power, the earth would erelong be depopulated.

I was shown that Satan's power is especially exercised upon the people of God. Many were presented before me in a doubting despairing condition. The infirmities of the body affect the mind. A cunning and powerful enemy attends our steps, and employs his strength and skill in trying to turn us out of the right way. And it is too often the case that the people of God are not on their watch, therefore are ignorant of his devices. He works by means which will best conceal himself from view, and he often gains his object.—*Testimonies for the Church*, vol. 1, p. 304 (1862).

The Violation of Physical Law

Man came from the hand of his Creator perfect in organization and beautiful in form. The fact that he has for six thousand years withstood the ever-increasing weight of disease and crime is conclusive proof of the power of endurance with which he was first endowed. And although the antediluvians generally gave themselves up to sin without restraint, it was more than two thousand years before the violation of natural law was sensibly felt. Had Adam originally possessed no greater physical power than men now have, the race would ere this have become extinct.

Through the successive generations since the Fall, the tendency has been continually downward. Disease has been transmitted from parents to children, generation after generation. Even infants in the cradle suffer from afflictions caused by the sins of their parents. . . .

The patriarchs from Adam to Noah, with few exceptions, lived nearly a thousand years. Since then the average length of life has been decreasing.

At the time of Christ's first advent, the race had already so degenerated that not only the old, but the middle-aged and the young, were brought from every city to the Saviour, to be healed of their diseases. Many labored under a weight of misery inexpressible.

The violation of physical law, with its consequent suffering and premature death, has so long prevailed that these results are regarded as the appointed lot of humanity; but God did not create the race in such a feeble condition. This state of things is not the work of Providence, but of man. It has been brought about by wrong habits

---

Christian Temperance, pages 7-12 (1890).

—by violating the laws that God has made to govern man's existence. A continual transgression of nature's laws is a continual transgression of the law of God. Had men always been obedient to the law of the Ten Commandments, carrying out in their lives the principles of those precepts, the curse of disease now flooding the world would not exist. . . .

When men take any course which needlessly expends their vitality or beclouds their intellect, they sin against God; they do not glorify Him in their body and spirit, which are His. Yet despite the insult which man has offered Him, God's love is still extended to the race, and He permits light to shine, enabling man to see that in order to live a perfect life he must obey the natural laws which govern his being. How important, then, that man should walk in this light, exercising all his powers, both of body and mind, to the glory of God!

God's People to Stand in Purity

We are in a world that is opposed to righteousness or purity of character, and especially to growth in grace. Wherever we look, we see defilement and corruption, deformity and sin. How opposed is all this to the work that must be accomplished in us just previous to receiving the gift of immortality! God's elect must stand untainted amid the corruptions teeming around them in these last days. Their bodies must be made holy, their spirits pure. If this work is to be accomplished, it must be undertaken at once, earnestly and understandingly. The Spirit of God should have perfect control, influencing every action.

The health reform is one branch of the great work which is to fit a people for the coming of the Lord. It is as closely connected with the third angel's message as the hand is with the body. The law of Ten Commandments has been lightly regarded by man; yet the Lord will not come to punish the transgressors of that law without first sending them a message of warning. Men and women cannot violate natural law by indulging depraved appetites and lustful passions, without violating the law of God. Therefore He has permitted the light of health reform to shine upon us, that we may realize the sinfulness of breaking the laws which He has established in our very being.

Our heavenly Father sees the deplorable condition of men who, many of them ignorantly, are disregarding the principles of hygiene. And it is in love and pity to the race that He causes the light to shine upon health reform. He publishes His law and its penalties, in order that all may learn what is for their highest good. He proclaims His law so distinctly, and makes it so prominent, that it is like a city set on a hill. All intelligent beings can understand it if they will. None others are responsible.

The Folly of Ignorance

To make natural law plain, and to urge obedience to it, is a work that accompanies the third angel's message. Ignorance is no excuse now for the transgression of law. The light shines clearly, and none need be ignorant; for the great God Himself is man's instructor. All are bound by the most sacred obligations to heed the sound philosophy and genuine experience which God is now giving them in reference to health reform. He designs that the subject shall be agitated and the public mind deeply stirred to investigate it; for it is impossible for men and women, while under the power of sinful, health-destroying, brain-enervating habits, to appreciate sacred truth.

Those who are willing to inform themselves concerning the effect which sinful indulgence has upon the health and who begin the work of reform, even from selfish motives, may in so doing place themselves where the truth of God can reach their hearts. And, on the other hand, those who have been reached by the presentation of Scripture truth, are in a position where the conscience may be aroused upon the subject of health. They see and feel the necessity of breaking away from the tyrannizing habits and appetites which have ruled them so long. There are many who would receive the truths of God's word, their judgment having been convinced by the clearest evidence; but the carnal desires, clamoring for gratification, control the intellect, and they reject truth because it conflicts with their lustful desires. The minds of many take so low a level that God cannot work either for them or with them. The current of their thoughts must be changed, their moral sensibilities must be aroused, before they can feel the claims of God.

The apostle Paul exhorts the church, "I beseech you therefore, brethren, by the mercies of God, that ye present your bodies a living sacrifice, holy, acceptable unto God, which is your reasonable service." Romans 12:1. Sinful indulgence defiles the body and unfits men for spiritual worship. He who cherishes the light which God has given him upon health reform has an important aid in the work of becoming sanctified through the truth, and fitted for immortality. But if he disregards that light and lives in violation of natural law, he must pay the penalty; his spiritual powers are benumbed, and how can he perfect holiness in the fear of God?

Men have polluted the soul temple, and God calls upon them to awake and to strive with all their might to win back their God-given manhood. Nothing but the grace of God can convict and convert the heart; from Him alone can the slaves of custom obtain power to break the shackles that bind them. It is impossible for a man to present his body a living sacrifice, holy, acceptable to God, while continuing to indulge habits that are depriving him of physical, mental, and moral vigor. Again the apostle says, "Be not conformed to this world: but be ye transformed by the renewing of your mind, that ye may prove what is that good, and acceptable, and perfect, will of God." Romans 12:2.

As in the Days of Noah

Jesus, seated on the Mount of Olives, gave instruction to His disciples concerning the signs which should precede His coming: "As the days of Noah were, so shall also the coming of the Son of man be. For as in the days that were before the Flood they were eating and drinking, marrying and giving in marriage, until the day that Noah entered into the ark, and knew not until the Flood came, and took them all away; so shall also the coming of the Son of man be." Matthew 24:37-39. The same sins that brought judgments upon the world in the days of Noah exist in our day. Men and women now carry their eating and drinking so far that it ends in gluttony and drunkenness. This prevailing sin, the indulgence of perverted appetite inflamed the passions of men in the days of Noah, and led to widespread corruption. Violence and sin reached to heaven. This moral pollution was finally swept from the earth by means of the Flood.

The same sins of gluttony and drunkenness benumbed the moral sensibilities of the inhabitants of Sodom, so that crime seemed to be the delight of the men and women of that wicked city. Christ thus warns the world: "Likewise also as it was in the days of Lot; they did eat, they drank, they bought, they sold, they planted, they builded; but the same day that Lot went out of Sodom it rained fire and brimstone from heaven, and destroyed them all. Even thus shall it be in the day when the Son of man is revealed." Luke 17:28-30.

Christ has left us here a most important lesson. He would lay before us the danger of making our eating and drinking paramount. He presents the result of unrestrained indulgence of appetite. The moral powers are enfeebled, so that sin does not appear sinful. Crime is lightly regarded, and passion controls the mind, until good principles and impulses are rooted out, and God is blasphemed. All this is the result of eating and drinking to excess. This is the very condition of things which Christ declares will exist at His second coming.

The Saviour presents to us something higher to toil for than merely what we shall eat and drink, and wherewithal we shall be clothed. Eating, drinking and dressing are carried to such excess that they become crimes. They are among the marked sins of the last days, and constitute a sign of Christ's soon coming. Time, money, and strength, which belong to the Lord, but which He has entrusted to us, are wasted in superfluities of dress and luxuries for the perverted appetite, which lessen vitality and bring suffering and decay. It is impossible to present our bodies a living sacrifice to God when we continually fill them with corruption and disease by our own sinful indulgence. Knowledge must be gained in regard to how to eat and drink and dress so as to preserve health. Sickness is the result of violating nature's law. Our first duty, one which we owe to God, to ourselves, and to our fellow men, is to obey the laws of God. These include the laws of health.

A Work of Reformation Needed

We are living in the midst of an "epidemic of crime," at which thoughtful, God-fearing men everywhere stand aghast. The corruption that prevails, it is beyond the power of the human pen to describe. Every day brings fresh revelations of political strife, bribery, and fraud. Every day brings its heart-sickening record of violence and lawlessness, of indifference to human suffering, of brutal, fiendish destruction of human life. Every day testifies to the increase of insanity, murder, and suicide. Who can doubt that satanic agencies are at work among men with increasing activity to distract and corrupt the mind, and defile and destroy the body?

And while the world is filled with these evils, the gospel is too often presented in so indifferent a manner as to make but little impression upon the consciences or the lives of men. Everywhere there are hearts crying out for something which they have not. They long for a power that will give them mastery over sin, a power that will deliver them from the bondage of evil, a power that will give health and life and peace. Many who once knew the power of God's word have dwelt where there is no recognition of God, and they long for the divine presence.

The world needs today what it needed nineteen hundred years ago—a revelation of Christ. A great work of reform is demanded, and it is only through the grace of Christ that the work of restoration, physical, mental, and spiritual, can be accomplished.—*The Ministry of Healing,* pages 142, 143 (1905).

The Outlook

The world is out of joint. As we look at the picture, the outlook seems discouraging. But Christ greets with hopeful assurance the very men and women who cause us discouragement. In them He sees qualifications that will enable them to take a place in His vineyard. If they will constantly be learners, through His providence He will make them men and women fitted to do a work that is not beyond their capabilities; through the impartation of the Holy Spirit, He will give them power of utterance.

Many of the barren, unworked fields must be entered by beginners. The brightness of the Saviour's view of the world will inspire confidence in many workers, who, if they begin in humility, and put their hearts into the work, will be found to be the right men for the time and place. Christ sees all the misery and despair of the world, the sight of which would bow down some of our workers of large capabilities with a weight of discouragement so great that they would not know how even to begin the work of leading men and women to the first round of the ladder. Their precise methods are of little value. They would stand above the lower rounds of the ladder, saying, "Come up where we are." But the poor souls do not know where to put their feet.

Christ's heart is cheered by the sight of those who are poor in every sense of the term; cheered by His view of the ill-used ones who are meek; cheered by the seemingly unsatisfied hungering after righteousness, by the inability of many to begin. He welcomes, as it were, the very condition of things that would discourage many ministers. He corrects our erring piety, giving the burden of the

Testimonies for the Church, vol. 7, pp. 271, 272 (1902).

(26)

work for the poor and needy in the rough places of the earth, to men and women who have hearts that can feel for the ignorant and for those that are out of the way. The Lord teaches these workers how to meet those whom He wishes them to help. They will be encouraged as they see doors opening for them to enter places where they can do medical missionary work. Having little self-confidence, they give God all the glory. Their hands may be rough and unskilled, but their hearts are susceptible to pity; they are filled with an earnest desire to do something to relieve the woe so abundant; and Christ is present to help them. He works through those who discern mercy in misery, gain in the loss of all things. When the Light of the world passes by, privileges appear in all hardships, order in confusion, the success and wisdom of God in that which has seemed to be a failure.

My brethren and sisters, in your ministry come close to the people. Uplift those who are cast down. Treat of calamities as disguised blessings, of woes as mercies. Work in a way that will cause hope to spring up in the place of despair. . . .

God the Source of Wisdom and Power

To every worker I would say: Go forth in humble faith, and the Lord will go with you. But watch unto prayer. This is the science of your labor. The power is of God. Work in dependence upon Him, remembering that you are laborers together with Him. He is your Helper. Your strength is from Him. He will be your wisdom, your righteousness, your sanctification, your redemption.

2—C.O.H.

Religion and Health

The view held by some that spirituality is a detriment to health, is the sophistry of Satan. The religion of the Bible is not detrimental to the health of either body or mind. The influence of the Spirit of God is the very best medicine for disease. Heaven is all health; and the more deeply heavenly influences are realized, the more sure will be the recovery of the believing invalid. The true principles of Christianity open before all a source of inestimable happiness. Religion is a continual wellspring, from which the Christian can drink at will and never exhaust the fountain.

The relation which exists between the mind and the body is very intimate. When one is affected, the other sympathizes. The condition of the mind affects the health of the physical system. If the mind is free and happy, from a consciousness of rightdoing and a sense of satisfaction in causing happiness to others, it creates a cheerfulness that will react upon the whole system, causing a freer circulation of the blood and a toning up of the entire body. The blessing of God is a healing power, and those who are abundant in benefiting others will realize that wondrous blessing in both heart and life.

When men who have indulged in wrong habits and sinful practices yield to the power of divine truth, the application of that truth to the heart revives the moral powers, which had seemed to be paralyzed. The receiver possesses stronger, clearer understanding than before he riveted his soul to the eternal Rock. Even his physical health improves by the realization of his security in Christ.

Christian Temperance, pages 13, 14 (1890).

The special blessing of God resting upon the receiver is of itself health and strength.

Those who walk in the path of wisdom and holiness find that "godliness is profitable unto all things, having promise of the life that now is, and of that which is to come." 1 Timothy 4:8. They are alive to the enjoyment of life's real pleasures, and are not troubled with vain regrets over misspent hours, nor with gloomy forebodings, as the worldling too often is when not diverted by some exciting amusement. Godliness does not conflict with the laws of health, but is in harmony with them. The fear of the Lord is the foundation of all real prosperity.

Christ's Love a Healing Power

When the gospel is received in its purity and power, it is a cure for the maladies that originated in sin. The Sun of Righteousness arises, "with healing in His wings." Malachi 4:2. Not all that this world bestows can heal a broken heart or impart peace of mind or remove care or banish disease. Fame, genius, talent—all are powerless to gladden the sorrowful heart or to restore the wasted life. The life of God in the soul is man's only hope.

The love which Christ diffuses through the whole being is a vitalizing power. Every vital part—the brain, the heart, the nerves—it touches with healing. By it the highest energies of the being are aroused to activity. It frees the soul from the guilt and sorrow, the anxiety and care, that crush the life forces. With it come serenity and composure. It implants in the soul joy that nothing earthly can destroy,—joy in the Holy Spirit,—health-giving, life-giving joy.—*The Ministry of Healing,* page 115 (1905).

Christ's Manner of Healing

This world is a vast lazar house, but Christ came to heal the sick, to proclaim deliverance to the captives of Satan. He was in Himself health and strength. He imparted His life to the sick, the afflicted, those possessed of demons. He turned away none who came to receive His healing power. He knew that those who petitioned Him for help had brought disease upon themselves, yet He did not refuse to heal them. And when virtue from Christ entered into these poor souls they were convicted of sin, and many were healed of their spiritual disease as well as of their physical maladies. The gospel still possesses the same power, and why should we not today witness the same results?

Christ feels the woes of every sufferer. When evil spirits rend a human frame, Christ feels the curse. When fever is burning up the life current, He feels the agony. And He is just as willing to heal the sick now as when He was personally on earth. Christ's servants are His representatives, the channels for His working. He desires through them to exercise His healing power.

In the Saviour's manner of healing there were lessons for His disciples. On one occasion He anointed the eyes of a blind man with clay and bade him, "Go, wash in the pool of Siloam. . . . He went his way therefore, and washed, and came seeing." John 9:7. The cure could be wrought only by the power of the Great Healer, yet Christ made use of the simple agencies of nature. While He did not give countenance to drug medication, He sanctioned the use of simple and natural remedies.

To many of the afflicted ones who received healing

The Desire of Ages, pages 823-825 (1898),

Christ said, "Sin no more, lest a worse thing come unto thee." John 5:14. Thus He taught that disease is the result of violating God's laws, both natural and spiritual. The great misery in the world would not exist, did men but live in harmony with the Creator's plan. . . .

These lessons are for us. There are conditions to be observed by all who would preserve health. All should learn what these conditions are. The Lord is not pleased with ignorance in regard to His laws, either natural or spiritual. We are to be workers together with God for the restoration of health to the body as well as to the soul.

And we should teach others how to preserve and to recover health. For the sick we should use the remedies which God has provided in nature, and we should point them to Him who alone can restore. It is our work to present the sick and suffering to Christ in the arms of our faith. We should teach them to believe in the Great Healer. We should lay hold on His promise and pray for the manifestation of His power. The very essence of the gospel is restoration, and the Saviour would have us bid the sick, the hopeless, and the afflicted take hold upon His strength.

The power of love was in all Christ's healing, and only by partaking of that love, through faith, can we be instruments for His work. If we neglect to link ourselves in divine connection with Christ, the current of life-giving energy cannot flow in rich streams from us to the people. There were places where the Saviour Himself could not do many mighty works because of their unbelief. So now unbelief separates the church from her divine Helper. Her hold upon eternal realities is weak. By her lack of faith, God is disappointed and robbed of His glory.

The Christian Physician as a Missionary

Those who have Christ abiding in the heart will have a love for the souls for whom He died. Those who have true love for Him will have an earnest desire to make His love comprehended by others.

I feel sad to see so few that have any real burden for their fellow men who are in darkness. Let not any truly converted soul settle down as a careless idler in the Master's vineyard. All power is given to Christ, in heaven and in earth, and He will impart strength to His followers for the great work of drawing men to Himself. He is constantly urging His human instrumentalities on their Heaven-appointed ways, in all the world, promising to be always with them. Heavenly intelligences—"ten thousand times ten thousand, and thousands of thousands" (Revelation 5:11)—are sent as messengers to the world, to unite with human agencies for the salvation of souls. Why does not our faith in the great truths that we bear, kindle a burning ardor upon the altar of our hearts? Why, I ask, in view of the greatness of these truths, are not all who profess to believe them inspired with missionary zeal, a zeal that must come to all who are laborers together with God?

Who Will Say, "Send Me"?

Christ's work is to be done. Let those who believe the truth consecrate themselves to God. Where there are now a few who are engaged in missionary work, there should be hundreds. Who will feel the importance, the divine greatness, of the call? Who will deny self? When the Saviour calls for workers, who will answer, "Here am I, send me"?

Medical Missionary, January, 1891.

There is need of both home and foreign missionaries. There is work right at hand that is strangely neglected by many. All who have tasted "the good word of God, and the powers of the world to come" (Hebrews 6:5), have a work to do for those in their homes and among their neighbors. The gospel of salvation must be proclaimed to others. Every man who has felt the converting power of God becomes in a sense a missionary. There are friends to whom he can speak of the love of God. He can tell in the church what the Lord is to him, even a personal Saviour; and the testimony given in simplicity may do more good than the most eloquent discourse. There is a great work to be done, too, in dealing justly with all and walking humbly with God. Those who are doing the work nearest them are gaining an experience that will fit them for a wider sphere of usefulness. There must be an experience in home missionary work as a preparation for foreign work.

The Care of the Sick

How shall the Lord's work be done? How can we gain access to souls buried in midnight darkness? Prejudice must be met; corrupt religion is hard to deal with. The very best ways and means of work must be prayerfully considered. There is a way in which many doors will be opened to the missionary. Let him become intelligent in the care of the sick, as a nurse, or learn how to treat disease, as a physician; and if he is imbued with the spirit of Christ, what a field of usefulness is opened before him!

Christ was the Saviour of the world. During His life on earth, the sick and afflicted were objects of His special compassion. When He sent out His disciples, He commissioned them to heal the sick as well as to preach the gospel. When He sent forth the seventy, He commanded them to heal the sick, and next to preach that the kingdom of God had come nigh unto them. Their physical health was to be first cared for, in order that the way might be prepared for the truth to reach their minds.

Christ's Method of Evangelism

The Saviour devoted more time and labor to healing the afflicted of their maladies than to preaching. His last injunction to His apostles, His representatives on earth, was to lay hands on the sick that they might recover. When the Master shall come, He will commend those who have visited the sick and relieved the necessities of the afflicted.

The tender sympathies of our Saviour were aroused for fallen and suffering humanity. If you would be His followers, you must cultivate compassion and sympathy. Indifference to human woes must give place to lively interest in the sufferings of others. The widow, the orphan, the sick and the dying, will always need help. Here is an opportunity to proclaim the gospel—to hold up Jesus, the hope and consolation of all men. When the suffering body has been relieved, and you have shown a lively interest in the afflicted, the heart is opened, and you can pour in the heavenly balm. If you are looking to Jesus and drawing from Him knowledge and strength and grace, you can impart His consolation to others, because the Comforter is with you.

You will meet with much prejudice, a great deal of false zeal and miscalled piety, but in both the home and foreign field you will find more hearts that God has been preparing for the seed of truth than you imagine, and they will hail with joy the divine message when it is presented to them.

But there must be no duplicity, no crookedness, in the life of the worker. While error, even when held in sincerity, is dangerous to anyone, insincerity in the truth is fatal.

Work With Enthusiasm and Ardor

We are not to be idle spectators in the stirring scenes that will prepare the way of the Lord's second appearing. We must catch the enthusiasm and ardor of the Christian soldier. Everyone who is not for Christ is against Him. "He that gathereth not with Me scattereth abroad." Matthew 12:30. Inactivity is registered in the books of heaven as opposition to Christ's work, because it produces the same kind of fruit as positive hostility. God calls for active workers.

The more clearly our eyes behold the attractions of the future world, the deeper will be our solicitude for the inhabitants of this world. We cannot be self-centered. We are living in the time of special conflict between the powers of light and those of darkness. Go forth; let your light shine; diffuse its rays to all the world. Christ and the heavenly messengers co-operating with human agencies, will bring the unfinished parts of the work to a perfect whole. Not to fill our place because we love our ease, because we would avoid care and weariness, is not to shine; and how terrible the guilt, how fearful the consequences!

There should be those who are preparing themselves to become Christian missionary physicians and nurses. Doors will then be opened into the families of the higher classes as well as among the lowly. All the influences that we can command must be consecrated to the work. From the home mission should extend a chain of living, burning light to belt the world, every voice and every influence echoing, "The Spirit and the bride say, Come. And let him that heareth say, Come. . . . And whosoever will, let him take the water of life freely." Revelation 22:17.

Effects of Wrong Habits

There is but little moral power in the professed Christian world. Wrong habits have been indulged, and physical and moral laws have been disregarded, until the general standard of virtue and piety is exceedingly low. Habits which lower the standard of physical health, enfeeble mental and moral strength. The indulgence of unnatural appetites and passions has a controlling influence upon the nerves of the brain. The animal organs are strengthened, while the moral are depressed. It is impossible for an intemperate man to be a Christian, for his higher powers are brought into slavery to the passions. —*Testimonies for the Church,* vol. 3, p. 51 (1871).

A World Unwarned

We have before us a great work—the closing work of giving God's last warning message to a sinful world. But what have we done to give this message? Look, I beg of you, at the many, many places that have never yet been even entered. Look at our workers treading over and over the same ground, while around them is a neglected world, lying in wickedness and corruption—a world as yet unwarned. To me this is an awful picture. What appalling indifference we manifest to the needs of a perishing world!—*Testimonies for the Church,* vol. 7, p. 103 (1902).

ESSENTIALS TO HEALTH

A Knowledge of First Principles

Many have inquired of me, "What course shall I take to best preserve my health?" My answer is, Cease to transgress the laws of your being; cease to gratify a depraved appetite; eat simple food; dress healthfully, which will require modest simplicity; work healthfully; and you will not be sick.

It is a sin to be sick, for all sickness is the result of transgression. Many are suffering in consequence of the transgression of their parents. They cannot be censured for their parents' sin; but it is nevertheless their duty to ascertain wherein their parents violated the laws of their being, which has entailed upon their offspring so miserable an inheritance; and wherein their parents' habits were wrong, they should change their course, and place themselves by correct habits in a better relation to health.

Men and women should inform themselves in regard to the philosophy of health. The minds of rational beings seem shrouded in darkness in regard to their own physical structure, and how to preserve it in a healthy condition. The present generation have trusted their bodies with the doctors and their souls with the ministers. Do they not pay the minister well for studying the Bible for them, that they need not be to the trouble? and is it not his business to tell them what they must believe, and to settle all doubtful questions of theology without special investiga-

---

Health Reformer, August, 1866, vol. 1, No. 1.

tion on their part? If they are sick, they send for the doctor—believe whatever he may tell, and swallow anything he may prescribe; for do they not pay him a liberal fee, and is it not his business to understand their physical ailments, and what to prescribe to make them well, without their being troubled with the matter? . . .

So closely is health related to our happiness, that we cannot have the latter without the former. A practical knowledge of the science of human life is necessary in order to glorify God in our bodies. It is therefore of the highest importance that among the studies selected for childhood, physiology should occupy the first place. How few know anything about the structure and functions of their own bodies and of nature's laws! Many are drifting about without knowledge, like a ship at sea without compass or anchor; and what is more, they are not interested to learn how to keep their bodies in a healthy condition and prevent disease.

Self-Denial Essential

The indulgence of animal appetites has degraded and enslaved many. Self-denial and a restraint upon the animal appetites are necessary to elevate and establish an improved condition of health and morals, and purify corrupted society. Every violation of principle in eating and drinking blunts the perceptive faculties, making it impossible for them to appreciate or place the right value upon eternal things. It is of the greatest importance that mankind should not be ignorant in regard to the consequences of excess. Temperance in all things is necessary to health and the development and growth of a good Christian character.

Those who transgress the laws of God in their physical organism will not be less slow to violate the law of God spoken from Sinai. Those who will not, after the light has come to them, eat and drink from principle instead of being controlled by appetite, will not be tenacious in regard to being governed by principle in other things. The agitation of the subject of reform in eating and drinking will develop character and will unerringly bring to light those who make a "god of their bellies."

Responsibility of Parents

Parents should arouse and in the fear of God inquire, What is truth? A tremendous responsibility rests upon them. They should be practical physiologists, that they may know what are and what are not correct physical habits, and be enabled thereby to instruct their children. The great mass are as ignorant and indifferent in regard to the physical and moral education of their children as the animal creation. And yet they dare assume the responsibilities of parents.

Every mother should acquaint herself with the laws that govern physical life. She should teach her children that the indulgence of animal appetites produces a morbid action in the system and weakens their moral sensibilities. Parents should seek for light and truth, as for hid treasures. To parents is committed the sacred charge of forming the characters of their children in childhood. They should be to their children both teacher and physician. They should understand nature's wants and nature's laws. A careful conformity to the laws God has implanted in our being will ensure health, and there will not be a breaking of the constitution which will tempt the afflicted to call for a physician to patch them up again.

Many seem to think they have a right to treat their own bodies as they please, but they forget that their bodies are not their own. Their Creator, who formed them, has claims upon them that they cannot rightly throw off. Every needless transgression of the laws which God has established in our being is virtually a violation of the law of God, and is as great a sin in the sight of Heaven as to break the Ten Commandments. Ignorance upon this important subject is sin; the light is now beaming upon us, and we are without excuse if we do not cherish the light and become intelligent in regard to these things, which it is our highest earthly interest to understand.

The Wisdom of God's Works

Lead the people to study the manifestation of God's love and wisdom in the works of nature. Lead them to study that marvelous organism, the human system, and the laws by which it is governed. Those who perceive the evidences of God's love, who understand something of the wisdom and beneficence of His laws and the results of obedience, will come to regard their duties and obligations from an altogether different point of view. Instead of looking upon an observance of the laws of health as a matter of sacrifice or self-denial, they will regard it, as it really is, as an inestimable blessing.

Every gospel worker should feel that the giving of instruction in the principles of healthful living is a part of his appointed work. Of this work there is great need, and the world is open for it.—*The Ministry of Healing,* page 147 (1905).

Govern the Body

Life is a gift of God. Our bodies have been given us to use in God's service, and He desires that we shall care for and appreciate them. We are possessed of physical as well as mental faculties. Our impulses and passions have their seat in the body, and therefore we must do nothing that would defile this entrusted possession. Our bodies must be kept in the best possible condition physically, and under the most spiritual influences, in order that we may make the best use of our talents. Read 1 Corinthians 6:13.

A misuse of the body shortens that period of time which God designs shall be used in His service. By allowing ourselves to form wrong habits, by keeping late hours, by gratifying appetite at the expense of health, we lay the foundation for feebleness. By neglecting to take physical exercise, by overworking mind or body, we unbalance the nervous system. Those who thus shorten their lives by disregarding nature's laws are guilty of robbery toward God. We have no right to neglect or misuse the body, the mind, or the strength, which should be used to offer God consecrated service.

All should have an intelligent knowledge of the human frame, that they may keep their bodies in the condition necessary to do the work of the Lord. Those who form habits that weaken the nerve power and lessen the vigor of mind or body, make themselves inefficient for the work God has given them to do. On the other hand, a pure, healthy life is most favorable for the perfection of Christian character and for the development of the powers of mind and body.

Review and Herald, Dec. 1, 1896.

The law of temperance must control the life of every Christian. God is to be in all our thoughts; His glory is ever to be kept in view. We must break away from every influence that would captivate our thoughts and lead us from God. We are under sacred obligations to God so to govern our bodies and rule our appetites and passions that they will not lead us away from purity and holiness, or take our minds from the work God requires us to do. Read Romans 12:1.

Adherence to a Simple Diet

If ever there was a time when the diet should be of the most simple kind, it is now. Meat should not be placed before our children. Its influence is to excite and strengthen the lower passions and has a tendency to deaden the moral powers. Grains and fruits prepared free from grease, and in as natural a condition as possible, should be the food for the tables of all who claim to be preparing for translation to heaven. The less feverish the diet, the more easily can the passions be controlled. Gratification of taste should not be consulted irrespective of physical, intellectual, or moral health.

Indulgence of the baser passions will lead very many to shut their eyes to the light; for they fear that they will see sins which they are unwilling to forsake. All may see if they will. If they choose darkness rather than light, their criminality will be none the less. Why do not men and women read and become intelligent upon these things, which so decidedly affect their physical, intellectual, and moral strength?—*Testimonies for the Church,* vol. 2, p. 352 (1869).

Purchased of God

"Know ye not that your body is the temple of the Holy Ghost which is in you, which ye have of God, and ye are not your own? For ye are bought with a price: therefore glorify God in your body, and in your spirit, which are God's." 1 Corinthians 6:19, 20.

We are not our own. We have been purchased with a dear price, even the sufferings and death of the Son of God. If we could understand this and fully realize it, we would feel a great responsibility resting upon us to keep ourselves in the very best condition of health, that we might render to God perfect service. But when we take any course which expends our vitality, decreases our strength, or beclouds the intellect, we sin against God. In pursuing this course we are not glorifying Him in our bodies and spirits which are His, but are committing a great wrong in His sight.

Has Jesus given Himself for us? Has a dear price been paid to redeem us? And is it so, that we are not our own? Is it true that all the powers of our being, our bodies, our spirits, all that we have, and all we are, belong to God? It certainly is. And when we realize this, what obligation does it lay us under to God to preserve ourselves in that condition that we may honor Him upon the earth in our bodies and in our spirits which are His?

The Reward of Holiness

We believe without a doubt that Christ is soon coming. This is not a fable to us; it is a reality. We have no doubt, neither have we had a doubt for years, that the doctrines we hold today are present truth, and that we are nearing the judgment. We are preparing to meet Him who, escorted by a retinue of holy angels, is to appear in the clouds of heaven to give the faithful and the just the finishing touch of immortality. When He comes He is not to cleanse us of our sins, to remove from us the defects in our character, or to cure us of the infirmities of our tempers and dispositions. If wrought for us at all, this work will all be accomplished before that time. When the Lord comes, those who are holy will be holy still. Those who have preserved their bodies and spirits in holiness, in sanctification and honor, will then receive the finishing touch of immortality. But those who are unjust, unsanctified, and filthy, will remain so forever. No work will then be done for them to remove their defects, and give them holy characters. The Refiner does not then sit to pursue His refining process and remove their sins and their corruption. This is all to be done in these hours of probation. It is *now* that this work is to be accomplished for us. . . .

We are now in God's workshop. Many of us are rough stones from the quarry. But as we lay hold upon the truth of God, its influence affects us. It elevates us and removes from us every imperfection and sin, of whatever nature. Thus we are prepared to see the King in His beauty and finally to unite with the pure and heavenly angels in the kingdom of glory. It is here that this work is to be accomplished for us, here that our bodies and spirits are to be fitted for immortality.

The Work of Sanctification

We are in a world that is opposed to righteousness and purity of character and to a growth in grace. Wherever we look, we see corruption and defilement, deformity and sin. And what is the work that we are to undertake here just previous to receiving immortality? It is to preserve our bodies holy, our spirits pure, that we may stand forth unstained amid the corruptions teeming around us in these last days. And if this work is accomplished, we need to engage in it at once, heartily and understandingly. Selfishness should not come in here to influence us. The Spirit of God should have perfect control of us, influencing us in all our actions. If we have a right hold on Heaven, a right hold of the power that is from above, we shall feel the sanctifying influence of the Spirit of God upon our hearts.

When we have tried to present the health reform to our brethren and sisters, and have spoken to them of the importance of eating and drinking and doing all that they do to the glory of God, many by their actions have said, "It is nobody's business whether I eat this or that. Whatever we do, we are to bear the consequences ourselves." Dear friends, you are greatly mistaken. You are not the only sufferers from a wrong course. The society you are in bears the consequences of your wrongs, in a great degree, as well as yourselves.

If you suffer from your intemperance in eating or drinking, we that are around you or associated with you are also affected by your infirmities. We have to suffer on account of your wrong course. If it has an influence to lessen your powers of mind or body, we feel it when in your society and are affected by it. If, instead of having a buoyancy of spirit, you are gloomy, you cast a shadow upon the spirits of all around you. If we are sad and depressed and in trouble, you could, if in a right condition of health, have a clear brain to show us the way out, and speak a comforting word to us. But if your brain is so benumbed by your wrong course of living that you cannot give us the right counsel, do we not meet with a loss? Does not your influence seriously affect us? We may have a good degree of confidence in our own judgment, yet we want to have counselors; for "in the multitude of counselors there is safety." Proverbs 11:14.

We desire that our course should look consistent to those we love, and we wish to seek their counsel and have them able to give it with a clear brain. But what care we for your judgment if your brain nerve power has been taxed to the utmost, and the vitality withdrawn from the brain to take care of the improper food placed in your stomachs, or of an enormous quantity of even healthful food? What care we for the judgment of such persons? They see through a mass of undigested food. Therefore your course of living affects us. It is impossible for you to pursue any wrong course without causing others to suffer.

The Christian Race

"Know ye not that they which run in a race run all, but one receiveth the prize? So run, that ye may obtain. And every man that striveth for the mastery is temperate in all things. Now they do it to obtain a corruptible crown; but we an incorruptible. I therefore so run, not as uncertainly; so fight I, not as one that beateth the air: but I keep under my body, and bring it into subjection: lest that by any means, when I have preached to others, I myself should be a castaway." 1 Corinthians 9:24-27. Those who engaged in running the race to obtain that laurel which was considered a special honor were temperate in all things, so that their muscles, their brains, and every part of them might be in the very best condition to run. If they were not temperate in all things, they would not have that elasticity that they would have if they were. If temperate, they could run that race more successfully; they were more sure of receiving the crown.

But notwithstanding all their temperance, all their efforts to subject themselves to a careful diet in order to be in the best condition, those who ran the earthly race only ran a venture. They might do the very best they could, and yet after all not receive the token of honor; for another might be a little in advance of them and take the prize. Only one received the prize. But in the heavenly race we can all run, and all receive the prize. There is no uncertainty, no risk, in the matter. We must put on the heavenly graces, and, with the eye directed upward to the crown of immortality, keep the Pattern ever before us. He was a Man of Sorrows, and acquainted with grief. The humble, self-denying life of our divine Lord we are to keep constantly in view. And then as we seek to imitate Him, keeping our eye upon the mark of the prize, we can run this race with certainty, knowing that if we do the very best we can, we shall certainly secure the prize.

Men would subject themselves to self-denial and discipline in order to run and obtain a corruptible crown, one that would perish in a day and which was only a token of honor from mortals here. But we are to run the race, at the end of which is a crown of immortality and everlasting life. Yes, a far more exceeding and eternal weight of glory will be awarded to us as the prize when the race is run. "We," says the apostle, "an incorruptible."

And if those who engaged in this race here upon the earth for a temporal crown, could be temperate in all things, cannot we, who have in view an incorruptible crown, an eternal weight of glory, and a life which measures with the life of God? When we have this great inducement before us, cannot we "run with patience the race that is set before us, looking unto Jesus the Author and Finisher of our faith"? Hebrews 12:1, 2. He has pointed out the way for us and marked it all along by His own footsteps. It is the path that He traveled, and we may, with Him, experience the self-denial and the suffering, and walk in this pathway imprinted by His own blood.

Develop Ability

Be not satisfied with reaching a low standard. We are not what we might be, or what it is God's will that we should be. God has given us reasoning powers, not to remain inactive or to be perverted to earthly and sordid pursuits, but that they may be developed to the utmost, refined, sanctified, ennobled, and used in advancing the interests of His kingdom.

None should consent to be mere machines, run by another man's mind. God has given us ability to think and to act, and it is by acting with carefulness, looking to Him for wisdom, that you will become capable of bearing burdens. Stand in your God-given personality. Be no other person's shadow. Expect that the Lord will work in and by and through you.—*The Ministry of Healing,* pages 498, 499 (1905)

Temperance in All Things

The health reform is an important part of the third angel's message; and as a people professing this reform, we should not retrograde, but make continual advancement. It is a great thing to ensure health by placing ourselves in right relations to the laws of life, and many have not done this. A large share of the sickness and suffering among us is the result of the transgression of physical law, is brought upon individuals by their own wrong habits.

Our ancestors have bequeathed to us customs and appetites which are filling the world with disease. The sins of the parents, through perverted appetite, are with fearful power visited upon the children to the third and fourth generations. The bad eating of many generations, the gluttonous and self-indulgent habits of the people, are filling our poorhouses, our prisons, and our insane asylums. Intemperance, in drinking tea and coffee, wine, beer, rum, and brandy, and the use of tobacco, opium, and other narcotics, has resulted in great mental and physical degeneracy, and this degeneracy is constantly increasing.

Are these ills visited upon the race through God's providence? No; they exist because the people have gone contrary to His providence, and still continue to rashly disregard His laws. In the words of the apostle, I would entreat those who are not blinded and paralyzed by wrong teaching and practices, those who would render to God the best service of which they are capable: "I beseech you therefore, brethren, by the mercies of God, that ye present your bodies a living sacrifice, holy, acceptable unto God, which is your reasonable service. And be not conformed to this world: but be ye transformed by the renewing of

Review and Herald, July 29, 1884.

your mind, that ye may prove what is that good, and acceptable, and perfect, will of God." Romans 12:1, 2. We have no right to wantonly violate a single principle of the laws of health. Christians should not follow the customs and practices of the world.

The history of Daniel is placed upon record for our benefit. He chose to take a course that would make him singular in the king's court. He did not conform to the habits of the courtiers in eating and drinking, but purposed in his heart that he would not eat of the king's meat nor drink of his wines. This was not a hastily formed, wavering purpose, but one that was intelligently formed and resolutely carried out. Daniel honored God; and the promise was fulfilled to him. "Them that honor Me I will honor." 1 Samuel 2:30. The Lord gave him "knowledge and skill in all learning and wisdom," and he had "understanding in all visions and dreams" (Daniel 1:17); so that he was wiser than all in the king's courts, wiser than all the astrologers and magicians in the kingdom.

Those who serve God in sincerity and truth will be a peculiar people, unlike the world, separate from the world. Their food will be prepared, not to encourage gluttony or gratify a perverted taste, but to secure to themselves the greatest physical strength, and consequently the best mental conditions. . . .

Excessive indulgence in eating and drinking is sin. Our heavenly Father has bestowed upon us the great blessing of health reform, that we may glorify Him by obeying the claims He has upon us. It is the duty of those who have received the light upon this important subject to manifest greater interest for those who are still suffering for want of knowledge. Those who are looking for the soon appearing of their Saviour should be the last to manifest a lack of interest in this great work of reform. The harmonious, healthy action of all the powers of body and mind results in happiness; the more elevated and refined the powers, the more pure and unalloyed the happiness. An aimless life is a living death. The mind should dwell upon themes relating to our eternal interests. This will be conducive to health of body and mind.

Our faith requires us to elevate the standard of reform, and take advance steps. The condition of our acceptance with God is a practical separation from the world. The Lord calls upon us as a people, "Come out from among them, and be ye separate," "and touch not the unclean thing; and I will receive you." The world may despise you because you do not meet their standard, engage in their dissipating amusements, and follow their pernicious ways; but the God of heaven promises to receive you, and to be a Father unto you. "Ye shall be My sons and daughters, saith the Lord Almighty." 2 Corinthians 6:17, 18.

The World No Criterion

The world should be no criterion for us. It is fashionable to indulge the appetite in luxurious food and unnatural stimulus, thus strengthening the animal propensities and crippling the growth and development of the moral faculties. There is no encouragement given to any of the sons or daughters of Adam that they may become victorious overcomers in the Christian warfare unless they decide to practice temperance in all things. If they do this, they will not fight as one that beateth the air.—*Testimonies for the Church*, vol. 4, p. 35 (1876).

Physical Exercise

Another precious blessing is proper exercise. There are many indolent, inactive ones who are disinclined to physical labor or exercise because it wearies them. What if it does weary them? The reason why they become weary is that they do not strengthen their muscles by exercise, therefore they feel the least exertion. Invalid women and girls are better pleased to busy themselves with light employment, as crocheting, embroidering, or making tatting, than to engage in physical labor. If invalids would recover health, they should not discontinue physical exercise; for they will thus increase muscular weakness and general debility. Bind up the arm and permit it to remain useless, even for a few weeks, then free it from its bondage, and you will discover that it is weaker than the one you have been using moderately during the same time. Inactivity produces the same effect upon the whole muscular system. The blood is not enabled to expel the impurities as it would if active circulation were induced by exercise.

When the weather will permit, all who can possibly do so ought to walk in the open air every day, summer and winter. But the clothing should be suitable for the exercise, and the feet should be well protected. A walk, even in winter, would be more beneficial to the health than all the medicine the doctors may prescribe. For those who can walk, walking is preferable to riding. The muscles and veins are enabled better to perform their work. There will be increased vitality, which is so necessary to health. The lungs will have needful action; for it is impossible to go out in the bracing air of a winter's morning without inflating the lungs.

Testimonies for the Church, vol. 2, pp. 528-533 (1870).

Riches and idleness are thought by some to be blessings indeed. But when some persons have acquired wealth, or inherited it unexpectedly, their active habits have been broken up, their time is unemployed, they live at ease, and their usefulness seems at an end; they become restless, anxious, and unhappy, and their lives soon close. Those who are always busy, and go cheerfully about the performance of their daily tasks, are the most happy and healthy. The rest and composure of night brings to their wearied frames unbroken slumber. . . .

Exercise will aid the work of digestion. To walk out after a meal, hold the head erect, put back the shoulders, and exercise moderately, will be a great benefit. The mind will be diverted from self to the beauties of nature. The less the attention is called to the stomach after a meal, the better. If you are in constant fear that your food will hurt you, it most assuredly will. Forget self, and think of something cheerful.

Colds and Fresh Air

Many labor under the mistaken idea that if they have taken cold, they must carefully exclude the outside air and increase the temperature of their room until it is excessively hot. The system may be deranged, the pores closed by waste matter, and the internal organs suffering more or less inflammation, because the blood has been chilled back from the surface and thrown upon them. At this time, of all others, the lungs should not be deprived of pure, fresh air. If pure air is ever necessary, it is when any part of the system, as the lungs or stomach, is diseased. Judicious exercise would induce the blood to the surface and thus relieve the internal organs. Brisk, yet not violent, exercise in the open air, with cheerfulness of spirits, will promote the circulation, giving a healthful glow to the skin, and sending the blood, vitalized by the pure air, to the extremities. The diseased stomach will find relief by exercise. Physicians frequently advise invalids to visit foreign countries, to go to the springs, or to ride upon the ocean, in order to regain health; when, in nine cases out of ten, if they would eat temperately and engage in healthful exercise with a cheerful spirit, they would regain health and save time and money. Exercise and a free and abundant use of the air and sunlight—blessings which Heaven has freely bestowed upon all—would give life and strength to the emaciated invalid. . . .

Inaction and Weakness

Those who do not use their limbs every day will realize a weakness when they do attempt to exercise. The veins and muscles are not in a condition to perform their work and keep all the living machinery in healthful action, each organ in the system doing its part. The limbs will strengthen with use. Moderate exercise every day will impart strength to the muscles, which without exercise become flabby and enfeebled. By active exercise in the open air every day, the liver, kidneys, and lungs also will be strengthened to perform their work. Bring to your aid the power of the will, which will resist cold and will give energy to the nervous system. In a short time you will so realize the benefit of exercise and pure air that you would not live without these blessings. Your lungs, deprived of air, will be like a hungry person deprived of food. Indeed, we can live longer without food than without air, which is the food that God has provided for the lungs. Therefore do not regard it as an enemy, but as a precious blessing from God.

Pure Air and Sunlight

In no case should sick persons be deprived of a full supply of fresh air in pleasant weather. Their rooms may not always be so constructed as to allow the windows or doors to be opened, without the draft coming directly upon them, thus exposing them to the taking of cold. In such cases windows and doors should be opened in an adjoining room, thus letting fresh air enter the room occupied by the sick. Fresh air will prove far more beneficial to sick persons than medicine, and is far more essential to them than their food. They will do better, and will recover sooner, when deprived of food, than when deprived of fresh air.

Many invalids have been confined for weeks and even for months in close rooms, with the light and the pure, invigorating air of heaven shut out, as if air were a deadly enemy, when it was just the medicine they needed to make them well. . . . These valuable remedies which Heaven has provided, without money and without price, were cast aside and considered not only as worthless, but even as dangerous enemies, while poisons, prescribed by physicians, were in blind confidence taken.

Thousands have died for want of pure water and pure air who might have lived. And thousands of invalids, who are a burden to themselves and others, think that their lives depend upon taking medicines from the doctors. They are continually guarding themselves against the air and avoiding the use of water. These blessings they need in order to become well. If they would become enlightened and let medicine alone, and accustom themselves to outdoor exercise and to air in their houses, summer and winter, and use soft water for drinking and

How to Live, part 4, pp. 55-62. Published in 1865.

bathing purposes, they would be comparatively well and happy instead of dragging out a miserable existence.

The Health of the Nurse to Be Considered

It is the duty of attendants and nurses to take special care of their own health, especially in critical cases of fever and consumption. One person should not be kept closely confined to the sickroom. It is safer to have two or three to depend upon, who are careful and understanding nurses, these changing and sharing the care and confinement of the sickroom. Each should have exercise in the open air as often as possible. This is important to sickbed attendants, especially if the friends of the sick are among the class that continue to regard air, if admitted into the sickroom, as an enemy, and will not allow the windows raised or the doors opened. In such cases the sick and the attendants are compelled to breathe the poisonous atmosphere from day to day because of the inexcusable ignorance of the friends of the sick.

In very many cases the attendants are ignorant of the needs of the system, and of the relation that the breathing of fresh air sustains to health, and of the life-destroying influence of inhaling the impure air of a sickroom. In this case the life of the sick is endangered, and the attendants themselves are liable to take on disease, and lose health, and perhaps life. . . .

The sickroom, if possible, should have a draft of air through it, day and night. The draft should not come directly upon the invalid. While burning fevers are raging, there is but little danger of taking cold. But special care is needful when the crisis comes and the fever is passing away. Then constant watching may be necessary to keep vitality in the system. The sick must have pure, invigorating air. If no other way can be devised, the sick, if possible, should be removed to another room and another bed, while the sickroom, the bed and bedding, are being purified by ventilation. If those who are well need the blessings of light and air and need to observe habits of cleanliness in order to remain well, the need of the sick is still greater in proportion to their debilitated condition.

Some houses are furnished expensively, more to gratify pride and to receive visitors than for the comfort, convenience, and health of the family. The best rooms are kept dark. The light and air are shut out lest the light of heaven should injure the rich furniture, fade the carpets, or tarnish the picture frames. When visitors are seated in these rooms they are in danger of taking cold because of the cellarlike atmosphere pervading them. Parlor chambers and bedrooms are kept closed in the same manner and for the same reasons. And whoever occupies these beds which have not been freely exposed to light and air does so at the expense of health, and often of life itself.

Rooms that are not exposed to light and air become damp. Beds and bedding gather dampness, and the atmosphere in these rooms is poisonous, because it has not been purified by light and air. . . .

Sleeping rooms especially should be well ventilated, and the atmosphere made healthy by light and air. Blinds should be left open several hours each day, and the curtains put aside, and the rooms thoroughly aired. Nothing should remain, even for a short time, which would destroy the purity of the atmosphere. . . .

Sleeping apartments should be large and so arranged as to have circulation of air through them day and night. Those who have excluded the air from their sleeping rooms should begin to change their course immediately.

They should let in air by degrees and increase its circulation until they can bear it winter and summer, with no danger of taking cold. The lungs, in order to be healthy, must have pure air.

Those who have not had a free circulation of air in their rooms through the night generally awake feeling exhausted and feverish, and know not the cause. It was air, vital air, that the whole system required, but which it could not obtain. Upon rising in the morning, most persons would be benefited by taking a sponge bath, or, if more agreeable, a hand bath, with merely a washbowl of water. This will remove impurities from the skin. Then the clothing should be removed piece by piece from the bed, and exposed to the air. The windows should be opened, the blinds fastened back, and the air allowed to circulate freely for several hours, if not all day, through the sleeping apartments. In this manner the bed and clothing will become thoroughly aired, and the impurities will be removed from the room.

Shade trees and shrubbery too close and dense around a house are unhealthful; for they prevent a free circulation of air and shut out the rays of the sun. In consequence of this, dampness gathers in the house. Especially in wet seasons the sleeping rooms become damp, and those who occupy them are troubled with rheumatism, neuralgia, and lung complaints which generally end in consumption. Numerous shade trees cast off many leaves, which, if not immediately removed, decay and poison the atmosphere. A yard beautified with trees and shrubbery, at a proper distance from the house, has a happy, cheerful influence upon the family, and, if well taken care of, will prove no injury to health. Dwellings, if possible, should be built upon high and dry ground. If a house is built where water settles around it, remaining for a time, and then drying away, a poisonous miasma arises, and fever and ague, sore throat, lung diseases, and fevers will be the result.

Many have expected that God would keep them from sickness merely because they have asked Him to do so. But God did not regard their prayers, because their faith was not made perfect by works. God will not work a miracle to keep those from sickness who have no care for themselves, but are continually violating the laws of health and make no efforts to prevent disease. When we do all we can on our part to have health, then may we expect that the blessed results will follow, and we can ask God in faith to bless our efforts for the preservation of health. He will then answer our prayer, if His name can be glorified thereby. But let all understand that they have a work to do. God will not work in a miraculous manner to preserve the health of persons who by their careless inattention to the laws of health are taking a sure course to make themselves sick.

Deep Breathing

In order to have good blood, we must breathe well. Full, deep inspirations of pure air which fill the lungs with oxygen, purify the blood. They impart to it a bright color, and send it, a life-giving current, to every part of the body. A good respiration soothes the nerves; it stimulates the appetite and renders digestion more perfect; and it induces sound, refreshing sleep.—*The Ministry of Healing,* page 272 (1905).

Superstitions Concerning Night Air

Many have been taught from childhood that night air is positively injurious to health, and therefore must be

3—C.O.H.

excluded from their rooms. To their own injury they close the windows and doors of their sleeping apartments, to protect themselves from the night air which they say is so dangerous to health. In this they are deceived. In the cool of the evening it may be necessary to guard from chilliness by extra clothing; but they should give their lungs air. . . . Many are suffering from disease because they refuse to receive into their rooms at night the pure night air. The free, pure air of heaven is one of the richest blessings we can enjoy.—*Testimonies for the Church,* vol. 2, pp. 527, 528 (1870).

The Influence of Fresh Air

Air, air, the precious boon of heaven, which all may have, will bless you with its invigorating influence, if you will not refuse it entrance. Welcome it, cultivate a love for it, and it will prove a precious soother of the nerves. Air must be in constant circulation to be kept pure. The influence of pure, fresh air is to cause the blood to circulate healthfully through the system. It refreshes the body and tends to render it strong and healthy, while at the same time its influence is decidedly felt upon the mind, imparting a degree of composure and serenity. It excites the appetite, and renders the digestion of food more perfect, and induces sound and sweet sleep.—*Testimonies for the Church,* vol. 1, p. 702 (1870).

Scrupulous Sanitation

When severe sickness enters a family, there is great need of each member's giving strict attention to personal cleanliness and diet, to preserve himself in a healthful condition, thus fortifying himself against disease. It is also of the greatest importance that the sickroom, from the first, be properly ventilated. This is beneficial to the afflicted, and highly necessary to keep those well who are compelled to remain a length of time in the sickroom. . . .

A great amount of suffering might be saved if all would labor to prevent disease, by strictly obeying the laws of health. Strict habits of cleanliness should be observed. Many, while well, will not take the trouble to keep in a healthy condition. They neglect personal cleanliness, and are not careful to keep their clothing pure. Impurities are constantly and imperceptibly passing from the body, through the pores, and if the surface of the skin is not kept in a healthy condition, the system is burdened with impure matter. If the clothing worn is not often washed and frequently aired, it becomes filthy with impurities which are thrown off from the body by sensible and insensible perspiration. And if the garments worn are not frequently cleansed from these impurities, the pores of the skin absorb again the waste matter thrown off. The impurities of the body, if not allowed to escape, are taken back into the blood and forced upon the internal organs. Nature, to relieve herself of poisonous impurities, makes an effort to free the system. This effort produces fevers

First published in *How to Live,* part 4, pp. 54-61; reproduced in *Review and Herald,* Dec. 5, 12, 1899.

and what is termed disease. But even then, if those who are afflicted would assist nature in her efforts by the use of pure, soft water, much suffering would be prevented. But many, instead of doing this, and seeking to remove the poisonous matter from the system, take a more deadly poison into the system, to remove a poison already there.

If every family realized the beneficial results of thorough cleanliness, they would make special efforts to remove every impurity from their persons and from their houses, and would extend their efforts to their premises. Many suffer decayed vegetable matter to remain about their premises. They are not awake to the influence of these things. There is constantly arising from these decaying substances an effluvium that is poisoning the air. By inhaling the impure air, the blood is poisoned, the lungs become affected, and the whole system is diseased. Disease of almost every description will be caused by inhaling the atmosphere affected by these decaying substances.

Families have been afflicted with fevers, some of their members have died, and the remaining portion of the family circle have almost murmured against their Maker because of their distressing bereavements, when the sole cause of all their sickness and death has been the result of their own carelessness. The impurities about their own premises have brought upon them contagious diseases and the sad afflictions which they charge upon God. Every family that prizes health should cleanse their houses and their premises of all decaying substances.

God commanded that the children of Israel should in no case allow impurities of their persons or of their clothing. Those who had any personal uncleanness were shut out of the camp until evening, and then were required to cleanse themselves and their clothing before they could enter the camp. Also they were commanded of God to have no impurities upon their premises within a great distance of the encampment, lest the Lord should pass by and see their uncleanness.

In regard to cleanliness, God requires no less of His people now than He did of ancient Israel. A neglect of cleanliness will induce disease. Sickness and premature death do not come without cause. Stubborn fevers and violent diseases have prevailed in neighborhoods and towns that had formerly been considered healthy, and some persons have died, while others have been left with broken constitutions, to be crippled with disease for life. In many instances their own yards contained the agent of destruction, which sent forth deadly poison into the atmosphere, to be inhaled by the family and the neighborhood. The slackness and recklessness sometimes witnessed is beastly, and the ignorance of the results of such things upon health is astonishing. Such places should be purified, especially in summer, by lime or ashes, or by a daily burial with earth.

Use Simple Food

In order to render to God perfect service, you must have clear conceptions of His requirements. You should use the most simple food, prepared in the most simple manner, that the fine nerves of the brain be not weakened, benumbed, or paralyzed, making it impossible for you to discern sacred things, and to value the atonement, the cleansing blood of Christ, as of priceless worth.—*Testimonies for the Church,* vol. 2, p. 46 (1868).

Physical Habits and Spiritual Health

The character of Daniel is presented to the world as a striking example of what God's grace can make of men fallen by nature and corrupted by sin. The record of his noble, self-denying life is an encouragement to our common humanity. From it we may gather strength to nobly resist temptation, and firmly, and in the grace of meekness, stand for the right under the severest trial.

Daniel's Experience

Daniel might have found a plausible excuse to depart from his strictly temperate habits; but the approbation of God was dearer to him than the favor of the most powerful earthly potentate—dearer even than life itself. Having by his courteous conduct obtained favor with Melzar, the officer in charge of the Hebrew youth, Daniel made a request that they might not eat of the king's meat or drink of his wine. Melzar feared that should he comply with this request, he might incur the displeasure of the king and thus endanger his own life. Like many at the present day, he thought that an abstemious diet would render these youth pale and sickly in appearance and deficient in muscular strength, while the luxurious food from the king's table would make them ruddy and beautiful and would impart superior physical activity.

Daniel requested that the matter be decided by a ten days' trial—the Hebrew youth during this brief period being permitted to eat of simple food, while their companions partook of the king's dainties. The request was finally granted, and then Daniel felt assured, that he had gained his case. Although but a youth, he had seen the injurious effects of wine and luxurious living upon physical and mental health.

At the end of the ten days the result was found to be quite the opposite of Melzar's expectations. Not only in personal appearance, but in physical activity and mental vigor, those who had been temperate in their habits exhibited a marked superiority over their companions who had indulged appetite. As a result of this trial, Daniel and his associates were permitted to continue their simple diet during the whole course of their training for the duties of the kingdom.

The Lord regarded with approval the firmness and self-denial of these Hebrew youth, and His blessing attended them. He "gave them knowledge and skill in all learning and wisdom: and Daniel had understanding in all visions and dreams." At the expiration of the three years of training, when their ability and acquirements were tested by the king, he "found none like Daniel, Hananiah, Mishael, and Azariah: therefore stood they before the king. And in all matters of wisdom and understanding, that the king inquired of them, he found them ten times better than all the magicians and astrologers that were in all his realm." Daniel 1:17, 19, 20.

Here is a lesson for all, but especially for the young. A strict compliance with the requirements of God is beneficial to the health of body and mind. In order to reach the highest standard of moral and intellectual attainments, it is necessary to seek wisdom and strength from God, and to observe strict temperance in all the habits of life. In the experience of Daniel and his companions we have an instance of the triumph of principle over temptation to indulge the appetite. It shows us that through religious principle young men may triumph over the lusts of the flesh and remain true to God's requirements, even though it cost them a great sacrifice.

What if Daniel and his companions had made a compromise with those heathen officers, and had yielded to the pressure of the occasion by eating and drinking as was customary with the Babylonians? That single instance of departure from principle would have weakened their sense of right and their abhorrence of wrong. Indulgence of appetite would have involved the sacrifice of physical vigor, clearness of intellect, and spiritual power. One wrong step would probably have led to others, until, their connection with Heaven being severed, they would have been swept away by temptation. . . .

The life of Daniel is an inspired illustration of what constitutes a sanctified character. Bible sanctification has to do with the whole man. . . . It is impossible for any to enjoy the blessing of sanctification while they are selfish and gluttonous. These groan under a burden of infirmities because of wrong habits of eating and drinking, which do violence to the laws of life and health. Many are enfeebling their digestive organs by indulging perverted appetite. The power of the human constitution to resist the abuses put upon it is wonderful; but persistent wrong habits in excessive eating and drinking will enfeeble every function of the body. Let these feeble ones consider what they might have been had they lived temperately and promoted health instead of abusing it. In the gratification of perverted appetite and passion, even professed Christians cripple nature in her work and lessen physical, mental, and moral power. Some who are doing this, claim to be sanctified to God; but such a claim is without foundation. . . .

Sanctification a Living Principle

We should consider the words of the apostle Paul, in which he appeals to his brethren, by the mercies of God, to present their bodies "a living sacrifice, holy, acceptable unto God." . . . Sanctification is not merely a theory, an emotion, or a form of words, but a living, active principle, entering into the everyday life. It requires that our habits of eating, drinking, and dressing be such as to secure the preservation of physical, mental, and moral health, that we may present to the Lord our bodies—not an offering corrupted by wrong habits but—"a living sacrifice, holy, acceptable unto God." Romans 12:1.

Let none who profess godliness regard with indifference the health of the body, and flatter themselves that intemperance is no sin and will not affect their spirituality. A close sympathy exists between the physical and the moral nature. The standard of virtue is elevated or degraded by the physical habits. Excessive eating of the best of food will produce a morbid condition of the moral feelings. And if the food is not the most healthful, the effects will be still more injurious. Any habit which does not promote healthful action in the human system degrades the higher and nobler faculties. Wrong habits of eating and drinking lead to errors in thought and action. Indulgence of appetite strengthens the animal propensities, giving them the ascendancy over the mental and spiritual powers.

"Abstain from fleshly lusts, which war against the soul" (1 Peter 2:11), is the language of the apostle Peter. Many regard this warning as applicable only to the licentious; but it has a broader meaning. It guards against every injurious gratification of appetite or passion. It is a most forcible warning against the use of such stimulants and narcotics as tea, coffee, tobacco, alcohol, and morphine. These indulgences may well be classed among the lusts that exert a pernicious influence upon moral character. The earlier these hurtful habits are formed, the more firmly will they hold their victims in slavery to lust, and the more certainly will they lower the standard of spirituality.

Bible teaching will make but a feeble impression upon those whose faculties are benumbed by indulgence of appetite. Thousands will sacrifice not only health and life, but their hope of heaven, before they will wage war against their own perverted appetites. One lady, who for many years claimed to be sanctified, made the statement that if she must give up her pipe or heaven she would say, "Farewell, heaven; I cannot overcome my love for my pipe." This idol had been enshrined in the soul, leaving to Jesus a subordinate place. Yet this woman claimed to be wholly the Lord's!

Wherever they may be, those who are truly sanctified will elevate the moral standard by preserving correct physical habits, and, like Daniel, presenting to others an example of temperance and self-denial. Every depraved appetite becomes a warring lust. Everything that conflicts with natural law creates a diseased condition of the soul. The indulgence of appetite produces a dyspeptic stomach, a torpid liver, a clouded brain, and thus perverts the temper and the spirit of the man. And these enfeebled powers are offered to God, who refused to accept the victims for sacrifice unless they were without a blemish. It is our duty to bring our appetite and our habits of life into conformity to natural law. If the bodies offered upon Christ's altar were examined with the close scrutiny to which the Jewish sacrifices were subjected, who with our present habits would be accepted?

With what care should Christians regulate their habits, that they may preserve the full vigor of every faculty to give to the service of Christ. If we would be sanctified in soul, body, and spirit, we must live in conformity to the divine law. The heart cannot preserve consecration to God while the appetites and passions are indulged at the expense of health and life. . . .

Paul's inspired warnings against self-indulgence are sounding along the line down to our time. . . . He presents for our encouragement the freedom enjoyed by the truly sanctified. "There is therefore now no condemnation to them which are in Christ Jesus, who walk not after the flesh, but after the Spirit." Romans 8:1. He charges the Galatians to "walk in the Spirit, and ye shall not fulfill the lust of the flesh. For the flesh lusteth against the Spirit, and the Spirit against the flesh." Galatians 5:16, 17. He names some of the forms of fleshly lusts—idolatry, drunkenness, and such like. After mentioning the fruits of the Spirit, among which is temperance, he adds, "And they that are Christ's have crucified the flesh with the affections and lusts." Verse 24.

There are many among professed Christians today who would decide that Daniel was too particular and would pronounce him narrow and bigoted. They consider the matter of eating and drinking of too little consequence to require such a decided stand—one involving the probable sacrifice of every earthly advantage. But those who reason thus will find in the day of judgment that they turned from God's express requirements and set up their own opinion as a standard of right and wrong. They will find that what seemed to them unimportant was not so regarded of God. His requirements should be sacredly obeyed. Those who accept and obey one of His precepts because it is convenient to do so, while they reject another because its observance would require a sacrifice, lower the standard of right, and by their example lead others to lightly regard the holy law of God. "Thus saith the Lord" is to be our rule in all things.

Nonuse of Flesh Meats

Will the people who are preparing to become holy, pure, and refined, that they may be introduced into the society of heavenly angels, continue to take the life of God's creatures and subsist on their flesh and enjoy it as a luxury? From what the Lord has shown me, this order of things will be changed, and God's peculiar people will exercise temperance in all things. . . .

The liability to take disease is increased tenfold by meat eating. The intellectual, the moral, and the physical powers are depreciated by the habitual use of flesh meats. Meat eating deranges the system, beclouds the intellect, and blunts the moral sensibilities. . . . Your safest course is to let meat alone.—*Testimonies for the Church,* vol. 2, pp. 63, 64 (1868).

Avoid Gluttony

Some do not exercise control over their appetites, but indulge taste at the expense of health. As the result, the brain is clouded, their thoughts are sluggish, and they fail to accomplish what they might if they were self-denying and abstemious. These rob God of the physical and mental strength which might be devoted to His service if temperance were observed in all things. . . .

The word of God places the sin of gluttony in the same catalogue with drunkenness. So offensive was this sin in the sight of God that He gave directions to Moses that a child who would not be restrained on the point of appetite, but would gorge himself with anything his taste might crave, should be brought by his parents before the rulers in Israel and should be stoned to death. The condition of the glutton was considered hopeless. He would be of no use to others and was a curse to himself. No dependence could be placed upon him in anything. His influence would be ever contaminating others, and the world would be better without such a character for his terrible defects would be perpetuated.

None who have a sense of their accountability to God will allow the animal propensities to control reason. Those who do this are not Christians, whoever they may be and however exalted their profession. The injunction of Christ is, "Be ye therefore perfect, even as your Father which is in heaven is perfect." Matthew 5:48. He here shows us that we may be as perfect in our sphere as God is in His sphere.—*Testimonies for the Church*, vol. 4, pp. 454, 455 (1880).

Lessons From the Experience of John the Baptist

For years the Lord has been calling the attention of His people to health reform. This is one of the great branches of the work of preparation for the coming of the Son of man.

John the Baptist went forth in the spirit and power of Elijah to prepare the way of the Lord and to turn the people to the wisdom of the just. He was a representative of those living in these last days, to whom God has entrusted sacred truths to present before the people, to prepare the way for the second appearing of Christ. John was a reformer. The angel Gabriel, direct from heaven, gave a discourse upon health reform to the Father and mother of John. He said that he should not drink wine or strong drink, and that he should be filled with the Holy Ghost from his birth.

John separated himself from friends, and from the luxuries of life. The simplicity of his dress, a garment woven of camel's hair, was a standing rebuke to the extravagance and display of the Jewish priests, and of the people generally. His diet, purely vegetable, of locusts and wild honey, was a rebuke to the indulgence of appetite, and the gluttony that everywhere prevailed.

The prophet Malachi declares, "Behold, I will send you Elijah the prophet before the coming of the great and dreadful day of the Lord: and he shall turn the heart of the fathers to the children, and the heart of the children to their fathers." Malachi 4:5, 6. Here the prophet describes the character of the work. Those who are to

_____

Testimonies for the Church, vol. 3, pp. 61-64 (1871).

prepare the way for the second coming of Christ, are represented by faithful Elijah, as John came in the spirit of Elijah to prepare the way for Christ's first advent. The great subject of reform is to be agitated, and the public mind is to be stirred. Temperance in all things is to be connected with the message, to turn the people of God from their idolatry, their gluttony, and their extravagance in dress and other things. The self-denial, humility, and temperance required of the righteous, whom God especially leads and blesses, is to be presented to the people in contrast to the extravagant, health-destroying habits of those who live in this degenerate age.

God has shown that health reform is as closely connected with the third angel's message as the hand is with the body. There is nowhere to be found so great a cause of physical and moral degeneracy as a neglect of this important subject. Those who indulge appetite and passion and close their eyes to the light for fear they will see sinful indulgences which they are unwilling to forsake, are guilty before God. Whoever turns from the light in one instance hardens his heart to disregard the light upon other matters. Whoever violates moral obligations in the matter of eating and dressing, prepares the way to violate the claims of God in regard to eternal interests.

Our bodies are not our own. God has claims upon us to take care of the habitation He has given us, that we may present our bodies to Him a living sacrifice, holy and acceptable. Our bodies belong to Him who made them, and we are in duty bound to become intelligent in regard to the best means of preserving them from decay. If we enfeeble the body by self-gratification, by indulging the appetite, and by dressing in accordance with health-destroying fashions, in order to be in harmony with the world, we become enemies of God. . . .

Providence has been leading the people of God out from the extravagant habits of the world, away from the indulgence of appetite and passion, to take their stand upon the platform of self-denial and temperance in all things. The people whom God is leading will be peculiar. They will not be like the world. But if they follow the leadings of God, they will accomplish His purposes, and will yield their will to His will. Christ will dwell in the heart. The temple of God will be holy. Your body, says the apostle, is the temple of the Holy Ghost. God does not require His children to deny themselves to the injury of physical strength. He requires them to obey natural law, to preserve physical health. Nature's path is the road He marks out, and it is broad enough for any Christian. God has, with a lavish hand, provided us with rich and varied bounties for our sustenance and enjoyment. But in order for us to enjoy the natural appetite, which will preserve health and prolong life, He restricts the appetite. He says, Beware; restrain, deny, unnatural appetite. If we create a perverted appetite, we violate the laws of our being, and assume the responsibility of abusing our bodies and of bringing disease upon ourselves. . . .

Self-denial is essential to genuine religion. Those who have not learned to deny themselves are destitute of vital, practical godliness. We cannot expect anything else than that the claims of religion will come in contact with the natural affections and worldly interests. There is work for everyone in the vineyard of the Lord.

Benevolence and Rectitude in Married Life

Those professing to be Christians should not enter the marriage relation until the matter has been carefully and prayerfully considered from an elevated standpoint, to see if God can be glorified by the union. Then they should duly consider the result of every privilege of the marriage relation, and sanctified principle should be the basis of every action. Before increasing their family, they should take into consideration whether God would be glorified or dishonored by their bringing children into the world. They should seek to glorify God by their union from the first, and during every year of their married life. They should calmly consider what provision can be made for their children. They have no right to bring children into the world to be a burden to others. Have they a business that they can rely upon to sustain a family, so that they need not become a burden to others? If they have not, they commit a crime in bringing children into the world to suffer for want of proper care, food, and clothing. In this fast, corrupt age these things are not considered. Lustful passion bears sway, and will not submit to control, although feebleness, misery, and death are the result of its reign. Women are forced to a life of hardship, pain, and suffering, because of the uncontrollable passions of men who bear the name of husband—more rightly could they be called brutes. Mothers drag out a miserable existence, with children in their arms nearly all the time, managing every way to put bread into their mouths and clothes upon their backs. Such accumulated misery fills the world.

Testimonies for the Church, vol. 2, pp. 380-383 (1868).

Passion Is Not Love

There is but little real, genuine, devoted, pure love. This precious article is very rare. Passion is termed love. Many a woman has had her fine and tender sensibilities outraged, because the marriage relation allowed him whom she called husband to be brutal in his treatment of her. His love she found to be of so base a quality that she became disgusted.

Very many families are living in a most unhappy state, because the husband and father allows the animal in his nature to predominate over the intellectual and moral. The result is that a sense of languor and depression is frequently felt, but the cause is seldom divined as being the result of their own improper course of action. We are under solemn obligations to God to keep the spirit pure and the body healthy, that we may be a benefit to humanity, and render to God perfect service. The apostle utters these words of warning: "Let not sin therefore reign in your mortal body, that ye should obey it in the lusts thereof." Romans 6:12. He urges us onward by telling us that "every man that striveth for the mastery is temperate in all things." 1 Corinthians 9:25. He exhorts all who call themselves Christians to present their bodies "a living sacrifice, holy, acceptable unto God." Romans 12:1. He says, "I keep under my body, and bring it into subjection: lest that by any means, when I have preached to others, I myself should be a castaway." 1 Corinthians 9:27.

Care of the Wife

It is an error generally committed to make no difference in the life of a woman previous to the birth of her children. At this important period the labor of the mother should be lightened. Great changes are going on in her system. It requires a greater amount of blood, and therefore an increase of food of the most nourishing quality to convert into blood. Unless she has an abundant supply of nutritious food, she cannot retain her physical strength, and her offspring is robbed of vitality. Her clothing also demands attention. Care should be taken to protect the body from a sense of chilliness. She should not call vitality unnecessarily to the surface to supply the want of sufficient clothing. If the mother is deprived of an abundance of wholesome, nutritious food, she will lack in the quantity and quality of blood. Her circulation will be poor, and her child will lack in the very same things. There will be inability in the offspring to appropriate food which it can convert into good blood to nourish the system. The prosperity of mother and child depends much upon good, warm clothing, and a supply of nourishing food. The extra draft upon the vitality of the mother must be considered and provided for.

Control of Appetite Important

But, on the other hand, the idea that women, because of their special condition, may let the appetite run riot, is a mistake based on custom, but not on sound sense. The appetite of women in this condition may be variable, fitful, and difficult to gratify; and custom allows her to have anything she may fancy, without consulting reason as to whether such food can supply nutrition for her body and for the growth of her child. The food should be nutritious, but should not be of an exciting quality. Custom says that if she wants flesh meats, pickles, spiced food, or mince pies, let her have them; appetite alone is to be consulted. This is a great mistake, and does much harm. The harm cannot be estimated. If ever there is need of simplicity of diet and special care as to the quality of food eaten, it is in this important period.

Women who possess principle and who are well instructed will not depart from simplicity of diet at this time of all others. They will consider that another life is dependent upon them and will be careful in all their habits, and especially in diet. They should not eat that which is innutritious and exciting, simply because it tastes good. There are too many counselors ready to persuade them to do things which reason would tell them they ought not to do.

Diseased children are born because of the gratification of appetite by the parents. The system did not demand the variety of food upon which the mind dwelt. Because once in the mind it must be in the stomach, is a great error, which Christian women should reject. Imagination should not be allowed to control the wants of the system. Those who allow the taste to rule, will suffer the penalty of transgressing the laws of their being. And the matter does not end here; their innocent offspring also will be sufferers. . . .

Pleasant Surroundings Essential

Great care should be exercised to have the surroundings of the mother pleasant and happy. The husband and father is under special responsibility to do all in his power to lighten the burden of the wife and mother. He should bear, as much as possible, the burden of her condition. He should be affable, courteous, kind, and tender, and especially attentive to all her wants.

Counsels Regarding Motherhood

Every woman about to become a mother whatever may be her surroundings, should encourage constantly a happy, contented disposition, knowing that for all her efforts in this direction she will be repaid tenfold in the physical, as well as in the moral, character of her offspring. Nor is this all. By habit she can accustom herself to cheerful thinking, and thus encourage a happy state of mind, and cast a cheerful reflection of her own happiness of spirit upon her family and those with whom she associates.

And in a very great degree her physical health will be improved. A force will be imparted to the life springs; the blood will not move sluggishly, as would be the case if she were to yield to despondency and gloom. Her mental and moral health are invigorated by the buoyancy of her spirits. The power of the will can resist impressions of the mind and will prove a grand soother of the nerves. Children who are robbed of that vitality which they should have inherited from their parents should have the utmost care. By close attention to the laws of their being a much better condition may be established.

The Feeding of Infants

The period in which the infant receives its nourishment from its mother is critical. Many a mother, while nursing her infant, has been permitted to overwork, heating her blood over the cookstove; and the nursling has been seriously affected, not only with fevered nourishment from the mother's breast, but its blood has been poisoned by the unhealthy diet of the mother, which has fevered her whole system, thereby affecting the food of the infant. The in-

---

Review and Herald, July 25, 1899.

fant is also affected by the condition of the mother's mind. If she is unhappy, easily agitated, irritable, giving vent to outbursts of passion, the nourishment the infant receives from its mother will be inflamed, often producing colic, spasms, and, in some instances, causing convulsions, or fits.

The character also of the child is more or less affected by the nature of the nourishment received from the mother. How important, then, that the mother, while nursing her infant, should preserve a happy state of mind, having perfect control of her own spirit. By thus doing, the food of the child is not injured, and the calm, self-possessed course the mother pursues in the treatment of her child has much to do in molding the mind of the infant. If it is nervous and easily agitated, the mother's careful, unhurried manner will have a soothing and correcting influence, and the health of the infant will be much improved.

Infants have been greatly abused by improper treatment. If fretful, they have generally been fed to keep them quiet, when, in most cases, receiving too much food, made injurious by the wrong habits of the mother, was the very cause of their fretfulness. More food only made the matter worse; for the stomach was already overloaded. . . .

The mother often plans to accomplish a certain amount of work during the day; and when the children trouble her, instead of taking time to soothe their little sorrows, and divert them, something is given them to eat, to keep them still. This accomplishes the purpose for a short time, but eventually makes things worse. The children's stomachs are pressed with food when they have not the least want of food. All that is required is a little of the mother's time and attention.

Refuse Tobacco Defilement

Tobacco, in whatever form it is used, tells upon the constitution. It is a slow poison. It affects the brain and benumbs the sensibilities, so that the mind cannot clearly discern spiritual things, especially those truths which would have a tendency to correct this filthy indulgence. Those who use tobacco in any form are not clear before God. In such a filthy practice it is impossible for them to glorify God in their bodies and spirits which are His. And while they are using slow and sure poisons, which are ruining their health and debasing the faculties of the mind, God cannot approbate them. He may be merciful to them while they indulge in this pernicious habit in ignorance of the injury it is doing them, but when the matter is set before them in its true light, then they are guilty before God if they continue to indulge this gross appetite.

God required the children of Israel to observe habits of strict cleanliness. In any case of the least impurity they were to remain out of the camp until evening, then to wash themselves and come into the camp. There was not a tobacco user in that vast army. If there had been, he would have been required to choose to remain out of the camp or cease the use of the filthy weed. And after cleansing his mouth from the least of its filthy remains, he might have been permitted to mingle with the congregation of Israel.

Tobacco Defilement an Offense to God

The priests, who ministered in sacred things, were commanded to wash their feet and their hands before entering the tabernacle in the presence of God to importune for

Israel, that they might not desecrate the sanctuary. If the priests had entered the sanctuary with their mouths polluted, they would have shared the fate of Nadab and Abihu. And yet professed Christians bow before God in their families to pray with their mouths defiled with the filth of tobacco. . . .

Strict Cleanliness Required

Men who have been set apart by the laying on of hands, to minister in sacred things, often stand in the desk with their mouths polluted, their lips stained, and their breath tainted with the defilements of tobacco. They speak to the people in Christ's stead. How can such a service be acceptable to a holy God, who required the priests of Israel to make such special preparations before coming into His presence, lest His sacred holiness should consume them for dishonoring Him, as in the case of Nadab and Abihu? These may be assured that the mighty God of Israel is still a God of cleanliness. They profess to be serving God while they are committing idolatry, by making a god of their appetite. Tobacco is their cherished idol. To it every high and sacred consideration must bow. They profess to be worshiping God, while at the same time they are violating the first commandment. They have other gods before the Lord. "Be ye clean, that bear the vessels of the Lord." Isaiah 52:11.

God requires purity of heart and personal cleanliness now, as when He gave the special directions to the children of Israel. If God was so particular to enjoin cleanliness upon those journeying in the wilderness, who were in the open air nearly all the time, He requires no less of us who live in ceiled houses, where impurities are more observable and have a more unhealthful influence.

Tobacco Using Contrary to Godliness

As I have seen men who claimed to enjoy the blessing of entire satisfaction, while they were slaves to tobacco, spitting and defiling everything around them, I have thought, How would heaven appear with tobacco users in it? The lips that were taking the precious name of Christ were defiled by tobacco spittle, the breath was polluted with the stench, and even the linen was defiled; the soul that loved this uncleanness and enjoyed this poisonous atmosphere must also be defiled. The sign was hung upon the outside, testifying of what was within.

Men professing godliness offer their bodies upon Satan's altar, and burn the incense of tobacco to his satanic majesty. Does this statement seem severe? The offering must be presented to some deity. As God is pure and holy, and will accept nothing defiling in its character, He refuses this expensive, filthy, and unholy sacrifice; therefore we conclude that Satan is the one who claims the honor.

Man the Property of Christ

Jesus died to rescue man from the grasp of Satan. He came to set us free by the blood of His atoning sacrifice. The man who has become the property of Jesus Christ, and whose body is the temple of the Holy Ghost, will not be enslaved by the pernicious habit of tobacco using. His powers belong to Christ, who has bought him with the price of blood. His property is the Lord's. How, then, can he be guiltless in expending every day the Lord's entrusted capital to gratify an appetite which has no foundation in nature?

Review and Herald, Jan. 25, 1881.

A Sad Misuse of Means

An enormous sum is yearly squandered for this indulgence, while souls are perishing for the word of life. How can Christians who are enlightened upon this subject continue to rob God in tithes and offerings used to sustain the gospel, while they offer on the altar of destroying lust, in the use of tobacco, more than they give to relieve the poor or to supply the wants of God's cause? If they are truly sanctified, every hurtful lust will be overcome. Then all these channels of needless expense will be turned to the Lord's treasury, and Christians will take the lead in self-denial, self-sacrifice, and in temperance. Then they will be the light of the world. . . .

Natural Sensibilities Are Deadened

To a tobacco user, everything is insipid and lifeless without the darling indulgence. Its use has deadened the natural sensibilities of body and mind, and he is not susceptible of the influence of the Spirit of God. In the absence of the usual stimulant, he has a hungering and yearning of body and soul not for righteousness, not for holiness, not for God's presence, but for his cherished idol. In the indulgence of hurtful lusts, professed Christians are daily enfeebling their powers, making it impossible to glorify God.

A Deceitful Poison

Tobacco is a poison of the most deceitful and malignant kind, having an exciting, then a paralyzing influence upon the nerves of the body. It is all the more dangerous because its effects upon the system are so slow, and at first scarcely perceivable. Multitudes have fallen victims to its poisonous influence.—*Spiritual Gifts,* vol. 4, p. 128 (1864).

Abstinence From Narcotics

Our people are constantly retrograding upon health reform. Satan sees that he cannot have such a controlling power over them as he could if appetite were indulged. Under the influence of unhealthful food, the conscience becomes stupefied, the mind becomes darkened, and its susceptibility to impressions is blunted. But because violated conscience is benumbed and becomes insensible, the guilt of the transgressor is not lessened.

Satan is corrupting minds and destroying souls through his subtle temptations. Will our people see and feel the sin of indulging perverted appetite? Will they discard tea, coffee, flesh meats, and all stimulating food, and devote the means expended for these hurtful indulgences to spreading the truth? These stimulants do only harm, and yet we see that a large number of those who profess to be Christians are using tobacco. These very men will deplore the evil of intemperance, and while speaking against the use of liquors, will eject the juice of tobacco. While a healthy state of mind depends upon the normal condition of the vital forces, what care should be exercised that neither stimulants nor narcotics be used.

Tobacco is a slow, insidious poison, and its effects are more difficult to cleanse from the system than those of liquor. What power can the tobacco devotee have to stay the progress of intemperance? There must be a revolution in our world upon the subject of tobacco before the ax is laid at the root of the tree. We press the subject still closer. Tea and coffee are fostering the appetite which is developing for stronger stimulants, as tobacco and liquor.

Testimonies for the Church, vol. 3, pp. 569, 570 (1875).

And we come still closer home, to the daily meals, the tables spread in Christian households. Is temperance practiced in all things? Are the reforms which are essential to health and happiness carried out there? Every true Christian will have control of his appetite and passions. Unless he is free from the bondage and slavery of appetite, he cannot be a true, obedient servant of Christ. It is the indulgence of appetite and passion which makes the truth of none effect upon the heart. It is impossible for the spirit and power of the truth to sanctify a man, soul, body, and spirit, when he is controlled by appetite and passion.

Self-Denial and Prayer

When Christ was the most fiercely beset by temptation, he ate nothing. He committed Himself to God, and through earnest prayer and perfect submission to the will of His Father, came off conqueror. Those who profess the truth for these last days, above every other class of professed Christians, should imitate the great Exemplar in prayer. . . .

Jesus sought earnestly for strength from His Father. This the divine Son of God considered of more value even for Himself, than to sit at the most luxurious table. He has given us evidence that prayer is essential in order to receive strength to contend with the powers of darkness, and to do the work allotted us. Our own strength is weakness, but that which God gives is mighty, and will make everyone who obtains it more than conqueror. —*Testimonies for the Church,* vol. 2, pp. 202, 203 (1869).

Evil Effects of Tea and Coffee

The use of tea and coffee is also injurious to the system. To a certain extent, tea produces intoxication. It enters into the circulation and gradually impairs the energy of body and mind. It stimulates, excites, and quickens the motion of the living machinery, forcing it to unnatural action, and thus gives the tea drinker the impression that it is doing him great service, imparting to him strength. This is a mistake. Tea draws upon the strength of the nerves, and leaves them greatly weakened. When its influence is gone and the increased action caused by its use is abated, then what is the result? Languor and debility corresponding to the artificial vivacity the tea imparted.

When the system is already overtaxed and needs rest, the use of tea spurs up nature by stimulation to perform unwonted, unnatural action, and thereby lessens her power to perform, and her ability to endure; and her powers give out long before Heaven designed they should. Tea is poisonous to the system. Christians should let it alone.

The influence of coffee is in a degree the same as tea, but the effect upon the system is still worse. Its influence is exciting, and just in the degree that it elevates above par, it will exhaust and bring prostration below par. Tea and coffee drinkers carry the marks upon their faces. The skin becomes sallow and assumes a lifeless appearance. The glow of health is not seen upon the countenance.

Tea and Coffee Do Not Nourish

Tea and coffee do not nourish the system. The relief obtained from them is sudden, before the stomach has

Testimonies for the Church, vol. 2, pp. 64, 65 (1868).

(87)

time to digest them. This shows that what the users of these stimulants call strength, is only received by exciting the nerves of the stomach, which convey the irritation to the brain, and this in turn is aroused to impart increased action to the heart, and short-lived energy to the entire system. All this is false strength, that we are the worse for having. They do not give a particle of natural strength. The second effect of tea drinking is headache, wakefulness, palpitation of the heart, indigestion, trembling of the nerves, with many other evils.

Self-Indulgence Displeasing to God

"I beseech you therefore, brethren, by the mercies of God, that ye present your bodies a living sacrifice, holy, acceptable unto God, which is your reasonable service." Romans 12:1. God calls for a living sacrifice, not a dead or dying one. When we realize the requirements of God, we shall see that He requires us to be temperate in all things. The end of our creation is to glorify God in our bodies and spirits which are His. How can we do this when we indulge the appetite to the injury of the physical and moral powers? God requires that we present our bodies a living sacrifice. Then the duty is enjoined on us to preserve that body in the very best condition of health, that we may comply with His requirements. "Whether therefore ye eat, or drink, or whatsoever ye do, do all to the glory of God." 1 Corinthians 10:31.

Avoid the Use of Poisonous Drugs

A practice that is laying the foundation of a vast amount of disease and of even more serious evils, is the free use of poisonous drugs. When attacked by disease, many will not take the trouble to search out the cause of their illness. Their chief anxiety is to rid themselves of pain and inconvenience. So they resort to patent nostrums, of whose real properties they know little, or they apply to a physician for some remedy to counteract the result of their misdoing, but with no thought of making a change in their unhealthful habits. If immediate benefit is not realized, another medicine is tried, and then another. Thus the evil continues.

Drugs Do Not Cure Disease

People need to be taught that drugs do not cure disease. It is true that they sometimes afford present relief, and the patient appears to recover as the result of their use; this is because nature has sufficient vital force to expel the poison and to correct the conditions that caused the disease. Health is recovered in spite of the drug. But in most cases the drug only changes the form and location of the disease. Often the effect of the poison seems to be overcome for a time, but the results remain in the system, and work great harm at some later period.

By the use of poisonous drugs, many bring upon themselves lifelong illness, and many lives are lost that might be saved by the use of natural methods of healing. The poisons contained in many so-called remedies create habits and appetites that mean ruin to both soul and body. Many of the popular nostrums called patent medicines, and even

The Ministry of Healing, pages 126, 127 (1905).

some of the drugs dispensed by physicians, act a part in laying the foundation of the liquor habit, the opium habit, the morphine habit, that are so terrible a curse to society.

Restorative Power in Nature

The only hope of better things is in the education of the people in right principles. Let physicians teach the people that restorative power is not in drugs, but in nature. Disease is an effort of nature to free the system from conditions that result from a violation of the laws of health. In case of sickness, the cause should be ascertained. Unhealthful conditions should be changed, wrong habits corrected. Then nature is to be assisted in her effort to expel impurities and to re-establish right conditions in the system.

Natural Remedies

Pure air, sunlight, abstemiousness, rest, exercise, proper diet, the use of water, trust in divine power—these are the true remedies. Every person should have a knowledge of nature's remedial agencies and how to apply them. It is essential both to understand the principles involved in the treatment of the sick and to have a practical training that will enable one rightly to use this knowledge.

The use of natural remedies requires an amount of care and effort that many are not willing to give. Nature's process of healing and upbuilding is gradual, and to the impatient it seems slow. The surrender of hurtful indulgences requires sacrifice. But in the end it will be found that nature, untrammeled, does her work wisely and well. Those who persevere in obedience to her laws will reap the reward in health of body and health of mind.

Healthful Dress

In all respects the dress should be healthful. "Above all things," God desires us to "be in health"—health of body and of soul. And we are to be workers together with Him for the health of both soul and body. Both are promoted by healthful dress. . . .

It was the adversary of all good who instigated the invention of the ever-changing fashions. He desires nothing so much as to bring grief and dishonor to God by working the misery and ruin of human beings. One of the means by which he most effectually accomplishes this is the devices of fashion, that weaken the body, as well as enfeeble the mind and belittle the soul.

Women are subject to serious maladies, and their sufferings are greatly increased by their manner of dress. Instead of preserving their health for the trying emergencies that are sure to come, they by their wrong habits too often sacrifice not only health but life, and leave to their children a legacy of woe, in a ruined constitution, perverted habits, and false ideas of life.

One of fashion's wasteful and mischievous devices is the skirt that sweeps the ground. Uncleanly, uncomfortable, inconvenient, unhealthful—all this and more is true of the trailing skirt. It is extravagant, both because of the superfluous material required, and because of the needless wear on account of its length. And whoever has seen a woman in a trailing skirt, with hands filled with parcels, attempt to go up or down stairs, to enter a streetcar, to walk through a crowd, to walk in the rain, or on a muddy road, needs no other proof of its inconvenience and discomfort.

Another serious evil is the wearing of skirts so that

The Ministry of Healing, pages 288-294 (1905).

4—C.O.H.

their weight must be sustained by the hips. This heavy weight, pressing upon the internal organs, drags them downward and causes weakness of the stomach and a feeling of lassitude, inclining the wearer to stoop, which further cramps the lungs, making correct breathing more difficult.

Of late years the dangers resulting from compression of the waist have been so fully discussed that few can be ignorant in regard to them; yet so great is the power of fashion that the evil continues. By this practice, women and young girls are doing themselves untold harm. It is essential to health that the chest have room to expand to its fullest extent, in order that the lungs may be enabled to take full inspiration. When the lungs are restricted, the quantity of oxygen received into them is lessened. The blood is not properly vitalized, and the waste, poisonous matter which should be thrown off through the lungs, is retained. In addition to this, the circulation is hindered; and the internal organs are so cramped and crowded out of place that they cannot perform their work properly.

Tight lacing does not improve the form. One of the chief elements in physical beauty is symmetry, the harmonious proportion of parts. And the correct model for physical development is to be found, not in the figures displayed by French modistes, but in the human form as developed according to the laws of God in nature. God is the author of all beauty, and only as we conform to His ideal shall we approach the standard of true beauty.

Another evil which custom fosters is the unequal distribution of the clothing, so that while some parts of the body have more than is required, others are insufficiently clad. The feet and limbs, being remote from the vital organs, should be especially guarded from cold by abundant clothing. It is impossible to have health when the extremities are habitually cold; for if there is too little blood in them there will be too much in other portions of the body. Perfect health requires a perfect circulation; but this cannot be had while three or four times as much clothing is worn upon the body, where the vital organs are situated, as upon the feet and limbs.

A multitude of women are nervous and careworn, because they deprive themselves of the pure air that would make pure blood, and of the freedom of motion that would send the blood bounding through the veins, giving life, health, and energy. Many women have become confirmed invalids when they might have enjoyed health, and many have died of consumption and other diseases when they might have lived their allotted term of life, had they dressed in accordance with health principles and exercised freely in the open air.

In order to secure the most healthful clothing, the needs of every part of the body must be carefully studied. The character of the climate, the surroundings, the condition of health, the age and the occupation must all be considered. Every article of dress should fit easily, obstructing neither the circulation of the blood, nor a free, full, natural respiration. Everything worn should be so loose that when the arms are raised, the clothing will be correspondingly lifted.

Women who are in failing health can do much for themselves by sensible dressing and exercise. When suitably dressed for outdoor enjoyment, let them exercise in the open air, carefully at first, but increasing the amount of exercise as they can endure it. By taking this course many might regain health and live to take their share in the world's work.

The Power of the Will

The power of the will is not valued as it should be. Let the will be kept awake and rightly directed, and it will impart energy to the whole being, and will be a wonderful aid in the maintenance of health. It is a power also in dealing with disease. Exercised in the right direction, it would control the imagination, and be a potent means of resisting and overcoming disease of both mind and body. By the exercise of the will power in placing themselves in right relation to life, patients can do much to co-operate with the physician's efforts for their recovery. There are thousands who can recover health if they will. The Lord does not want them to be sick. He desires them to be well and happy, and they should make up their minds to be well. Often invalids can resist disease simply by refusing to yield to ailments and settle down in a state of inactivity. Rising above their aches and pains, let them engage in useful employment suited to their strength. By such employment and the free use of air and sunlight, many an emaciated invalid might recover health and strength.—*The Ministry of Healing,* page 246 (1905).

Suitable Employment

Inactivity is the greatest curse that could come upon most invalids. Light employment in useful labor, while it does not tax mind and body, has a happy influence upon both. It strengthens the muscles, improves the circulation, and gives the invalid the satisfaction of knowing that he is not wholly useless in this busy world. He may be able to do but little at first, but he will soon find his strength increasing and the amount of work done can be increased accordingly.—*The Ministry of Healing,* page 240 (1905).

Control the Imagination

In the creation of man, the Lord designed that he should be active and useful. Yet many live in this world as useless machines, as though they hardly existed. They brighten the path of none, they are a blessing to none. They live only to burden others. So far as their influence on the side of right is concerned, they are mere ciphers; but they tell with weight upon the wrong side. Search the lives of such closely, and scarcely an act of disinterested benevolence can be found. When they die, their memory dies with them. Their names soon perish; for they cannot live, even in the affections of their friends, by means of true goodness and virtuous acts. With such persons, life has been a mistake. They have not been faithful stewards. They have forgotten that their Creator has claims upon them, and that He designs them to be active in doing good and in blessing others with their influence. Selfish interests attract the mind and lead to forgetfulness of God and of the purpose of their Creator.

All who profess to be followers of Jesus should feel that a duty rests upon them to preserve their bodies in the best condition of health, that their minds may be clear to comprehend heavenly things. The mind needs to be controlled; for it has a most powerful influence upon the health. The imagination often misleads, and when indulged, brings severe forms of disease upon the afflicted. Many die of diseases which are mostly imaginary. . . .

Some are so afraid of air that they will muffle up their heads and bodies until they look like mummies. They sit in the house, generally inactive, fearing they shall

Testimonies for the Church, vol. 2, pp. 522-525, (1870).

weary themselves and get sick if they exercise either indoors or out in the open air. They could take habitual exercise in the open air every pleasant day, if they only thought so. Continued inactivity is one of the greatest causes of debility of body and feebleness of mind. Many are sick who ought to be in very good health and thus in possession of one of the richest blessings they could enjoy.

I have been shown that many who are apparently feeble, and are ever complaining, are not so badly off as they imagine themselves to be. Some of these have a powerful will, which, exercised in the right direction, would be a potent means of controlling the imagination and thus resisting disease. But it is too frequently the case that the will is exercised in a wrong direction, and stubbornly refuses to yield to reason. That will has settled the matter; invalids they are, and the attention due to invalids they will have irrespective of the judgment of others.

I have been shown mothers who are governed by a diseased imagination, the influence of which is felt upon husband and children. The windows must be kept closed because the mother feels the air. If she is at all chilly, and a change is made in her clothing, she thinks her children must be treated in the same manner, and thus the entire family are robbed of physical stamina. All are affected by one mind, physically and mentally injured through the diseased imagination of one woman who considers herself a criterion for the whole family. The body is clothed in accordance with the caprices of a diseased imagination, and smothered under an amount of wrappings which debilitate the system. The skin cannot perform its office; the studied habit of shunning the air and avoiding exercise, closes the pores, the little mouths through which the body breathes,—making it impossible to throw off impurities through that channel. The burden of labor is thrown upon the liver, lungs, kidneys, etc., and these internal organs are compelled to do the work of the skin.

Thus persons bring disease upon themselves by their wrong habits; yet, in the face of light and knowledge, they will adhere to their own course. They reason thus: "Have we not tried the matter? and do we not understand it by experience?" But the experience of a person whose imagination is at fault should not have much weight with anyone.

The season most to be dreaded by any going among these invalids is winter. It is winter indeed, not only outdoors, but in, to those who are compelled to live in the same house and sleep in the same room. These victims of a diseased imagination shut themselves indoors and close the windows; for the air affects their lungs and their heads. Imagination is active; they expect to take cold, and they will have it. No amount of reasoning can make them believe that they do not understand the philosophy of the whole matter. Have they not proved it? they will argue. It is true that they have proved one side of the question, —by persisting in their own course,—and yet they do take cold if in the least exposed. Tender as babies, they cannot endure anything; yet they live on, and continue to close the windows and doors, and hover over the stove, and enjoy their misery. They have surely proved that their course has not made them well, but has increased their difficulties. Why will not such allow reason to influence the judgment and control the imagination? Why not now try an opposite course, and in a judicious manner obtain exercise and air out of doors?

Moderation in Work

In order to gain a little money, many deliberately arrange their business matters so that it necessarily brings a great amount of hard work upon those laboring out of doors, and upon their families in the house. The bone, muscle, and brain of all are taxed to the utmost: a great amount of work is before them to be done, and the excuse is, they must accomplish just all that they possibly can, or there will be a loss, something will be wasted. Everything *must* be saved, let the result be what it may.

What have such gained? Perhaps they have been able to keep the principal good, and add to it. But on the other hand, what have they lost? Their capital of health, which is invaluable to the poor as well as the rich, has been steadily diminishing. The mother and the children have made repeated drafts upon their fund of health and strength, thinking that such an extravagant expenditure would never exhaust their capital, until they are surprised at last to find their vigor of life exhausted. They have nothing left to draw upon in case of emergency. The sweetness and happiness of life are embittered by racking pains and sleepless nights. Both physical and mental vigor are gone. The husband and father who, for the sake of gain, made the unwise arrangement of his business, it may be with the full sanction of the wife and mother, may, as the result, bury the mother and one or more of the children. Health and life were sacrificed for the love of money. (Read 1 Timothy 6:10.)—*Testimonies for the Church,* vol, 1, p. 478 (1865).

Temperance in Labor

Intemperance in eating and drinking, intemperance in labor, intemperance in almost everything, exists on every hand. Those who make great exertions to accomplish just so much work in a given time, and continue to labor when their judgment tells them they should rest, are never gainers. They are living on borrowed capital. They are expending the vital force which they will need at a future time. And when the energy they have so recklessly used is demanded, they fail for want of it. The physical strength is gone, the mental powers fail. They realize that they have met with a loss, but do not know what it is. Their time of need has come, but their physical resources are exhausted. Everyone who violates the laws of health must sometime be a sufferer to a greater or less degree. God has provided us with constitutional force, which will be needed at different periods of our life. If we recklessly exhaust this force by continual overtaxation, we shall sometime be losers. Our usefulness will be lessened, if not our life itself destroyed.

As a rule, the labor of the day should not be prolonged into the evening. If all the hours of the day are well improved, the work extended into the evening is so much extra, and the overtaxed system will suffer from the burden imposed upon it. I have been shown that those who do this often lose much more than they gain, for their energies are exhausted and they labor on nervous excitement. They may not realize any immediate injury, but they are surely undermining their constitution.

Christian Temperance, pages 64-66 (1890).

Let parents devote the evenings to their families. Lay off care and perplexity with the labors of the day. The husband and father would gain much if he would make it a rule not to mar the happiness of his family by bringing his business troubles home to fret and worry over. He may need the counsel of his wife in difficult matters, and they may both obtain relief in their perplexities by unitedly seeking wisdom of God; but to keep the mind constantly strained upon business affairs will injure the health of both mind and body.

Let the evenings be spent as happily as possible. Let home be a place where cheerfulness, courtesy, and love exist. This will make it attractive to the children. If the parents are continually borrowing trouble, are irritable and faultfinding, the children partake of the same spirit of dissatisfaction and contention, and home is the most miserable place in the world. The children find more pleasure among strangers, in reckless company, or in the streets, than at home. All this might be avoided if temperance in all things were practiced, and patience cultivated. Self-control on the part of all the members of the family will make home almost a paradise. Make your rooms as cheerful as possible. Let the children find home the most attractive place on earth. Throw about them such influences that they will not seek for street companions, nor think of the haunts of vice except with horror. If the home life is what it should be, the habits formed there will be a strong defense against the assaults of temptation when the young shall leave the shelter of home for the world.

Order and Cleanliness

Order is heaven's first law, and the Lord desires His people to give in their homes a representation of the order and harmony that pervade the heavenly courts. Truth never places her delicate feet in a path of uncleanness or impurity. Truth does not make men and women coarse or rough and untidy. It raises all who accept it to a high level. Under Christ's influence, a work of constant refinement goes on.

Special direction was given to the armies of Israel that everything in and around their tents should be clean and orderly, lest the angel of the Lord, passing through the encampment, should see their uncleanness. Would the Lord be particular to notice these things? He would; for the fact is stated, lest in seeing their uncleanness, He could not go forward with their armies to battle.

He who was so particular that the children of Israel should cherish habits of cleanliness, will not sanction any impurity in the homes of His people today. God looks with disfavor on uncleanness of any kind. How can we invite Him into our homes unless all is neat and clean and pure?

An Outward Sign of Purity Within

Believers should be taught that even though they may be poor, they need not be uncleanly or untidy in their persons or in their homes. Help must be given in this line to those who seem to have no sense of the meaning and importance of cleanliness. They are to be taught that those who are to represent the high and holy God must keep their souls pure and clean, and that this purity must extend to their dress, and to everything in the home, so

Review and Herald, June 10, 1902.

that the ministering angels will have evidence that the truth has wrought a change in the life, purifying the soul and refining the tastes. Those who, after receiving the truth, make no change in word or deportment, in dress or surroundings, are living to themselves, not to Christ. They have not been created anew in Christ Jesus unto purification and holiness.

Some are very untidy in person. They need to be guided by the Holy Spirit to prepare for a pure and holy heaven. God declared that when the children of Israel came to the mount, to hear the proclamation of the law, they were to come with clean bodies and clean clothes. Today His people are to honor Him by habits of scrupulous neatness and purity.

Christians will be judged by the fruit they bear. The true child of God will be neat and clean. While we are to guard against needless adornment and display, we are in no case to be careless and indifferent in regard to outward appearance. All about our persons and our homes is to be neat and attractive. The youth are to be taught the importance of presenting an appearance above criticism, an appearance that honors God and the truth.

The Mother's Example

The mother's dress should be simple, but neat and tasty. The mother who wears torn, untidy clothes, who thinks any dress good enough for home wear, no matter how soiled or dilapidated it may be, gives her children an example that encourages them in untidiness. And more than this, she loses her influence over them. They cannot help seeing the difference between her appearance and the appearance of those who dress neatly; and their respect for her is weakened. Mothers, make yourselves attractive, not by wearing elaborately trimmed garments, but by wearing those that are neat and well fitting. Let your appearance teach a lesson of neatness. You cannot afford to lose the respect of your children.

From their infancy, children should be taught lessons of purity. Mothers cannot too early begin to fill the minds of their children with pure, holy thoughts. And one way of doing this is to keep everything about them clean and pure. Mothers, if you desire your children's thoughts to be pure, let their surroundings be pure. Let their sleeping rooms be scrupulously neat and clean. Teach them to care for their clothing. Each child should have a place of his own to care for his clothes. Few parents are so poor that they cannot afford to provide for this purpose a large box, which may be fitted with shelves and tastefully covered.

Teaching Spiritual Truths

To teach children habits of order will take some time each day; but this time is not lost. In the future, the mother will be more than repaid for her efforts in this direction.

See that the children have a daily bath, followed by friction till their bodies are aglow. Tell them that God does not like to see His children with unclean bodies and ragged garments. Then go further, and speak of inward purity. Let it be your constant effort to uplift and ennoble your children.

We are living in the last days. Soon Christ is coming for His people to take them to the mansions He is preparing for them. But nothing that defiles can enter those mansions. Heaven is pure and holy, and those who pass through the gates of the City of God must here be clothed with inward and outward purity.

Frequent Bathing

Persons in health should on no account neglect bathing. They should by all means bathe as often as twice a week. Those who are not in health have impurities in the blood, and the skin is not in a healthy condition. The multitude of pores, or little mouths, through which the body breathes, become clogged and filled with waste matter. The skin needs to be carefully and thoroughly cleansed, that the pores may do their work in freeing the body from impurities; therefore feeble persons who are diseased surely need the advantages and blessings of bathing as often as twice a week, and frequently even more than this is positively necessary. Whether a person is sick or well, respiration is more free and easy if bathing is practiced. By it, the muscles become more flexible, the mind and body are alike invigorated, the intellect is made brighter, and every faculty becomes livelier. The bath is a soother of the nerves. It promotes general perspiration, quickens the circulation, overcomes obstructions in the system, and acts beneficially on the kidneys and urinary organs. Bathing helps the bowels, stomach, and liver, giving energy and new life to each. It also promotes digestion, and instead of the system being weakened, it is strengthened. Instead of increasing the liability to cold, a bath, properly taken, fortifies against cold, because the circulation is improved, and the uterine organs, which are more or less congested are relieved; for the blood is brought to the surface, and a more easy and regular flow of the blood through all the blood vessels is obtained.— *Testimonies for the Church,* vol. 3, pp. 70, 71 (1871).

How to Preserve Our Sensibilities

God created man a little lower than the angels and bestowed upon him attributes that will, if properly used, make him a blessing to the world and cause him to reflect the glory to the Giver. But although made in the image of God, man has, through intemperance, violated principle and God's law in his physical nature. Intemperance of any kind benumbs the perceptive organs and so weakens the brain nerve power that eternal things are not appreciated, but placed upon a level with the common. The higher powers of the mind, designed for elevated purposes, are brought into slavery to the baser passions. If our physical habits are not right, our mental and moral powers cannot be strong; for great sympathy exists between the physical and the moral. The apostle Peter understood this and raised his voice of warning to his brethren: "Dearly beloved, I beseech you as strangers and pilgrims, abstain from fleshly lusts, which war against the soul." 1 Peter 2:11. . . .

Those who have had the light upon the subjects of eating and dressing with simplicity, in obedience to physical and moral laws, and who turn from the light which points out their duty, will shun duty in other things. If they blunt their consciences to avoid the cross which they will have to take up to be in harmony with natural law, they will, in order to shun reproach, violate the Ten Commandments. There is a decided unwillingness with some to endure the cross and despise the shame. Some will be laughed out of their principles. Conformity to the world is gaining ground among God's people, who profess to be pilgrims and strangers, waiting and watching for the

Testimonies for the Church, vol. 3, pp. 50-52 (1871).

Lord's appearing. There are many among professed Sabbathkeepers in ———— who are more firmly wedded to
worldly fashions and lusts than they are to healthy bodies, sound minds, or sanctified hearts. . . .

The Lord, by close and pointed truths for these last
days, is cleaving out a people from the world and purifying them unto Himself. Pride and unhealthful fashions,
the love of display, the love of approbation—all must be
left with the world, if we would be renewed in knowledge after the image of Him who created us. "For the
grace of God that bringeth salvation hath appeared to all
men, teaching us that, denying ungodliness and worldly
lusts, we should live soberly, righteously and godly, in
this present world; looking for that blessed hope, and the
glorious appearing of the great God and our Saviour Jesus
Christ; who gave Himself for us, that He might redeem
us from all iniquity, and purify unto Himself a peculiar
people, zealous of good works." Titus 2:11-14.

To a Brother

Said the angel, "Abstain from fleshly lusts which war
against the soul." You have stumbled at the health reform. It appears to you to be a needless appendix to the
truth. It is not so; it is a part of the truth. Here is a work
before you which will come closer and be more trying
than anything which has yet been brought to bear upon
you. While you hesitate and stand back, failing to lay
hold upon the blessing which it is your privilege to receive, you suffer loss.—*Testimonies for the Church,* vol.
1, p. 546 (1890).

DIET AND HEALTH

Relation of Diet to Health and Morals

Only one lease of life is granted us; and the inquiry with everyone should be, "How can I invest my powers so that they may yield the greatest profit? How can I do most for the glory of God and the benefit of my fellow men?" For life is valuable only as it is used for the attainment of these ends.

Self-Development a Duty

Our first duty toward God and our fellow beings is that of self-development. Every faculty with which the Creator has endowed us should be cultivated to the highest degree of perfection, that we may be able to do the greatest amount of good of which we are capable. Hence that time is spent to good account which is used in the establishment and preservation of physical and mental health. We cannot afford to dwarf or cripple any function of body or mind. As surely as we do this we must suffer the consequences.

Every man has the opportunity, to a great extent, of making himself whatever he chooses to be. The blessings of this life, and also of the immortal state, are within his reach. He may build up a character of solid worth, gaining new strength at every step. He may advance daily in knowledge and wisdom, conscious of new delights as he progresses, adding virtue to virtue, grace to grace. His faculties will improve by use; the more wisdom he gains,

Christian Temperance, pages 41-53 (1890).

the greater will be his capacity for acquiring. His intelligence, knowledge, and virtue will thus develop into greater strength and more perfect symmetry.

On the other hand, he may allow his powers to rust out for want of use, or to be perverted through evil habits, lack of self-control or moral and religious stamina. His course then tends downward; he is disobedient to the law of God and to the laws of health. Appetite conquers him; inclination carries him away. It is easier for him to allow the powers of evil, which are always active, to drag him backward, than to struggle against them, and go forward. Dissipation, disease, and death follow. This is the history of many lives that might have been useful in the cause of God and humanity.

Temptation Through Appetite

One of the strongest temptations that man has to meet is upon the point of appetite. In the beginning the Lord made man upright. He was created with a perfectly balanced mind, the size and strength of all his organs being fully and harmoniously developed. But through the seductions of the wily foe the prohibition of God was disregarded, and the laws of nature wrought out their full penalty.

Adam and Eve were permitted to eat of all the trees in their Eden home save one. The Lord said to the holy pair, In the day that ye eat of the tree of knowledge of good and evil, ye shall surely die. Eve was beguiled by the serpent and made to believe that God would not do as He had said. She ate, and, thinking she felt the sensation of a new and more exalted life, she bore the fruit to her husband. The serpent had said that she should not die, and she felt no ill effects from eating the fruit, nothing which could be interpreted to mean death, but, instead, a pleasurable sensation, which she imagined was as the angels felt. Her experience stood arrayed against the positive command of Jehovah, yet Adam permitted himself to be seduced by it.

Thus we often find it, even in the religious world. God's expressed commands are transgressed; and "because sentence against an evil work is not executed speedily, therefore the heart of the sons of men is fully set in them to do evil." Ecclesiastes 8:11. In the face of the most positive commands of God, men and women will follow their own inclinations, and then dare to pray over the matter, to prevail upon God to allow them to go contrary to His expressed will. Satan comes to the side of such persons, as he did to Eve in Eden, and impresses them. They have an exercise of mind, and this they relate as a most wonderful experience which the Lord has given them. But true experience will be in harmony with natural and divine law; false experience arrays itself against the laws of life and the precepts of Jehovah.

Appetite Ruled Antediluvians

Since the first surrender to appetite, mankind have been growing more and more self-indulgent, until health has been sacrificed on the altar of appetite. The inhabitants of the antediluvian world were intemperate in eating and drinking. They would have flesh meats, although God had at that time given man no permission to eat animal food. They ate and drank till the indulgence of their depraved appetite knew no bounds, and they became so corrupt that God could bear with them no longer. Their cup of iniquity was full, and He cleansed the earth of its moral pollution by a flood.

Intemperance After the Flood

As men multiplied upon the earth after the Flood, they again forgot God and corrupted their ways before Him. Intemperance in every form increased, until almost the whole world was given up to its sway. Entire cities have been swept from the face of the earth because of the debasing crimes and revolting iniquity that made them a blot upon the fair field of God's created works. The gratification of unnatural appetite led to the sins that caused the destruction of Sodom and Gomorrah. God ascribes the fall of Babylon to her gluttony and drunkenness. Indulgence of appetite and passion was the foundation of all their sins.

Esau's Experience

Esau had a strong desire for a particular article of food, and he had so long gratified himself that he did not feel the necessity of turning from the tempting, coveted dish. He allowed his imagination to dwell upon it until the power of appetite bore down every other consideration and controlled him. He thought he would suffer great inconvenience, and even death, if he could not have that particular dish. The more he reflected upon it, the more his desire strengthened, until his birthright lost its value and sacredness in his sight, and he bartered it away. He flattered himself that he could dispose of his birthright at will and buy it back at pleasure; but when he sought to regain it, even at a great sacrifice, he was not able to do so. He then bitterly repented of his rashness, his folly, his madness, but it was all in vain. He had despised the blessing, and the Lord had removed it from him forever.

Israel Desired the Fleshpots of Egypt

When the God of Israel brought His people out of Egypt, He withheld flesh meats from them in a great measure, but gave them bread from heaven and water from the flinty rock. With this they were not satisfied. They loathed the food given them and wished themselves back in Egypt, where they could sit by the fleshpots. They preferred to endure slavery, and even death, rather than to be deprived of flesh. God granted their desire, giving them flesh, and leaving them to eat till their gluttony produced a plague, from which many of them died.

Example after example might be cited to show the effects of yielding to appetite. It seemed a small matter to our first parents to transgress the command of God in that one act,—the eating from a tree that was so beautiful to the sight and so pleasant to the taste,—but it broke their allegiance to God and opened the gates to a flood of guilt and woe that has deluged the world.

Intemperance and Crime

Crime and disease have increased with every succeeding generation. Intemperance in eating and drinking, and the indulgence of the baser passions, have benumbed the nobler faculties of man. Reason, instead of being the ruler, has come to be the slave of appetite to an alarming extent. An increasing desire for rich food has been indulged, until it has become the fashion to crowd all the delicacies possible into the stomach. Especially at parties of pleasure is the appetite indulged with but little restraint. Rich dinners and late suppers are served, consisting of highly seasoned meats, with rich sauces, cakes, pies, ices, tea, coffee, etc. No wonder that with such a diet people have sallow complexions and suffer untold agonies from dyspepsia.

Against every transgression of the laws of life, nature will utter her protest. She bears abuse as long as she can; but finally the retribution comes, and it falls upon the mental as well as the physical powers. Nor does it end with the transgressor; the effects of his indulgence are seen in his offspring, and thus the evil is passed down from generation to generation.

Our Youth Lack Self-Control

The youth of today are a sure index to the future of society; and as we view them, what can we hope for that future? The majority are fond of amusement and averse to work. They lack moral courage to deny self and to respond to the claims of duty. They have but little self-control and become excited and angry on the slightest occasion. Very many in every age and station of life are without principle or conscience; and with their idle, spend-thrift habits they are rushing into vice and are corrupting society, until our world is becoming a second Sodom. If the appetites and passions were under the control of reason and religion, society would present a widely different aspect. God never designed that the present woeful condition of things should exist; it has been brought about through the gross violation of nature's laws.

The character is formed, to a great extent, in early years. The habits then established have more influence than any natural endowment, in making men either giants or dwarfs in intellect; for the very best talents may, through wrong habits, become warped and enfeebled. The earlier in life one contracts hurtful habits, the more firmly will they hold their victim in slavery, and the more certainly will they lower his standard of spirituality. On the other hand, if correct and virtuous habits are formed in youth, they will generally mark the course of the possessor through life. In most cases, it will be found that those who in later life reverence God and honor the right, learned that lesson before there was time for the world to stamp its image of sin upon the soul. Those of mature age are generally as insensible to new impressions as is the hardened rock; but youth is impressible. Youth is the time to acquire knowledge for daily practice through life; a right character may then be easily formed. It is the time to establish good habits, to gain and to hold the power of self-control. Youth is the sowing time, and the seed sown determines the harvest, both for this life and the life to come.

Responsibility of Parents

Parents should make it their first object to become intelligent in regard to the proper manner of dealing with their children, that they may secure to them sound minds in sound bodies. The principles of temperance should be carried out in all the details of home life. Self-denial should be taught to children and enforced upon them, so far as is consistent, from babyhood. Teach the little ones that they should eat to live, not live to eat; that appetite must be held in abeyance to the will; and that the will must be governed by calm, intelligent reason.

If parents have transmitted to their children tendencies which will make more difficult the work of educating them to be strictly temperate, and of cultivating pure and virtuous habits, what a solemn responsibility rests upon the parents to counteract that influence by every means in their power! How diligently and earnestly should they strive to do their duty by their unfortunate offspring! To parents is committed the sacred trust of guarding the physical and moral constitution of their children. Those who indulge a child's appetite and do not teach him to control his passions may afterward see, in the tobacco-loving, liquor-drinking slave, whose senses are benumbed, and whose lips utter falsehood and profanity, the terrible mistake they have made.

It is impossible for those who give the reins to appetite to attain to Christian perfection. The moral sensibilities of your children cannot be easily aroused unless you are careful in the selection of their food. Many a mother sets a table that is a snare to her family. Flesh meats, butter, cheese, rich pastry, spiced foods, and condiments are freely partaken of by both old and young. These things do their work in deranging the stomach, exciting the nerves, and enfeebling the intellect. The blood-making organs cannot convert such things into good blood. The grease cooked in the food renders it difficult of digestion. The effect of cheese is deleterious. Fine-flour bread does not impart to the system the nourishment that is to be found in unbolted wheat bread. Its common use will not keep the system in the best condition. Spices at first irritate the tender coating of the stomach, but finally destroy the natural sensitiveness of this delicate membrane. The blood becomes fevered, the animal propensities are aroused, while the moral and intellectual powers are weakened and become servants to the baser passions.

The mother should study to set a simple yet nutritious diet before her family. God has furnished man with abundant means for the gratification of an unperverted appetite. He has spread before him the products of the earth—a bountiful variety of food that is palatable to the taste and nutritious to the system. Of these our benevolent heavenly Father says we may freely eat. Fruits, grains, and vegetables, prepared in a simple way, free from spice and grease of all kinds, make, with milk or cream, the most healthful diet. They impart nourishment to the body and give a power of endurance and vigor of intellect that are not produced by a stimulating diet.

Evils of Meat Eating

Those who use flesh meats freely do not always have an unclouded brain and an active intellect, because the use of the flesh of animals tends to cause a grossness of body and to benumb the finer sensibilities of the mind. The liability to disease is increased by flesh eating. We do not hesitate to say that meat is not essential to the maintenance of health and strength.

Those who subsist largely upon meat cannot avoid sometimes eating flesh which is more or less diseased. In many cases the process of fitting animals for market produces an unhealthy condition. Shut away from light and pure air, inhaling the atmosphere of filthy stables, the entire body soon becomes contaminated with foul matter; and when such flesh is received into the human body it corrupts the blood, and disease is produced. If the person already has impure blood, this unhealthful condition will be greatly aggravated. But few can be made to believe that it is the meat they have eaten which has poisoned their blood and caused their suffering. Many die of diseases wholly due to meat eating, when the real cause is scarcely suspected by themselves or others. Some do not immediately feel its effects, but this is no evidence that it does not hurt them. It may be doing its work surely upon the system, yet for the time being the victim may realize nothing of it.

Pork, although one of the most common articles of diet, is one of the most injurious. God did not prohibit the Hebrew from eating swine's flesh merely to show His authority, but because it is not a proper article of food for man. God never created the swine to be eaten under any circumstances. It is impossible for the flesh of any living creature to be healthful when filth is its natural element, and when it feeds upon every detestable thing.

It is not the chief end of man to gratify his appetite. There are physical wants to be supplied; but because of this is it necessary that man shall be controlled by appetite? Will the people who are seeking to become holy, pure, refined, that they may be introduced into the society of heavenly angels, continue to take the life of God's creatures, and enjoy their flesh as a luxury? From what the Lord has shown me, this order of things will be changed, and God's peculiar people will exercise temperance in all things.

Proper Preparation of Food a Duty

There is a class who seem to think that whatever is eaten is lost, that anything tossed into the stomach to fill it, will do as well as food prepared with intelligence and care. But it is important that we relish the food we eat. If we cannot, and have to eat mechanically, we fail to receive the proper nourishment. Our bodies are constructed from what we eat; and in order to make tissues of good quality, we must have the right kind of food, and it must be prepared with such skill as will best adapt it to the wants of the system. It is a religious duty for those who cook, to learn how to prepare healthful food in a variety of ways, so that it may be both palatable and healthful. Poor cookery is wearing away the life energies of thousands. More souls are lost from this cause than many realize. It deranges the system and produces disease. In the condition thus induced, heavenly things cannot be readily discerned.

Some do not feel that it is a religious duty to prepare food properly; hence they do not try to learn how. They let the bread sour before baking, and the saleratus added to remedy the cook's carelessness makes it totally unfit for the human stomach. It requires thought and care to make good bread. But there is more religion in a good loaf of bread than many think. Food can be prepared simply and healthfully, but it requires skill to make it both palatable and nourishing. In order to learn how to cook, women should study, then patiently reduce what they learn to practice. People are suffering because they will not take the trouble to do this. I say to such, It is time for you to rouse your dormant energies and inform yourselves. Do not think the time wasted which is devoted to obtaining a thorough knowledge and experience in the preparation of healthful, palatable food. No matter how long an experience you have had in cooking, if you still have the responsibilities of a family, it is your duty to learn how to care for them properly. If necessary, go to some good cook and put yourself under her instruction until you are mistress of the art.

Wrong Eating Destroys Health

A wrong course of eating or drinking destroys health, and with it the sweetness of life. Oh, how many times has a good meal, as it is called, been purchased at the expense of sleep and quiet rest! Thousands, by indulging a perverted appetite, have brought on fever or some other acute disease, which has resulted in death. That was enjoyment purchased at an immense cost.

Because it is wrong to eat merely to gratify perverted taste, it does not follow that we should be indifferent in regard to our food. It is a matter of the highest importance. No one should adopt an impoverished diet. Many are debilitated from disease and need nourishing, well-cooked food. Health reformers, above all others, should be careful to avoid extremes. The body must have sufficient nourishment. The God who gives His beloved sleep has furnished them also suitable food to sustain the physical system in a healthy condition.

Many turn from light and knowledge, and sacrifice principle to taste. They eat when the system needs no food and at irregular intervals, because they have no moral stamina to resist inclination. As the result, the abused stomach rebels and suffering follows. Regularity in eating is very important for health of body and serenity of mind. Never should a morsel of food pass the lips between meals.

Too Frequent Eating a Cause of Dyspepsia

Many indulge in the pernicious habit of eating just before retiring. They may have taken their regular meals, yet because they feel a sense of faintness they think they must have a lunch. By indulging this wrong practice it becomes a habit, and they feel as though they could not sleep without food. In many cases this faintness comes because the digestive organs have been too severely taxed through the day in disposing of the great quantity of food forced upon them. These organs need a period of entire rest from labor, to recover their exhausted energies. A second meal should never be eaten until the stomach has had time to recover from the labor of digesting the preceding meal. When we lie down at night, the stomach should have its work all done, that it, as well as other portions of the body, may enjoy rest. But if more food is forced upon it, the digestive organs are put in motion again, to perform the same round of labor through the sleeping hours. The sleep of such is often disturbed with unpleasant dreams, and in the morning they awake unrefreshed. When this practice is followed, the digestive organs lose their natural vigor, and the person finds himself a miserable dyspeptic. And not only does the transgression of nature's laws affect the individual unfavorably, but others suffer more or less with him. Let anyone take a course that irritates him in any way, and see how quickly he manifests impatience. He cannot, without special grace, speak or act calmly. He casts a shadow wherever he goes. How can anyone say, then, "It is nobody's business what I eat or drink"?

Evils to be Avoided

It is possible to eat immoderately, even of wholesome food. It does not follow that because one has discarded the use of hurtful articles of diet he can eat just as much as he pleases. Overeating, no matter what the quality of the food, clogs the living machine and thus hinders it in its work.

Many make a mistake in drinking cold water with their meals. Food should not be washed down. Taken with meals, water diminishes the flow of the saliva; and the colder the water, the greater the injury to the stomach. Ice water or ice lemonade, taken with meals, will arrest digestion until the system has imparted sufficient warmth to the stomach to enable it to take up its work again. Masticate slowly, and allow the saliva to mingle with the food.

The more liquid there is taken into the stomach with the meals, the more difficult it is for the food to digest, for the liquid must first be absorbed. Do not eat largely of salt; give up spiced pickles; keep fiery food out of the stomach; eat fruit with the meals, and the irritation that calls for so much drink will cease to exist. But if anything is needed to quench the thirst, pure water is all that nature requires. Never take tea, coffee, beer, wine, or any spirituous liquor.

Eat Slowly

In order to secure healthy digestion, food should be eaten slowly. Those who wish to avoid dyspepsia, and those who realize their obligation to keep all their powers in a condition which will enable them to render the best service to God, will do well to remember this. If your time to eat is limited, do not bolt your food, but eat less, and masticate slowly. The benefit derived from food does not depend so much on the quantity eaten, as on its thorough digestion; nor the gratification of taste so much on the amount of food swallowed, as on the length of time it remains in the mouth. Those who are excited, anxious, or in a hurry would do well not to eat until they have found rest or relief, for the vital powers, already severely taxed, cannot supply the necessary digestive fluids. When traveling, some are almost constantly nibbling, if there is anything in their reach. This is a most pernicious practice. If travelers would eat regularly of the simplest and most nutritious kinds of food, they would not experience so great weariness, nor suffer so much from sickness.

In order to preserve health, temperance in all things

is necessary—temperance in labor, temperance in eating and drinking. Our heavenly Father sent the light of health reform to guard against the evils resulting from a debased appetite, that those who love purity and holiness may know how to use with discretion the good things He has provided for them, and that by exercising temperance in daily life, they may be sanctified through the truth.

At general meetings and camp meetings we should have good, wholesome, nourishing food, prepared in a simple manner. We should not turn these seasons into occasions for feasting. If we appreciate the blessings of God, if we are feeding on the bread of life, we will not be much concerned about gratifying the appetite. The great burden of our thoughts will be, How is it with my soul? There will be such a longing for spiritual food—something which will impart spiritual strength—that we will not complain if the diet is plain and simple.

God requires the body to be rendered a living sacrifice to Him, not a dead or a dying sacrifice. The offerings of the ancient Hebrews were to be without blemish, and will it be pleasing to God to accept a human offering that is filled with disease and corruption? He tells us that our body is the temple of the Holy Ghost; and He requires us to take care of this temple, that it may be a fit habitation for His Spirit. The apostle Paul gives us this admonition: "Ye are not your own; for ye are bought with a price; therefore glorify God in your body, and in your spirit, which are God's." 1 Corinthians 6:19, 20. All should be very careful to preserve the body in the best condition of health, that they may render to God perfect service and do their duty in the family and in society.

Reference for further study: *The Ministry of Healing,* pages 295-310, "Diet and Health."

The Power of Appetite

One of the strongest temptations that man has to meet is upon the point of appetite. Between the mind and the body there is a mysterious and wonderful relation. They react upon each other. To keep the body in a healthy condition to develop its strength, that every part of the living machinery may act harmoniously, should be the first study of our life. To neglect the body is to neglect the mind. It cannot be to the glory of God for His children to have sickly bodies or dwarfed minds. To indulge the taste at the expense of health is a wicked abuse of the senses. Those who engage in any species of intemperance, either in eating or drinking, waste their physical energies and weaken moral power. They will feel the retribution which follows the transgression of physical law.

The Redeemer of the world knew that the indulgence of appetite would bring physical debility and so deaden the perceptive organs that sacred and eternal things would not be discerned. Christ knew that the world was given up to gluttony, and that this indulgence would pervert the moral powers. If the indulgence of appetite was so strong upon the race that, in order to break its power, the divine Son of God, in behalf of man, was required to fast nearly six weeks, what a work is before the Christian in order that he may overcome even as Christ overcame! The strength of the temptation to indulge perverted appetite can be measured only by the inexpressible anguish of Christ in that long fast in the wilderness.

Christ knew that in order to successfully carry forward the plan of salvation He must commence the work of redeeming man just where the ruin began. Adam fell by the indulgence of appetite. In order to impress upon man his obligations to obey the law of God, Christ began His work of redemption by reforming the physical habits of man. The declension in virtue and the degeneracy of the race are chiefly attributable to the indulgence of perverted appetite.

A Solemn Responsibility

There is a solemn responsibility upon all, especially upon ministers who teach the truth, to overcome upon the point of appetite. Their usefulness would be much greater if they had control of their appetites and passions, and their mental and moral powers would be stronger if they combined physical labor with mental exertion. With strictly temperate habits, and with mental and physical labor combined, they could accomplish a far greater amount of labor and preserve clearness of mind. If they would pursue such a course, their thoughts and words would flow more freely, their religious exercises would be more energized, and the impressions made upon their hearers would be more marked.

Intemperance in eating, even of food of the right quality, will have a prostrating influence upon the system and will blunt the keener and holier emotions. Strict temperance in eating and drinking is highly essential for the healthy preservation and vigorous exercise of all the functions of the body. Strictly temperate habits, combined with exercise of the muscles as well as of the mind, will preserve both mental and physical vigor, and give power of endurance to those engaged in the ministry, to editors, and to all others whose habits are sedentary. . . .

The Effect of Stimulating Food

Intemperance commences at our tables, in the use of unhealthful food. After a time, through continued indulgence, the digestive organs become weakened and the food taken does not satisfy the appetite. Unhealthy conditions are established, and there is a craving for more stimulating food. Tea, coffee, and flesh meats produce an immediate effect. Under the influence of these poisons, the nervous system is excited, and, in some cases, for the time being, the intellect seems to be invigorated and the imagination to be more vivid.

Because these stimulants produce for the time being such agreeable results, many conclude that they really need them, and continue their use. But there is always a reaction. The nervous system, having been unduly excited, borrowed power for present use from its future resources of strength. All this temporary invigoration of the system is followed by depression. In proportion as these stimulants temporarily invigorate the system, will be the letting down of the power of the excited organs after the stimulus has lost its force. The appetite is educated to crave something stronger which will have a tendency to keep up and increase the agreeable excitement, until indulgence becomes habit, and there is a continual craving for stronger stimuli, as tobacco, wines, and liquors. The more the appetite is indulged, the more frequent will be its demands and the more difficult of control. The more debilitated the system becomes, and the less able to do without unnatural stimulus, the more the passion for these things increases, until the will is overborne and there seems to be no power to deny the unnatural craving for these indulgences.

The only safe course is to touch not, taste not, handle not, tea, coffee, wines, tobacco, opium, and alcoholic drinks. The necessity for the men of this generation to call to their aid the power of the will strengthened by the grace of God, in order to withstand the temptations of Satan and resist the least indulgence of perverted appetite, is twice as great as it was several generations ago. But the present generation have less power of self-control than had those who lived then. Those who have indulged the appetite for these stimulants have transmitted their depraved appetites and passions to their children, and greater moral power is required to resist intemperance in all its forms. The only perfectly safe course to pursue is to stand firmly on the side of temperance and not venture in the path of danger.

The great end for which Christ endured that long fast in the wilderness was to teach us the necessity of self-denial and temperance. This work should commence at our tables and should be strictly carried out in all the concerns of life. The Redeemer of the world came from heaven to help man in his weakness, that, in the power which Jesus came to bring him, he might become strong to overcome appetite and passion and might be victor on every point.

Many parents educate the tastes of their children and form their appetites. They indulge them in eating flesh meats and in drinking tea and coffee. The highly seasoned flesh meats and the tea and coffee, which some mothers encourage their children to use, prepare the way for them to crave stronger stimulants, as tobacco. The use of tobacco encourages the appetite for liquor, and the use of tobacco and liquor invariably lessens nerve power.

If the moral sensibilities of Christians were aroused

upon the subject of temperance in *all things,* they could, by their example, commencing at their tables, help those who are weak in self-control, who are almost powerless to resist the cravings of appetite. If we could realize that the habits we form in this life will affect our eternal interests, that our eternal destiny depends upon strictly temperate habits, we would work to the point of strict temperance in eating and drinking. By our example and personal effort we may be the means of saving many souls from the degradation of intemperance, crime, and death. Our sisters can do much in the great work for the salvation of others by spreading their tables with only healthful, nourishing food. They may employ their precious time in educating the tastes and appetites of their children, in forming habits of temperance in all things, and in encouraging self-denial and benevolence for the good of others.

Results of Indulgence

Notwithstanding the example that Christ gave us in the wilderness of temptation by denying appetite and overcoming its power, there are many Christian mothers, who, by their example and by the education which they are giving their children, are preparing them to become gluttons and winebibbers. Children are frequently indulged in eating what they choose and when they choose, without reference to health. There are many children who are educated gourmands from their babyhood. Through indulgence of appetite they are made dyspeptics at an early age. Self-indulgence and intemperance in eating grow with their growth and strengthen with their strength. Mental and physical vigor are sacrificed through the indulgence of parents.

Faithfulness in Health Reform

I am instructed to bear a message to all our people on the subject of health reform, for many have backslidden from their former loyalty to health-reform principles.

God's purpose for His children is that they shall grow up to the full stature of men and women in Christ. In order to do this, they must use aright every power of mind, soul, and body. They cannot afford to waste any mental or physical strength.

The question of how to preserve the health is one of primary importance. When we study this question in the fear of God, we shall learn that it is best, for both our physical and our spiritual advancement, to observe simplicity in diet. Let us patiently study this question. We need knowledge and judgment in order to move wisely in this matter. Nature's laws are not to be resisted, but obeyed.

Those who have received instruction regarding the evils of the use of flesh foods, tea and coffee, and rich and unhealthful food preparations, and who are determined to make a covenant with God by sacrifice, will not continue to indulge their appetite for food that they know to be unhealthful. God demands that the appetites be cleansed, and that self-denial be practiced in regard to those things which are not good. This is a work that will have to be done before His people can stand before Him a perfected people.

Personal Responsibility

The remnant people of God must be a converted people. The presentation of this message is to result in the

---

conversion and sanctification of souls. We are to feel the power of the Spirit of God in this movement. This is a wonderful, definite message; it means everything to the receiver, and it is to be proclaimed with a loud cry. We must have a true, abiding faith that this message will go forth with increasing importance till the close of time.

There are some professed believers who accept certain portions of the Testimonies as the message of God, while they reject those portions that condemn their favorite indulgences. Such persons are working contrary to their own welfare and the welfare of the church. It is essential that we walk in the light while we have the light. Those who claim to believe in health reform, and yet work counter to its principles in the daily life practice, are hurting their own souls and are leaving wrong impressions upon the minds of believers and unbelievers.

Strength Through Obedience

A solemn responsibility rests upon those who know the truth, that all their works shall correspond with their faith and that their lives shall be refined and sanctified, and they be prepared for the work that must rapidly be done in these closing days of the message. They have no time or strength to spend in the indulgence of appetite. The words should come to us now with impelling earnestness, "Repent ye therefore, and be converted, that your sins may be blotted out, when the times of refreshing shall come from the presence of the Lord." Acts 3:19. There are many among us who are deficient in spirituality, and who, unless they are wholly converted, will certainly be lost. Can you afford to run the risk?

Pride and weakness of faith are depriving many of the rich blessings of God. There are many who, unless they humble their hearts before the Lord, will be surprised and disappointed when the cry is heard, "Behold, the Bridegroom cometh." Matthew 25:6. They have the theory of the truth, but they have no oil in their vessels with their lamps. Our faith at this time must not stop with an assent to, or belief in, the theory of the third angel's message. We must have the oil of the grace of Christ that will feed the lamp and cause the light of life to shine forth, showing the way to those who are in darkness.

If we would escape having a sickly experience, we must begin in earnest without delay to work out our own salvation with fear and trembling. There are many who give no decided evidence that they are true to their baptismal vows. Their zeal is chilled by formality, worldly ambition, pride, and love of self. Occasionally their feelings are stirred, but they do not fall on the Rock Christ Jesus. They do not come to God with hearts that are broken in repentance and confession. Those who experience the work of true conversion in their lives will reveal the fruits of the Spirit in their lives. O that those who have so little spiritual life would realize that eternal life can be granted only to those who become partakers of the divine nature and escape the corruption that is in the world through lust!

The power of Christ alone can work the transformation in heart and mind that all must experience who would partake with Him of the new life in the kingdom of heaven. "Except a man be born again," the Saviour has said, "he cannot see the kingdom of God." John 3:3. The religion that comes from God is the only religion that can lead to God. In order to serve Him aright, we must be born of the divine Spirit. This will lead to watchfulness. It will purify the heart and renew the mind and give us a new capacity for knowing and loving God. It will give us willing obedience to all His requirements. This is true worship.

God requires of His people continual advancement. We need to learn that indulged appetite is the greatest hindrance to mental improvement and soul sanctification. With all our profession of health reform, many of us eat improperly. Indulgence of appetite is the greatest cause of physical and mental debility, and lies largely at the foundation of feebleness and premature death. Let the individual who is seeking to possess purity of spirit bear in mind that in Christ there is power to control the appetite.

Flesh Foods

If we could be benefited by indulging the desire for flesh foods, I would not make this appeal to you; but I know we cannot. Flesh foods are injurious to the physical well-being, and we should learn to do without them. Those who are in a position where it is possible to secure a vegetarian diet, but who choose to follow their own preferences in this matter, eating and drinking as they please, will gradually grow careless of the instruction the Lord has given regarding other phases of the present truth and will lose their perception of what is truth; they will surely reap as they have sown.

I have been instructed that the students in our schools are not to be served with flesh foods or with food preparations that are known to be unhealthful. Nothing that will serve to encourage a desire for stimulants should be placed on the tables. I appeal to old and young and to middle-

aged. Deny your appetite of those things that are doing
you injury. Serve the Lord by sacrifice.

Let the children have an intelligent part in this work.
We are all members of the Lord's family, and the Lord
would have His children, young and old, determine to
deny appetite and to save the means needed for the building of meetinghouses and the support of missionaries.

I am instructed to say to parents: Place yourselves,
soul and spirit, on the Lord's side of this question. We
need ever to bear in mind that in these days of probation
we are on trial before the Lord of the universe. Will
you not give up indulgences that are doing you injury?
Words of profession are cheap; let your acts of self-denial
testify that you will be obedient to the demands that God
makes of His peculiar people. Then put into the treasury
a portion of the means you save by your acts of self-denial,
and there will be that with which to carry on the work
of God.

There are many who feel that they cannot get along
without flesh foods; but if these would place themselves
on the Lord's side, resolutely resolved to walk in the way
of His guidance, they would receive strength and wisdom as did Daniel and his fellows. They would find that
the Lord would give them sound judgment. Many would
be surprised to see how much could be saved for the cause
of God by acts of self-denial. The small sums saved by
deeds of sacrifice will do more for the upbuilding of the
cause of God than larger gifts will accomplish that have
not called for denial of self.

Seventh-day Adventists are handling momentous
truths. More than forty years ago the Lord gave us special
light on health reform, but how are we walking in that

light? How many have refused to live in harmony with the counsels of God! As a people, we should make advancement proportionate to the light received. It is our duty to understand and respect the principles of health reform. On the subject of temperance we should be in advance of all other people; and yet there are among us well-instructed members of the church, and even ministers of the gospel, who have little respect for the light that God has given upon this subject. They eat as they please and work as they please.

Let those who are teachers and leaders in our cause take their stand firmly on Bible ground in regard to health reform and give a straight testimony to those who believe we are living in the last days of this earth's history. A line of distinction must be drawn between those who serve God and those who serve themselves.

I have been shown that the principles that were given us in the early days of the message are as important and should be regarded just as conscientiously today as they were then. There are some who have never followed the light given on the question of diet. It is now time to take the light from under the bushel and let it shine forth in clear, bright rays.

The principles of healthful living mean a great deal to us individually and as a people. When the message of health reform first came to me, I was weak and feeble, subject to frequent fainting spells. I was pleading with God for help, and He opened before me the great subject of health reform. He instructed me that those who are keeping His commandments must be brought into sacred relationship to Himself, and that by temperance in eating and drinking they must keep mind and body in the most favorable condition for service. This light has been a great blessing to me. I took my stand as a health reformer, knowing that the Lord would strengthen me. I have better health today, notwithstanding my age, than I had in my younger days.

It is reported by some that I have not followed the principles of health reform as I have advocated them with my pen; but I can say that I have been a faithful health reformer. Those who have been members of my family know that this is true.

"To the Glory of God"

We do not mark out any precise line to be followed in diet; but we do say that in countries where there are fruits, grains, and nuts in abundance, flesh food is not the right food for God's people. I have been instructed that flesh food has a tendency to animalize the nature, to rob men and women of that love and sympathy which they should feel for everyone, and to give the lower passions control over the higher powers of the being. If meat eating was ever healthful, it is not safe now. Cancers, tumors, and pulmonary diseases are largely caused by meat eating.

We are not to make the use of flesh food a test of fellowship, but we should consider the influence that professed believers who use flesh foods have over others. As God's messengers, shall we not say to the people, "Whether therefore ye eat, or drink, or whatsoever ye do, do all to the glory of God"? 1 Corinthians 10:31. Shall we not bear a decided testimony against the indulgence of perverted appetite? Will any who are ministers of the gospel, proclaiming the most solemn truth ever given to mortals, set an example in returning to the fleshpots of Egypt? Will those who are supported by the tithe from

God's storehouse permit themselves by self-indulgence to poison the life-giving current flowing through their veins? Will they disregard the light and warnings that God has given them? The health of body is to be regarded as essential for growth in grace and the acquirement of an even temper. If the stomach is not properly cared for, the formation of an upright, moral character will be hindered. The brain and nerves are in sympathy with the stomach. Erroneous eating and drinking result in erroneous thinking and acting.

All are now being tested and proved. We have been baptized into Christ, and if we will act our part by separating from everything that would drag us down and make us what we ought not to be, there will be given us strength to grow up into Christ, who is our living head, and we shall see the salvation of God.

Only when we are intelligent in regard to the principles of healthful living can we be fully aroused to see the evils resulting from improper diet. Those who, after seeing their mistakes, have courage to change their habits, will find that the reformatory process requires a struggle and much perseverance; but when correct tastes are once formed, they will realize that the use of the food which they formerly regarded as harmless was slowly but surely laying the foundation for dyspepsia and other diseases.

Fathers and mothers, watch unto prayer. Guard strictly against intemperance in every form. Teach your children the principles of true health reform. Teach them what things to avoid in order to preserve health. Already the wrath of God has begun to be visited upon the children of disobedience. What crimes, what sins, what iniquitous practices, are being revealed on every hand!

As a people, we are to exercise great care in guarding our children against depraved associates.

Teaching Health Principles

Greater efforts should be put forth to educate the people in the principles of health reform. Cooking schools should be established, and house-to-house instruction should be given in the art of cooking wholesome food. Old and young should learn how to cook more simply. Wherever the truth is presented, the people are to be taught how to prepare food in a simple yet appetizing way. They are to be shown that nourishing diet can be provided without the use of flesh foods.

Teach the people that it is better to know how to keep well than how to cure disease. Our physicians should be wise educators, warning all against self-indulgence and showing that abstinence from the things that God has prohibited is the only way to prevent ruin of body and mind.

Much tact and discretion should be employed in preparing nourishing food to take the place of that which has formerly constituted the diet of those who are learning to be health reformers. Faith in God, earnestness of purpose, and a willingness to help one another will be required. A diet lacking in the proper elements of nutrition brings reproach upon the cause of health reform. We are mortal and must supply ourselves with food that will give proper nourishment to the body.

Extremes in Diet

Some of our people, while conscientiously abstaining from eating improper foods, neglect to supply themselves with the elements necessary for the sustenance of the body. Those who take an extreme view of health reform are in danger of preparing tasteless dishes, making them so insipid that they are not satisfying. Food should be prepared in such a way that it will be appetizing as well as nourishing. It should not be robbed of that which the system needs. I use some salt, and always have, because salt, instead of being deleterious, is actually essential for the blood. Vegetables should be made palatable with a little milk or cream, or something equivalent.

While warnings have been given regarding the dangers of disease through butter, and the evil of the free use of eggs by small children, yet we should not consider it a violation of principle to use eggs from hens that are well cared for and suitably fed. Eggs contain properties that are remedial agencies in counteracting certain poisons.

Some, in abstaining from milk, eggs, and butter, have failed to supply the system with proper nourishment, and as a consequence have become weak and unable to work. Thus health reform is brought into disrepute. The work that we have tried to build up solidly is confused with strange things that God has not required, and the energies of the church are crippled. But God will interfere to prevent the results of these too strenuous ideas. The gospel is to harmonize the sinful race. It is to bring the rich and poor together at the feet of Jesus.

The time will come when we may have to discard some of the articles of diet we now use, such as milk and cream and eggs; but it is not necessary to bring upon ourselves perplexity by premature and extreme restrictions. Wait until the circumstances demand it, and the Lord prepares the way for it.

Those who would be successful in proclaiming the

principles of health reform must make the word of God their guide and counselor. Only as the teachers of health-reform principles do this can they stand on vantage ground. Let us never bear a testimony against health reform by failing to use wholesome, palatable food in place of the harmful articles of diet that we have discarded. Do not in any way encourage an appetite for stimulants. Eat only plain, simple, wholesome food, and thank God constantly for the principles of health reform. In all things be true and upright, and you will gain precious victories.

Diet in Different Countries

While working against gluttony and intemperance, we must recognize the condition to which the human family is subjected. God has made provision for those who live in the different countries of the world. Those who desire to be co-workers with God must consider carefully before they specify just what foods should and should not be eaten. We are to be brought into connection with the masses. Should health reform in its most extreme form be taught to those whose circumstances forbid its adoption, more harm than good would be done. As I preach the gospel to the poor, I am instructed to tell them to eat that food which is most nourishing. I cannot say to them: "You must not eat eggs, or milk, or cream. You must use no butter in the preparation of food." The gospel must be preached to the poor, but the time has not yet come to prescribe the strictest diet.

A Word to the Wavering

Those ministers who feel at liberty to indulge the appetite are falling far short of the mark. God wants them to be health reformers. He wants them to live up to the light that has been given on this subject. I feel sad when I see those who ought to be zealous for our health principles, not yet converted to the right way of living. I pray that the Lord may impress their minds that they are meeting with great loss. If things were as they should be in the households that make up our churches, we might do double work for the Lord.

In order to be purified and to remain pure, Seventh-day Adventists must have the Holy Spirit in their hearts and in their homes. The Lord has given me light that when the Israel of today humble themselves before Him, and cleanse the soul temple from all defilement, He will hear their prayers in behalf of the sick and will bless in the use of His remedies for disease. When in faith the human agent does all he can to combat disease, using the simple methods of treatment that God as provided, his efforts will be blessed of God.

If, after so much light has been given, God's people will cherish wrong habits, indulging self and refusing to reform, they will suffer the sure consequences of transgression. If they are determined to gratify perverted appetite at any cost, God will not miraculously save them from the consequences of their indulgence. They "shall lie down in sorrow." Isaiah 50:11.

Those who choose to be presumptuous, saying, "The Lord has healed me, and I need not restrict my diet; I can eat and drink as I please," will erelong need, in body and soul, the restoring power of God. Because the Lord has graciously healed you, you must not think you can link yourselves up with the self-indulgent practices of the world. Do as Christ commanded after His work of healing—"go, and sin no more." John 8:11. Appetite must not be your god.

The Lord gave His word to ancient Israel, that if they would cleave strictly to Him, and do all His requirements, He would keep them from all the diseases such as He had brought upon the Egyptians; but this promise was given on the condition of obedience. Had the Israelites obeyed the instruction they received, and profited by their advantages, they would have been the world's object lesson of health and prosperity. The Israelites failed of fulfilling God's purpose and thus failed of receiving the blessings that might have been theirs. But in Joseph and Daniel, in Moses and Elijah, and many others, we have noble examples of the results of the true plan of living. Like faithfulness today will produce like results. To us it is written, "Ye are a chosen generation, a royal priesthood, an holy nation, a peculiar people; that ye should show forth the praises of Him who hath called you out of darkness into His marvelous light." 1 Peter 2:9.

Oh, how many lose the richest blessings that God has in store for them in health and spiritual endowments! There are many souls who wrestle for special victories and special blessings that they may do some great thing. To this end they are always feeling that they must make an agonizing struggle in prayer and tears. When these persons search the Scriptures with prayer to know the expressed will of God, and then do His will from the heart without one reservation or self-indulgence, they will find rest. All the agonizing, all the tears and struggles, will not bring them the blessing they long for. Self must be entirely surrendered. They must do the work that presents itself, appropriating the abundance of the grace of God which is promised to all who ask in faith.

"If any man will come after Me," said Jesus, "let him

deny himself, and take up his cross daily, and follow Me."
Luke 9:23. Let us follow the Saviour in His simplicity
and self-denial. Let us lift up the Man of Calvary by word
and by holy living. The Saviour comes very near to those
who consecrate themselves to God. If ever there was a
time when we needed the working of the Spirit of God
upon our hearts and lives, it is now. Let us lay hold of
this divine power for strength to live a life of holiness and
self-surrender.

Partakers of the Divine Nature

Jesus rested upon the wisdom and strength of His heavenly Father. He declares, "The Lord God will help Me;
therefore shall I not be confounded: . . . and I know that
I shall not be ashamed. . . . Behold, the Lord God will
help Me." Pointing to His own example, He says to us,
"Who is among you that feareth the Lord, . . . that walketh in darkness, and hath no light? let him trust in the
name of the Lord, and stay upon his God."

"The prince of this world cometh," said Jesus, "and
hath nothing in Me." There was nothing in Him that
responded to Satan's sophistry. He did not consent to
sin. Not even by a thought did He yield to temptation.
So it may be with us. Christ's humanity was united with
divinity; He was fitted for the conflict by the indwelling
of the Holy Spirit. And He came to make us partakers
of the divine nature. So long as we are united to Him by
faith, sin has no more dominion over us. God reaches
for the hand of faith in us to direct it to lay fast hold upon
the divinity of Christ, that we may attain to perfection
of character.—*The Desire of Ages,* page 123 (1898).

Result of Disregarding Light

The sickness that has visited many families in ———— need not have been, if they had followed the light God has given them. Like ancient Israel, they have disregarded the light and could see no more necessity of restricting their appetite than did ancient Israel. The children of Israel would have flesh meats, and said, as many now say, We shall die without meat. God gave rebellious Israel flesh, but His curse was with it. Thousands of them died while the meat they desired was between their teeth. We have the example of ancient Israel, and the warning for us not to do as they did. . . . How can we pass on so indifferently, choosing our own course, following the sight of our own eyes, and departing farther and farther from God, as did the Hebrews? God cannot do great things for His people because of their hardness of heart and sinful unbelief.

God is no respecter of persons, but in every generation they that fear the Lord and work righteousness are accepted of Him, while those who are murmuring, unbelieving, and rebellious will not have His favor nor the blessings promised to those who love the truth and walk in it. Those who have the light and do not follow it, but disregard the requirements of God, will find that their blessings will be changed into curses and their mercies into judgments. God would have us learn humility and obedience as we read the history of ancient Israel, who were His chosen and peculiar people, but who brought their own destruction by following their own ways.— *Testimonies for the Church,* vol. 3, pp. 171, 172 (1872).

Faithfulness to the Laws of Health

I am convinced that none need to make themselves sick preparing for camp meeting, if they observe the laws of health in their cooking. If they make no cake or pies, but cook simple graham bread, and depend on fruit, canned or dried, they need not get sick in preparing for the meeting, and they need not be sick while at the meeting. None should go through the entire meeting without some warm food. . . .

Brethren and sisters must not be sick upon the encampment. If they clothe themselves properly in the chill of morning and night and are particular to vary their clothing according to the changing weather, so as to preserve proper circulation, and strictly observe regularity in sleeping and in eating of simple food, taking nothing between meals, they need not be sick. . . . Those who have been engaged in hard labor from day to day now cease their exercise; therefore they should not eat their average amount of food. If they do, their stomachs will be overtaxed. We wish to have the brain power especially vigorous at these meetings, and in the most healthy condition to hear the truth, appreciate it, and retain it, that all may practice it after their return from the meeting. If the stomach is burdened with too much food, even of a simple character, the brain force is called to the aid of the digestive organs. There is a benumbed sensation upon the brain. It is almost impossible to keep the eyes open. The very truths which should be heard, understood, and practiced are entirely lost through indisposition or because the brain is almost paralyzed in consequence of the amount of food eaten.—*Testimonies for the Church,* vol. 2, pp. 602, 603 (1871).

Healthful Cooking

Many do not feel that this is a matter of duty, hence they do not try to prepare food properly. This can be done in a simple, healthful, and easy manner, without the use of lard, butter, or flesh meats. Skill must be united with simplicity. To do this, women must read, and then patiently reduce what they read to practice. Many are suffering because they will not take the trouble to do this. I say to such, It is time for you to rouse your dormant energies and read up. Learn how to cook with simplicity, and yet in a manner to secure the most palatable and healthful food.

Because it is wrong to cook merely to please the taste or to suit the appetite, no one should entertain the idea that an impoverished diet is right. Many are debilitated with disease and need a nourishing, plentiful, well-cooked diet. We frequently find graham bread heavy, sour, and but partially baked. This is for want of interest to learn, and care to perform the important duty of cook. Sometimes we find gem cakes, or soft biscuit, dried, not baked, and other things after the same order. And then cooks will tell you they can do very well in the old style of cooking, but to tell the truth, their family do not like graham bread; that they would starve to live in this way.

I have said to myself, I do not wonder at it. It is your manner of preparing food that makes it so unpalatable. To eat such food would certainly give one the dyspepsia.

These poor cooks, and those who have to eat their food, will gravely tell you that the health reform does not agree with them. The stomach has not power to convert poor, heavy, sour bread into good; but this poor bread

Testimonies for the Church, vol. 1, pp. 681, 682 (1868).

will convert a healthy stomach into a diseased one. Those who eat such food know that they are failing in strength. Is there not a cause? Some of these persons call themselves health reformers, but they are not. They do not know how to cook. They prepare cakes, potatoes, and graham bread, but there is the same round, with scarcely a variation, and the system is not strengthened. They seem to think the time wasted which is devoted to obtaining a thorough experience in the preparation of healthful, palatable food.

Learn to Cook

Our sisters often do not know how to cook. To such I would say, I would go to the very best cook that could be found in the country, and remain there if necessary for weeks, until I had become mistress of the art—an intelligent, skillful cook. I would pursue this course if I were forty years old. It is your duty to know how to cook, and it is your duty to teach your daughters to cook. When you are teaching them the art of cookery, you are building around them a barrier that will preserve them from the folly and vice which they may otherwise be tempted to engage in. I prize my seamstress, I value my copyist; but my cook, who knows well how to prepare the food to sustain life and nourish brain, bone, and muscle, fills the most important place among the helpers in my family. —*Testimonies for the Church,* vol. 2, p. 370 (1869).

A Most Essential Accomplishment

It is a religious duty for those who cook to learn how to prepare healthful food in different ways, so that it may be eaten with enjoyment. Mothers should teach their children how to cook. What branch of the education of a young lady can be so important as this? The eating has to do with the life. Scanty, impoverished, ill-cooked food is constantly depraving the blood, by weakening the blood-making organs. It is highly essential that the art of cookery be considered one of the most important branches of education. There are but few good cooks. Young ladies consider that it is stooping to a menial office to become a cook. This is not the case. They do not view the subject from a right standpoint. Knowledge of how to prepare food healthfully, especially bread, is no mean science. . . .

Young ladies should be thoroughly instructed in cooking. Whatever may be their circumstances in life, here is knowledge which may be put to a practical use. It is a branch of education which has the most direct influence upon human life, especially the lives of those held most dear. Many a wife and mother who has not had the right education and lacks skill in the cooking department is daily presenting her family with ill-prepared food which is steadily and surely destroying the digestive organs, making a poor quality of blood and frequently bringing on acute attacks of inflammatory disease and causing premature death.

Many have been brought to their death by eating heavy, sour bread. An instance was related to me of a hired girl who made a batch of sour, heavy bread. In order to get rid of it and conceal the matter, she threw

Testimonies for the Church, vol. 1, pp. 682-687 (1868).

it to a couple of very large hogs. Next morning the man of the house found his swine dead, and upon examining the trough, found pieces of this heavy bread. He made inquiries, and the girl acknowledged what she had done She had not thought of the effect of such bread upon the swine. If heavy, sour bread will kill swine, which can devour rattlesnakes and almost every detestable thing, what effect will it have upon that tender organ, the human stomach?

It is a religious duty for every Christian girl and woman to learn at once to make good, sweet light bread from unbolted wheat flour. Mothers should take their daughters into the kitchen with them when very young and teach them the art of cooking. The mother cannot expect her daughters to understand the mysteries of housekeeping without education. She should instruct them patiently, lovingly, and make the work as agreeable as she can by her cheerful countenance and encouraging words of approval. If they fail once, twice, or thrice, censure not. Already discouragement is doing its work and tempting them to say, "It is of no use, I can't do it." This is not the time for censure. The will is becoming weakened. It needs the spur of encouraging, cheerful, hopeful words, as, "Never mind the mistakes you have made. You are but a learner, and must expect to make blunders. Try again. Put your mind on what you are doing. Be very careful, and you will certainly succeed."

Many mothers do not realize the importance of this branch of knowledge, and rather than have the trouble and care of instructing their children and bearing with their failings and errors while learning, they prefer to do all themselves. And when their daughters make a failure in their efforts, they send them away, with, "It is no use, you can't do this or that. You perplex and trouble me more than you help me."

Thus the first efforts of the learners are repulsed, and the first failure so cools their interest and ardor to learn that they dread another trial and will propose to sew, knit, clean house, anything but cook. . . .

Mothers should take their daughters with them into the kitchen and patiently educate them. Their constitution will be better for such labor; their muscles will gain tone and strength, and their meditations will be more healthy and elevated at the close of the day. They may be weary, but how sweet is rest after a proper amount of labor. Sleep, nature's sweet restorer, invigorates the weary body and prepares it for the next day's duties. Do not intimate to your children that it is no matter whether they labor or not. Teach them that their help is needed, that their time is of value, and that you depend on their labor.

Unwholesome Bread

When I have been from home sometimes, I have known that the bread upon the table, and the food generally, would hurt me; but I would be obliged to eat a little to sustain life. It is a sin in the sight of heaven to have such food. I have suffered for want of proper food. For a dyspeptic stomach, you may place upon your tables fruits of different kinds, but not too many at one meal. In this way you may have a variety, and it will taste good, and after you have eaten your meals, you will feel well.— *Testimonies for the Church,* vol. 2, p. 373 (1869).

Changing the Diet

Persons who have indulged their appetite to eat freely of meat, highly seasoned gravies, and various kinds of rich cakes and preserves cannot immediately relish a plain, wholesome, and nutritious diet. Their taste is so perverted they have no appetite for a wholesome diet of fruits, plain bread, and vegetables. They need not expect to relish at first food so different from that which they have been indulging themselves to eat. If they cannot at first enjoy plain food, they should fast until they can. That fast will prove to them of greater benefit than medicine, for the abused stomach will find that rest which it has long needed, and real hunger can be satisfied with a plain diet.

It will take time for the taste to recover from the abuses which it has received and to gain its natural tone. But perseverance in a self-denying course of eating and drinking will soon make plain, wholesome food palatable, and it will soon be eaten with greater satisfaction than the epicure enjoys over his rich dainties. The stomach is not fevered with meats and overtaxed, but is in a healthy condition and can readily perform its task. There should be no delay in reform. Efforts should be made to preserve carefully the remaining strength of the vital forces, by lifting off every overtaxing burden. The stomach may never recover health, but a proper course of diet will save further debility, and many will recover more or less, unless they have gone very far in gluttonous self-murder.—*Spiritual Gifts,* vol. 4, pp. 130, 131 (1864).

A Harmful Combination

In regard to milk and sugar: I know of persons who have become frightened at the health reform and said they would have nothing to do with it, because it has spoken against a free use of these things. Changes should be made with great care, and we should move cautiously and wisely. We want to take that course which will recommend itself to the intelligent men and women of the land. Large quantities of milk and sugar eaten together are injurious. They impart impurities to the system. . . . Sugar clogs the system. It hinders the working of the living machine.

There was one case in Montcalm County, Michigan, to which I will refer. The individual was a noble man. He stood six feet and was of fine appearance. I was called to visit him in his sickness. I had previously conversed with him in regard to his manner of living. "I do not like the looks of your eyes," said I. He was eating large quantities of sugar. I asked him why he did this. He said that he had left off meat, and did not know what would supply its place as well as sugar. . . .

Some of you send your daughters, who have nearly grown to womanhood, to school to learn the sciences before they know how to cook, when this should be made of the first importance. Here was a woman who did not know how to cook; she had not learned how to prepare healthful food. The wife and mother was deficient in this important branch of education, and as the result, poorly cooked food not being sufficient to sustain the demands of the system, sugar was eaten immoderately, which brought on a diseased condition of the entire system. . . .

Testimonies for the Church, vol. 2, pp. 368-370 (1869).

When I went to see the sick man, I tried to tell them as well as I could how to manage, and soon he began slowly to improve. But he imprudently exercised his strength when not able, ate a small amount not of the right quality, and was taken down again. This time there was no help for him. His system appeared to be a living mass of corruption. He died a victim to poor cooking. He tried to make sugar supply the place of good cooking, and it only made matters worse.

I frequently sit down to the tables of the brethren and sisters, and see that they use a great amount of milk and sugar. These clog the system, irritate the digestive organs, and affect the brain. Anything that hinders the active motion of the living machinery affects the brain very directly. And from the light given me, sugar, when largely used, is more injurious than meat.

Unpalatable Food

I am acquainted with families who have changed from a meat diet to one that is impoverished. Their food is so poorly prepared that the stomach loathes it, and such have told me that the health reform did not agree with them; that they were decreasing in physical strength. Here is one reason why some have not been successful in their efforts to simplify their food. They have a poverty-stricken diet. Food is prepared without painstaking, and there is a continual sameness. There should not be many kinds at one meal, but all meals should not be composed of the same kinds of food without variation. Food should be prepared with simplicity, yet with a nicety which will invite the appetite.—*Testimonies for the Church,* vol. 2, p. 63 (1868).

An Impoverished Diet

I have spoken of the importance of the quantity and quality of food being in strict accordance with the laws of health. But we would not recommend an impoverished diet. I have been shown that many take a wrong view of the health reform and adopt too poor a diet. They subsist upon a cheap, poor quality of food, prepared without care or reference to the nourishment of the system. It is important that the food should be prepared with care, that the appetite, when not perverted, can relish it. Because we from principle discard the use of meat, butter, mince pies, spices, lard, and that which irritates the stomach and destroys health, the idea should never be given that it is of but little consequence what we eat.

There are some who go to extremes. They must eat just such an amount and just such a quality, and confine themselves to two or three things. They allow only a few things to be placed before them or their families to eat. In eating a small amount of food, and that not of the best quality, they do not take into the stomach that which will suitably nourish the system. Poor food cannot be converted into good blood. An impoverished diet will impoverish the blood. . . .

Two classes were presented before me: First, those who were not living up to the light which God had given them. . . . There are many of you who profess the truth, who have received it because somebody else did, and for your life you could not give the reason. This is why you are as weak as water. Instead of weighing your motives in the light of eternity, instead of having a practical knowledge of the principles underlying all your actions, in-

Testimonies for the Church, vol. 2, pp. 367, 368 (1869).

stead of having dug down to the bottom, and built upon a right foundation for yourself, you are walking in the sparks kindled by somebody else. And you will fail in this, as you have failed in the health reform. Now if you had moved from principle, you would not have done this.

Some cannot be impressed with the necessity of eating and drinking to the glory of God. The indulgence of appetite affects them in all the relations of life. It is seen in their family, in their church, in the prayer meeting, and in the conduct of their children. It has been the curse of their lives. You cannot make them understand the truths for these last days. God has bountifully provided for the sustenance and happiness of all His creatures; and if His laws were never violated, and all acted in harmony with the divine will, health, peace, and happiness, instead of misery and continual evil, would be experienced.

Another class who have taken hold of the health reform are very severe. They take a position and stand stubbornly in that position and carry nearly everything over the mark. . . .

Flesh meats will depreciate the blood. Cook meat with spices, and eat it with rich cakes and pies, and you have a bad quality of blood. The system is too heavily taxed in disposing of this kind of food. The mince pies and the pickles, which should never find a place in any human stomach, will give a miserable quality of blood. And a poor quality of food, cooked in an improper manner and insufficient in quantity, cannot make good blood. Flesh meats and rich food, and an impoverished diet, will produce the same results.

Extremes in Diet

Many of the views held by Seventh-day Adventists differ widely from those held by the world in general. Those who advocate an unpopular truth should, above all others, seek to be consistent in their own life. They should not try to see how different they can be from others, but how near they can come to those whom they wish to influence, that they may help them to the positions they themselves so highly prize. Such a course will commend the truths they hold.

Those who are advocating a reform in diet should, by the provision they make for their own table, present the advantages of hygiene in the best light. They should so exemplify its principles as to commend it to the judgment of candid minds.

There is a large class who will reject any reform movement, however reasonable, if it lays a restriction upon the appetite. They consult taste, instead of reason and the laws of health. By this class, all who leave the beaten track of custom and advocate reform will be opposed and accounted radical, let them pursue ever so consistent a course.

But no one should permit opposition or ridicule to turn him from the work of reform or cause him to lightly regard it. He who is imbued with the spirit which actuated Daniel, will not be narrow or conceited, but he will be firm and decided in standing for the right. In all his associations, whether with his brethren or with others, he will not swerve from principle, while at the same time he will not fail to manifest a noble Christlike patience. When those who advocate hygienic reform carry the mat-

Christian Temperance, pages 55-59 (1890).

ter to extremes, people are not to blame if they become disgusted. Too often our religious faith is thus brought into disrepute, and in many cases those who witness such exhibitions of inconsistency can never afterward be brought to think that there is anything good in the reform. These extremists do more harm in a few months than they can undo in a lifetime. They are engaged in a work which Satan loves to see go on. . . .

Because we, from principle, discard the use of those things which irritate the stomach and destroy health, the idea should never be given that it is of little consequence what we eat. I do not recommend an impoverished diet. Many who need the benefits of healthful living and from conscientious motives adopt what they believe to be such, are deceived by supposing that a meager bill of fare, prepared without painstaking and consisting mostly of mushes and so-called gems, heavy and sodden, is what is meant by a reformed diet. Some use milk and a large amount of sugar on mush, thinking that they are carrying out health reform. But the sugar and milk combined are liable to cause fermentation in the stomach, and are thus harmful. The free use of sugar in any form tends to clog the system and is not unfrequently a cause of disease. Some think that they must eat only just such an amount, and just such a quality, and confine themselves to two or three kinds of food. But in eating too small an amount, and that not of the best quality, they do not receive sufficient nourishment.

There is real common sense in health reform. People cannot all eat the same things. Some articles of food that are wholesome and palatable to one person may be hurtful to another. Some cannot use milk, while others can subsist upon it. For some, dried beans and peas are wholesome, while others cannot digest them. Some stomachs have become so sensitive that they cannot make use of the coarser kind of graham flour. So it is impossible to make an unvarying rule by which to regulate everyone's dietetic habits.

Narrow ideas and overstraining of small points have been a great injury to the cause of hygiene. There may be such an effort at economy in the preparation of food, that, instead of a healthful diet, it becomes a poverty-stricken diet. What is the result? Poverty of the blood. I have seen several cases of disease most difficult to cure, which were due to impoverished diet. The persons thus afflicted were not compelled by poverty to adopt a meager diet, but did so in order to follow out their own erroneous ideas of what constitutes health reform. Day after day, meal after meal, the same articles of food were prepared without variation, until dyspepsia and general debility resulted.

Many who adopt the health reform complain that it does not agree with them; but after sitting at their tables I come to the conclusion that it is not the health reform that is at fault, but the poorly prepared food. I appeal to men and women to whom God has given intelligence: learn how to cook. I make no mistake when I say men, for they, as well as women, need to understand the simple, healthful preparation of food. Their business often takes them where they cannot obtain wholesome food. They may be called to remain days and even weeks in families that are entirely ignorant in this respect. Then, if they have the knowledge, they can use it to good purpose.

Investigate your habits of diet. Study from cause to effect, but do not bear false witness against health reform by ignorantly pursuing a course which militates against it. Do not neglect or abuse the body and thus unfit it to render to God that service which is His due. To my certain knowledge, some of the most useful workers in our cause have died through such neglect. To care for the body by providing for it food which is relishable and strengthening, is one of the first duties of the householder. Better by far have less expensive clothing and furniture, than to scrimp the supply of necessary articles for the table.

Most people enjoy better health while eating two meals a day than three; others, under their existing circumstances, may require something to eat at suppertime; but this meal should be very light. Let no one think himself a criterion for all—that everyone must do exactly as he does.

Never cheat the stomach out of that which health demands, and never abuse it by placing upon it a load which it should not bear. Cultivate self-control. Restrain appetite; keep it under the control of reason. Do not feel it necessary to load down your table with unhealthful food when you have visitors. The health of your family and the influence upon your children should be considered, as well as the habits and tastes of your guests. . . .

Health reform means something to us, and we must not belittle it by narrow views and practices. We must be true to our convictions of right. Daniel was blessed because he was steadfast in doing what he knew to be right, and we shall be blessed if we seek to honor God with full purpose of heart.

Reference for further study: *The Ministry of Healing*, pages 318-324, "Extremes in Diet."

Overeating

Many who have adopted the health reform have left off everything hurtful; but does it follow that because they have left off these things, they can eat just as much as they please? They sit down to the table, and instead of considering how much they should eat, they give themselves up to appetite and eat to great excess. And the stomach has all it can do, or all it should do the rest of that day, to worry away with the burden imposed upon it. All the food that is put into the stomach, from which the system cannot derive benefit, is a burden to nature in her work. It hinders the living machine. The system is clogged and cannot successfully carry on its work. The vital organs are unnecessarily taxed, and the brain nerve power is called to the stomach to help the digestive organs carry on their work of disposing of an amount of food which does the system no good.

Thus the power of the brain is lessened by drawing so heavily upon it to help the stomach get along with its heavy burden. And after it has accomplished the task, what are the sensations experienced as the result of this unnecessary expenditure of vital force? A feeling of goneness, a faintness, as though you must eat more. Perhaps this feeling comes just before mealtime. What is the cause of this? Nature has worried along with her work and it so thoroughly exhausted in consequence that you have this sensation of goneness. And you think that the stomach says, "More food," when, in its faintness, it is distinctly saying, "Give me rest."

Testimonies for the Church, vol. 2, pp. 362-364 (1869).

The Stomach Needs Periods of Rest

The stomach needs rest to gather up its exhausted energies for another work. But instead of allowing it any period of rest, you think it needs more food, and so heap another load upon nature and refuse it the needed rest. It is like a man laboring in the field all through the early part of the day until he is weary. He comes in at noon and says that he is weary and exhausted; but you tell him to go to work again and he will obtain relief. This is the way you treat the stomach. It is thoroughly exhausted. But instead of letting it rest, you give it more food, and then call the vitality from other parts of the system to the stomach to assist in the work of digestion.

Many of you have at times felt a numbness around the brain. You have felt disinclined to take hold of any labor which required either mental or physical exertion, until you have rested from the sense of this burden imposed upon your system. Then, again, there is this sense of goneness. But you say it is more food that is wanted, and place a double load upon the stomach for it to care for. Even if you are strict in the quality of your food, do you glorify God in your bodies and spirits, which are His, by partaking of such a quantity of food? Those who place so much food upon the stomach, and thus load down nature, could not appreciate the truth should they hear it dwelt upon. They could not arouse the benumbed sensibilities of the brain to realize the value of the atonement and the great sacrifice that has been made for fallen man. It is impossible for such to appreciate the great, the precious, and the exceedingly rich reward that is in reserve for the faithful overcomers. The animal part of our nature should never be left to govern the moral and intellectual.

And what influence does overeating have upon the stomach? It becomes debilitated, the digestive organs are weakened, and disease, with all its train of evils, is brought on as the result. If persons were diseased before, they thus increase the difficulties upon them and lessen their vitality every day they live. They call their vital powers into unnecessary action to take care of the food that they place in their stomachs.

Overworked Mothers

A great amount of hard labor is performed to obtain food for their tables which greatly injures the already overtaxed system. Women spend a great share of their time over a heated cookstove, preparing food, highly seasoned with spices to gratify the taste. As a consequence, the children are neglected and do not receive moral and religious instruction. The overworked mother neglects to cultivate a sweetness of temper, which is the sunshine of the dwelling. Eternal considerations become secondary. All the time has to be employed in preparing these things for the appetite which ruin health, sour the temper, and becloud the reasoning faculties.

A reform in eating would be a saving of expense and labor. The wants of a family can be easily supplied that is satisfied with plain, wholesome diet. Rich food breaks down the healthy organs of body and mind. And how many labor so very hard to accomplish this—*Spiritual Gifts,* vol. 4, pp. 131, 132 (1864).

Reference for further study: *Education,* pages 202-206, "Temperance and Dietetics."

Gluttony a Sin

It is sin to be intemperate in the quantity of food eaten, even if the quality is unobjectionable. Many feel that if they do not eat meat and the grosser articles of food, they may eat of simple food until they cannot well eat more. This is a mistake. Many professed health reformers are nothing less than gluttons. They lay upon the digestive organs so great a burden that the vitality of the system is exhausted in the effort to dispose of it. It also has a depressing influence upon the intellect, for the brain nerve power is called upon to assist the stomach in its work. Overeating, even of the simplest food, benumbs the sensitive nerves of the brain and weakens its vitality. Overeating has a worse effect upon the system than overworking; the energies of the soul are more effectually prostrated by intemperate eating than by intemperate working.

The digestive organs should never be burdened with a quantity or quality of food which it will tax the system to appropriate. All that is taken into the stomach, above what the system can use to convert into good blood, clogs the machinery, for it cannot be made into either flesh or blood, and its presence burdens the liver and produces a morbid condition of the system. The stomach is overworked in its efforts to dispose of it, and then there is a sense of languor which is interpreted to mean hunger, and without allowing the digestive organs time to rest from their severe labor, to recruit their energies, another immoderate amount is taken into the stomach, to set the weary machinery again in motion. The system receives less nourishment from too great a quantity of food, even of the right quality, than from a moderate quantity taken at regular periods. . . .

It is impossible to have clear conceptions of eternal things unless the mind is trained to dwell upon elevated themes. All the passions must be brought under perfect subjection to the moral powers. When men and women profess strong faith and earnest spirituality, I know that their profession is false if they have not brought all their passions under control. God requires this. The reason why such spiritual darkness prevails is that the mind is content to take a low level and is not directed upward in a pure, holy, and heavenly channel.

Avoid False Standards

While we would caution you not to overeat, even of the best quality of food, we would also caution those that are extremists not to raise a false standard and then endeavor to bring everybody to it. There are some who are starting out as health reformers who are not fit to engage in any other enterprise, and who have not sense enough to take care of their own families or keep their proper place in the church. And what do they do? Why, they fall back as health-reform physicians, as though they could make that a success. They assume the responsibilities of their practice and take the lives of men and women into their hands, when they really know nothing about the business.—*Testimonies for the Church*, vol. 2, pp. 374, 375 (1869).

OUTDOOR LIFE AND PHYSICAL ACTIVITY

The Example of Christ

The Saviour's life on earth was a life of communion with nature and with God. In this communion He revealed for us the secret of a life of power. . . . Working at the carpenter's bench, bearing the burdens of home life, learning the lessons of obedience and toil, He found recreation amidst the scenes of nature, gathering knowledge as He sought to understand nature's mysteries. He studied the word of God, and His hours of greatest happiness were found when He could turn aside from the scenes of His labors to go into the fields, to meditate in the quiet valleys, to hold communion with God on the mountainside or amid the trees of the forest. The early morning often found Him in some secluded place, meditating, searching the Scriptures, or in prayer. With the voice of singing He welcomed the morning light. With songs of thanksgiving He cheered His hours and brought heaven's gladness to the toilworn and disheartened.

During His ministry Jesus lived to a great degree an outdoor life. His journeys from place to place were made on foot, and much of His teaching was given in the open air. In training His disciples He often withdrew from the confusion of the city to the quiet of the fields, as more in harmony with the lessons of simplicity, faith, and self-abnegation He desired to teach them. . . .

Christ loved to gather the people about Him under

The Ministry of Healing, pages 51-58 (1905).

the blue heavens, on some grassy hillside, or on the beach beside the lake. Here, surrounded by the works of His own creation, He could turn their thoughts from the artificial to the natural. In the growth and development of nature were revealed the principles of His kingdom. As men should lift their eyes to the hills of God and behold the wonderful works of His hand, they could learn precious lessons of divine truth. In future days the lessons of the divine Teacher would thus be repeated to them by the things of nature. The mind would be uplifted and the heart would find rest. . . .

When Jesus said to His disciples that the harvest was great and the laborers were few, He did not urge upon them the necessity of ceaseless toil, but bade them, "Pray ye therefore the Lord of the harvest, that He will send forth laborers into His harvest." To His toil-worn workers today as really as to His first disciples He speaks these words of compassion, "Come ye yourselves apart, . . . and rest awhile."

All who are under the training of God need the quiet hour for communion with their own hearts, with nature, and with God. . . . We must individually hear Him speaking to the heart. When every other voice is hushed, and in quietness we wait before Him, the silence of the soul makes more distinct the voice of God. He bids us, "Be still, and know that I am God." This is the effectual preparation for all labor for God. Amidst the hurrying throng and the strain of life's intense activities, he who is thus refreshed will be surrounded with an atmosphere of light and peace. He will receive a new endowment of both physical and mental strength. His life will breathe out a fragrance and will reveal a divine power that will reach men's hearts.

Nature a Lesson Book

Christ taught His disciples by the lake, on the mountainside, in the fields and groves, where they could look upon the things of nature by which He illustrated His teachings. And as they learned of Christ they put their knowledge to use by co-operating with Him in His work.

So through the creation we are to become acquainted with the Creator. The book of nature is a great lesson book, which in connection with the Scriptures we are to use in teaching others of His character and guiding lost sheep back to the fold of God. As the works of God are studied, the Holy Spirit flashes conviction into the mind. It is not the conviction that logical reasoning produces, but unless the mind has become too dark to know God, the eye too dim to see Him, the ear too dull to hear His voice, a deeper meaning is grasped, and the sublime, spiritual truths of the written word are impressed on the heart.

In these lessons direct from nature there is a simplicity and purity that makes them of the highest value. All need the teaching to be derived from this source. In itself the beauty of nature leads the soul away from sin and worldly attractions and toward purity, peace, and God. Too often the minds of students are occupied with men's theories and speculations, falsely called science and philosophy. They need to be brought into close contact with nature. Let them learn that creation and Christianity have one God. Let them be taught to see the harmony of the natural with the spiritual. Let everything which their eyes see or their hands handle be made a lesson in character building. Thus the mental powers will be strength-

Christ's Object Lessons, pages 24-27 (1900).
(164)

ened, the character developed, the whole life ennobled.

Christ's purpose in parable teaching was in direct line with the purpose of the Sabbath. God gave to men the memorial of His creative power, that they might discern Him in the works of His hand. The Sabbath bids us behold in His created works the glory of the Creator. And it was because He desired us to do this that Jesus bound up His precious lessons with the beauty of natural things. On the holy rest day, above all other days, we should study the messages that God has written for us in nature. We should study the Saviour's parables where He spoke them, in the fields and groves, under the open sky, among the grass and flowers. As we come close to the heart of nature, Christ makes His presence real to us and speaks to our hearts of His peace and love.

And Christ has linked His teaching, not only with the day of rest, but with the week of toil. He has wisdom for him who drives the plow and sows the seed. . . . In every line of useful labor and every association of life He desires us to find a lesson of divine truth. Then our daily toil will no longer absorb our attention and lead us to forget God; it will continually remind us of our Creator and Redeemer. The thought of God will run like a thread of gold through all our homely cares and occupations. For us the glory of His face will again rest upon the face of nature. We shall ever be learning new lessons of heavenly truth and growing into the image of His purity. Thus shall we "be taught of the Lord," and in the lot wherein we are called we shall "abide with God."

Reference for further study: *The Ministry of Healing*, pages 51-58, "With Nature and With God."

In the Country

In August, 1901 while attending the Los Angeles camp meeting, I was, in the visions of the night, in a council meeting. The question under consideration was the establishment of a sanitarium in Southern California. By some it was urged that this sanitarium should be built in the city of Los Angeles, and the objections to establishing it out of the city were pointed out. Others spoke of the advantages of a country location.

There was among us One who presented this matter very clearly and with the utmost simplicity. He told us that it would be a mistake to establish a sanitarium within the city limits. A sanitarium should have the advantage of plenty of land, so that the invalids can work in the open air. For nervous, gloomy, feeble patients, outdoor work is invaluable. Let them have flower beds to care for. In the use of rake and hoe and spade, they will find relief for many of their maladies. Idleness is the cause of many diseases.

Life in the open air is good for body and mind. It is God's medicine for the restoration of health. Pure air, good water, sunshine, the beautiful surroundings of nature—these are His means for restoring the sick to health in natural ways. To the sick it is worth more than silver or gold to lie in the sunshine or in the shade of the trees.

In the country our sanitariums can be surrounded by flowers and trees, orchards and vineyards. Here it is easy for physicians and nurses to draw from the things of nature lessons teaching of God. Let them point the patients to Him whose hand has made the lofty trees,

Testimonies for the Church, vol. 7, pp. 85-87 (1901).

the springing grass, and the beautiful flowers, encouraging them to see in every opening bud and blossoming flower an expression of His love for His children.

It is the expressed will of God that our sanitariums shall be established as far from the cities as is consistent. So far as possible, these institutions should be located in quiet, secluded places, where opportunity will be afforded for giving the patients instruction concerning the love of God and the Eden home of our first parents, which, through the sacrifice of Christ, is to be restored to man.

In the effort made to restore the sick to health, use is to be made of the beautiful things of the Lord's creation. Seeing the flowers, plucking the ripe fruit, listening to the happy songs of the birds, has a peculiarly exhilarating effect on the nervous system. From outdoor life men, women, and children gain a desire to be pure and guileless. By the influence of the quickening, reviving, life-giving properties of nature's great medicinal resources, the functions of the body are strengthened, the intellect awakened, the imagination quickened, the spirits enlivened, and the mind prepared to appreciate the beauty of God's word.

Under these influences, combined with the influence of careful treatment and wholesome food, the sick find health. The feeble step recovers its elasticity. The eye regains its brightness. The hopeless become hopeful. The once despondent countenance wears an expression of cheerfulness. The complaining tones of the voice give place to tones of content. The words express the belief, "God is our refuge and strength, a very present help in trouble." Psalm 46:1. The clouded hope of the Christian is brightened. Faith returns. The word is heard, "Yea, though I walk through the valley of the shadow of death, I will fear no evil: for Thou art with me; Thy rod and Thy staff they comfort me." "My soul doth magnify the Lord, and my spirit hath rejoiced in God my Saviour." "He giveth power to the faint; and to them that have no might He increaseth strength." Psalm 23:4; Luke 1:46, 47; Isaiah 40:29. The acknowledgment of God's goodness in providing these blessings invigorates the mind. God is very near and is pleased to see His gifts appreciated.

The Source of Healing

Through the agencies of nature, God is working, day by day, hour by hour, moment by moment, to keep us alive, to build up and restore us. When any part of the body sustains injury, a healing process is at once begun; nature's agencies are set at work to restore soundness. But the power working through these agencies is the power of God. All life-giving power is from Him. When one recovers from disease, it is God who restores him.

Sickness, suffering, and death are work of an antagonistic power. Satan is the destroyer; God is the restorer.

The words spoken to Israel are true today to those who recover health of body or health of soul: "I am the Lord that healeth thee."

The desire of God for every human being is expressed in the words, "Beloved, I wish above all things that thou mayest prosper and be in health, even as thy soul prospereth."

He it is who "forgiveth all thine iniquities; who healeth all thy diseases; who redeemeth thy life from destruction; who crowneth thee with loving-kindness and tender mercies."—*The Ministry of Healing,* pages 112, 113 (1905).

The Value of Outdoor Life

The great medical institutions in our cities, called sanitariums do but a small part of the good they might do were they located where the patients could have the advantages of outdoor life. I have been instructed that sanitariums are to be established in many places in the country, and that the work of these institutions will greatly advance the cause of health and righteousness.

The things of nature are God's blessings, provided to give health to body, mind, and soul. They are given to the well to keep them well, and to the sick to make them well. Connected with water treatment, they are more effective in restoring health than all the drug medication in the world.

Nature, God's Physician

In the country the sick find many things to call their attention away from themselves and their sufferings. Everywhere they can look upon and enjoy the beautiful things of nature—the flowers, the fields, the fruit trees laden with their rich treasure, the forest trees casting their grateful shade, and the hills and valleys with their varied verdure and many forms of life.

And not only are they entertained by these surroundings, but at the same time they learn most precious spiritual lessons. Surrounded by the wonderful works of God, their minds are lifted from the things that are seen to the things that are unseen. The beauty of nature leads them to think of the matchless charms of the earth made new, where there will be nothing to mar the loveliness, noth-

Testimonies for the Church, vol. 7, pp. 76-79 (1902).

ing to taint or destroy, nothing to cause disease or death.

Nature is God's physician. The pure air, the glad sunshine, the beautiful flowers and trees, the orchards and vineyards, and outdoor exercise amid these surroundings, are health-giving—the elixir of life. Outdoor life is the only medicine that many invalids need. Its influence is powerful to heal sickness caused by fashionable life, a life that weakens and destroys the physical, mental, and spiritual powers.

How grateful to weary invalids accustomed to city life, the glare of many lights, and the noise of the streets are the quiet and freedom of the country! How eagerly do they turn to the scenes of nature! How glad would they be for the advantages of a sanitarium in the country, where they could sit in the open air, rejoice in the sunshine, and breathe the fragrance of tree and flower! There are life-giving properties in the balsam of the pine, in the fragrance of the cedar and the fir. And there are other trees that are health-promoting. Let no such trees be ruthlessly cut down. Cherish them where they are abundant, and plant more where there are but few.

For the chronic invalid nothing so tends to restore health and happiness as living amid attractive country surroundings. Here the most helpless ones can be left sitting or lying in the sunshine or in the shade of the trees. They have only to lift their eyes and they see above them the beautiful foliage. They wonder that they have never before noticed how gracefully the boughs bend, forming a living canopy over them, giving them just the shade they need. A sweet sense of restfulness and refreshing comes over them as they listen to the murmuring breezes. The drooping spirits revive. The waning strength is recruited. Unconsciously the mind becomes peaceful, the fevered pulse more calm and regular. As the sick grow stronger, they will venture to take a few steps to gather some of the lovely flowers—precious messengers of God's love to His afflicted family here below.

Healthful Exercise Will Work Miracles

Encourage the patients to be much in the open air. Devise plans to keep them out of doors, where, through nature, they can commune with God. Locate sanitariums on extensive tracts of land, where in the cultivation of the soil patients can have opportunity for healthful outdoor exercise. Such exercise, combined with hygienic treatment, will work miracles in restoring and invigorating the diseased body, and refreshing the worn and weary mind. Amid conditions so favorable the patients will not require so much care as if confined in a sanitarium in the city. Nor will they in the country be so much inclined to discontentment and repining. They will be ready to learn lessons in regard to the love of God—ready to acknowledge that He who cares so wonderfully for the birds and the flowers will care for the creatures formed in His own image. Thus opportunity is given physicians and helpers to reach souls, uplifting the God of nature before those who are seeking restoration to health.

A Small Country Sanitarium

In the night season I was given a view of a sanitarium in the country. The institution was not large, but it was complete. It was surrounded by beautiful trees and shrubbery, beyond which were orchards and groves. Connected with the place were gardens in which the lady patients, when they chose, could cultivate flowers of every description, each patient selecting a special plot for which to care. Outdoor exercise in these gardens was prescribed as a part of the regular treatment.

Scene after scene passed before me. In one scene a number of suffering patients had just come to one of our country sanitariums. In another I saw the same company, but, oh, how transformed their appearance! Disease had gone, the skin was clear, the countenance joyful; body and mind seemed animated with new life.

Living Object Lessons

I was also instructed that as those who have been sick are restored to health in our country sanitariums and return to their homes, they will be living object lessons, and many others will be favorably impressed by the transformation that has taken place in them. Many of the sick and suffering will turn from the cities to the country, refusing to conform to the habits, customs, and fashions of city life; they will seek to regain health in some one of our country sanitariums. Thus, though we are removed from the cities twenty or thirty miles, we shall be able to reach the people, and those who desire health will have opportunity to regain it under conditions most favorable.

God will work wonders for us if we will in faith cooperate with Him. Let us, then, pursue a sensible course, that our efforts may be blessed of heaven and crowned with success.

Reference for further study: *The Ministry of Healing,* pages 261-268, "In Contact With Nature."

Exercise, Air, and Sunlight

The chief if not the only reason why many become invalids is that the blood does not circulate freely, and the changes in the vital fluid, which are necessary to life and health, do not take place. They have not given their bodies exercise nor their lungs food, which is pure, fresh air; therefore it is impossible for the blood to be vitalized, and it pursues its course sluggishly through the system. The more we exercise, the better will be the circulation of the blood.

More people die for want of exercise than through overfatigue; very many more rust out than wear out. Those who accustom themselves to proper exercise in the open air, will generally have a good and vigorous circulation. We are more dependent upon the air we breathe than upon the food we eat. Men and women, young and old, who desire health, and who would enjoy active life should remember that they cannot have these without a good circulation. Whatever their business and inclinations, they should make up their minds to exercise in the open air as much as they can. They should feel it a religious duty to overcome the conditions of health which have kept them confined indoors, deprived of exercise in the open air.

Some invalids become willful in the matter and refuse to be convinced of the great importance of daily outdoor exercise, whereby they may obtain a supply of pure air. For fear of taking cold they persist, from year to year, in having their own way and living in an atmosphere almost destitute of vitality. It is impossible for this class to have a healthy circulation. The entire system suffers for want of exercise and pure air. The skin becomes debilitated and more sensitive to any change in the atmosphere. Additional clothing is put on, and the heat of the room increased. The next day they require a little more heat and a little more clothing in order to feel perfectly warm; and thus they humor every changing feeling until they have but little vitality to endure any cold.

Some may inquire, "What shall we do? Would you have us remain cold?" If you add clothing, let it be but little, and exercise, if possible, to regain the heat you need. If you positively cannot engage in active exercise, warm yourselves by the fire; but as soon as you are warm, lay off your extra clothing and remove from the fire. If those who can, would engage in some active employment to take the mind from themselves, they would generally forget that they were chilly, and would not receive harm. You should lower the temperature of your room as soon as you have regained your natural warmth. For invalids who have feeble lungs, nothing can be worse than an overheated atmosphere.

The Original Plan

It was not God's purpose that His people should be crowded into cities, huddled together in terraces and tenements. In the beginning He placed our first parents in a garden, amidst the beautiful sights and attractive sounds of nature, and these sights and sounds He desires men to rejoice in today. The more nearly we come into harmony with God's original plan, the more favorable will be our position for the recovery and the preservation of health.—*Testimonies for the Church,* vol. 7, p. 87 (1902).

Close Confinement at School

The system of education carried out for generations back has been destructive to health and even life itself. Many young children have passed five hours each day in schoolrooms not properly ventilated, nor sufficiently large for the healthful accommodation of the scholars. The air of such rooms soon becomes poison to the lungs that inhale it.

Little children, whose limbs and muscles are not strong, and whose brains are undeveloped, have been kept confined indoors to their injury. Many have but a slight hold on life to begin with. Confinement in school from day to day makes them nervous and diseased. Their bodies are dwarfed because of the exhausted condition of the nervous system. And if the lamp of life goes out, the parents and teachers do not consider that they had any direct influence in quenching the vital spark.

When standing by the graves of their children, the afflicted parents look upon their bereavement as a special dispensation of Providence, when, by inexcusable ignorance, their own course has destroyed the lives of their children. To then charge their death to Providence is blasphemy. God wanted the little ones to live and be disciplined, that they might have beautiful characters and glorify Him in this world and praise Him in the better world.

Ignorance of Nature's Requirements

Parents and teachers, in taking the responsibility of training these children, do not feel their accountability before God to become acquainted with the physical organ-

---

Testimonies for the Church, vol. 3, pp. 135-138 (1872).

ism, that they may treat the bodies of their children and pupils in a manner to preserve life and health. Thousands of children die because of the ignorance of parents and teachers. Mothers will spend hours over needless work upon their own dresses and those of their children, to fit them for display, and will then plead that they cannot find time to read up and obtain the information necessary to take care of the health of their children. They think it less trouble to trust their bodies to the doctors. In order to be in accordance with fashion and custom, many parents have sacrificed the health and lives of their children.

To become acquainted with the wonderful human organism, the bones, muscles, stomach, liver, bowels, heart, and pores of the skin, and to understand the dependence of one organ upon another for the healthful action of all, is a study in which most mothers take no interest. They know nothing of the influence of the body upon the mind, and of the mind upon the body. The mind, which allies finite to the infinite, they do not seem to understand. Every organ of the body was made to be servant to the mind. The mind is the capital of the body.

Children are allowed to eat flesh meats, spices, butter, cheese, pork, rich pastry, and condiments generally. They are also allowed to eat irregularly and between meals of unhealthful food. These things do their work of deranging the stomach, exciting the nerves to unnatural action, and enfeebling the intellect. Parents do not realize that they are sowing the seed which will bring forth disease and death.

Children Injured by Too Much Study

Many children have been ruined for life by urging the intellect and neglecting to strengthen the physical powers.

Many have died in childhood because of the course pursued by injudicious parents and schoolteachers in forcing their young intellects, by flattery or fear, when they were too young to see the inside of a schoolroom. Their minds have been taxed with lessons, when they should not have been called out, but kept back until the physical constitution was strong enough to endure mental effort. Small children should be left as free as lambs to run out of doors, to be free and happy, and should be allowed the most favorable opportunities to lay the foundation for sound constitutions.

Parents should be the only teachers of their children until they have reached eight or ten years of age. As fast as their minds can comprehend it, the parents should open before them God's great book of nature. The mother should have less love for the artificial in her house, and in the preparation of her dress for display, and should find time to cultivate, in herself and in her children, a love for the beautiful buds and opening flowers. By calling the attention of her children to their different colors and variety of forms, she can make them acquainted with God, who made all the beautiful things which attract and delight them. She can lead their minds up to their Creator and awaken in their young hearts a love for their heavenly Father, who has manifested so great love for them. Parents can associate God with all His created works. The only schoolroom for children from eight to ten years of age should be in the open air, amid the opening flowers and nature's beautiful scenery. And their only textbook should be the treasures of nature. These lessons, imprinted upon the minds of young children amid the pleasant, attractive scenes of nature, will not be soon forgotten.

In order for children and youth to have health, cheerfulness, vivacity, and well-developed muscles and brains, they should be much in the open air and have well-regulated employment and amusement. Children and youth who are kept at school and confined to books, cannot have sound physical constitutions. The exercise of the brain in study, without corresponding physical exercise, has a tendency to attract the blood to the brain, and the circulation of the blood through the system becomes unbalanced. The brain has too much blood, and the extremities too little. There should be rules regulating their studies to certain hours, and then a portion of their time should be spent in physical labor. And if their habits of eating, dressing, and sleeping are in accordance with physical law, they can obtain an education without sacrificing physical and mental health.

Simpler Methods

A return to simpler methods will be appreciated by the children and youth. Work in the garden and field will be an agreeable change from the wearisome routine of abstract lessons to which the young minds should never be confined. To the nervous child or youth, who finds lessons from books exhausting and hard to remember, it will be especially valuable. There is health and happiness for him in the study of nature; and the impressions made will not fade out of his mind, for they will be associated with objects that are continually before his eyes.—*Counsels to Teachers,* page 187 (1913).

A Proper Balance of Physical and Mental Labor

All the powers of the mind should be called into use and developed, in order for men and women to have well-balanced minds. The world is full of one-sided men and women, who have become such because one set of their faculties was cultivated, while others were dwarfed from inaction. The education of most youth is a failure. They overstudy, while they neglect that which pertains to practical business life. Men and women become parents without considering their responsibilities, and their offspring sink lower in the scale of human deficiency than they themselves. Thus the race is fast degenerating. The constant application to study, as the schools are now conducted, is unfitting youth for practical life. The human mind will have action. If it is not active in the right direction, it will be active in the wrong. In order to preserve the balance of the mind, labor and study should be united in the schools.

Provision should have been made in past generations for education upon a larger scale. In connection with the schools should have been agricultural and manufacturing establishments. There should also have been teachers of household labor. And a portion of the time each day should have been devoted to labor, that the physical and mental powers might be equally exercised. If schools had been established upon the plan we have mentioned, there would not now be so many unbalanced minds. . . .

I have been led to inquire, Must all that is valuable in our youth be sacrificed in order that they may obtain a school education? Had there been agricultural and manufacturing establishments connected with our schools, and had competent teachers been employed to educate the youth in the different branches of study and labor, devoting a portion of each day to mental improvement and a portion to physical labor, there would now be a more elevated class of youth to come upon the stage of action to have influence in molding society. Many of the youth who would graduate at such institutions would come forth with stability of character. They would have perseverance, fortitude, and courage to surmount obstacles, and such principles that they would not be swayed by a wrong influence, however popular. . . .

Young girls should have been instructed to manufacture wearing apparel, to cut, make, and mend garments, and thus become educated for the practical duties of life. For young men, there should be establishments where they could learn different trades, which would bring into exercise their muscles as well as their mental powers. If the youth can have but a one-sided education, which is of the greater consequence—a knowledge of the sciences, with all the disadvantages to health and life, or a knowledge of labor for practical life? We unhesitatingly answer, The latter. If one must be neglected, let it be the study of books.

There are very many girls who have married and have families, who have but little practical knowledge of the duties devolving upon a wife and mother. They can read and play upon an instrument of music, but they cannot cook. They cannot make good bread, which is very essential to the health of the family. They cannot cut and make garments, for they never learned how. They considered these things unessential, and in their married life they are as dependent upon someone to do these things for them as are their own little children. It is this inexcusable ignorance in regard to the most needful duties of life which makes very many unhappy families.

The impression that work is degrading to fashionable life has laid thousands in the grave who might have lived. Those who perform only manual labor, frequently work to excess without giving themselves periods of rest; while the intellectual class overwork the brain and suffer for want of the healthful vigor that physical labor gives. If the intellectual would to some extent share the burden of the laboring class and thus strengthen the muscles, the laboring class might do less and devote a portion of their time to mental and moral culture. Those of sedentary and literary habits should take physical exercise, even if they have no need to labor so far as means are concerned. Health should be a sufficient inducement to lead them to unite physical with mental labor.

Moral, intellectual, and physical culture should be combined in order to have well-developed, well-balanced men and women. Some are qualified to exercise greater intellectual strength than others, while others are inclined to love and enjoy physical labor. Both of these classes should seek to improve where they are deficient. . . .

The minds of thinking men labor too hard. They frequently use their mental powers prodigally; while there is another class whose highest aim in life is physical labor. The latter class do not exercise the mind. Their muscles are exercised, while their brains are robbed of intellectual strength; just as the minds of thinking men are worked, while their bodies are robbed of strength and vigor by their neglect to exercise the muscles. Those who are content to devote their lives to physical labor, and leave others to do the thinking for them, while they simply carry out what other brains have planned, will have strength of muscle, but feeble intellects. Their influence for good is small in comparison to what it might be if they would use their brains as well as their muscles. This class fall more readily if attacked by disease. The system is vitalized by the electrical force of the brain to resist disease.

Men who have good physical powers should educate themselves to think as well as to act, and not depend upon others to be brains for them. It is a popular error with a large class to regard work as degrading. Therefore young men are very anxious to educate themselves to become teachers, clerks, merchants, lawyers, and to occupy almost any position that does not require physical labor. Young women regard housework as demeaning. And although the physical exercise required to perform household labor, if not too severe, is calculated to promote health, yet they will seek for an education that will fit them to become teachers or clerks, or will learn some trade which will confine them indoors to sedentary employment. The bloom of health fades from their cheeks, and disease fastens upon them, because they are robbed of physical exercise and their habits are perverted generally. All this because it is fashionable! They enjoy delicate life, which is feebleness and decay.

True, there is some excuse for young women not choosing housework for employment, because those who hire kitchen girls generally treat them as servants. Frequently their employers do not respect them and treat them as though they were unworthy to be members of their families. They do not give them the privileges they do the seamstress, the copyist, and the teacher of music. But there can be no employment more important than that of housework. To cook well, to present healthful food upon the table in an inviting manner, requires intelligence and experience. The one who prepares the food that is to be placed in our stomachs, to be converted into blood to nourish the system, occupies a most important and elevated position. The position of copyist, dressmaker, or music teacher cannot equal in importance that of the cook.

The foregoing is a statement of what might have been done by a proper system of education. Time is too short now to accomplish that which might have been done in past generations; but we can do much, even in these last days, to correct the existing evils in the education of youth. And because time is short, we should be in earnest and work zealously to give the young that education which is consistent with our faith. We are reformers. We desire that our children should study to the best advantage. In order to do this, employment should be given them which will call the muscles into exercise. Daily, systematic labor should constitute a part of the education of the youth, even at this late period. Much can now be gained by connecting labor with schools. In following this plan, the students will realize elasticity of spirit and vigor of thought, and will be able to accomplish more mental labor in a given time than they could by study alone. And they can leave school with their constitutions unimpaired, and with strength and courage to persevere in any position in which the providence of God may place them.

The Results of Physical Inaction

With the present plan of education, a door of temptation is opened to the youth. Although they generally have too many hours of study, they have many hours without anything to do. These leisure hours are frequently spent in a reckless manner. The knowledge of bad habits is communicated from one to another, and vice is greatly increased. Very many young men who have been religiously instructed at home, and who go out to the schools comparatively innocent and virtuous, become corrupt by associating with vicious companions. They lose self-respect and sacrifice noble principles. Then they are prepared to pursue the downward path; for they have so abused their consciences that sin does not appear so exceeding sinful. These evils, which exist in the schools that are conducted according to the present plan, might be remedied in a great degree if study and labor could be combined. The same evils exist in the higher schools, only in a greater degree for many of the youth have educated themselves in vice, and their consciences are seared.

Many parents overrate the stability and good qualities of their children. They do not seem to consider that they will be exposed to the deceptive influences of vicious youth. Parents have their fears as they send them some distance away to school, but flatter themselves that as they have had good examples and religious instruction, they will be true to principle in their high-school life. Many parents have but a faint idea to what extent licentiousness exists in these institutions of learning. In many cases the parents have labored hard and suffered many privations for the

Testimonies for the Church, vol. 3, pp. 148-152 (1872).

cherished object of having their children obtain a finished education. And after all their efforts, many have the bitter experience of receiving their children from their course of studies with dissolute habits and ruined constitutions. And frequently they are disrespectful to their parents, unthankful, and unholy. These abused parents, who are thus rewarded by ungrateful children, lament that they sent their children from them, to be exposed to temptations and come back to them physical, mental, and moral wrecks. With disappointed hopes and almost broken hearts, they see their children, of whom they had high hopes, follow in a course of vice and drag out a miserable existence. . . .

Inordinate Study

Some students put their whole being into their studies and concentrate their mind upon the object of obtaining an education. They work the brain, but allow the physical powers to remain inactive. The brain is overworked, and the muscles become weak because they are not exercised. When these students graduate it is evident that they have obtained their education at the expense of life. They have studied day and night, year after year, keeping their minds continually upon the stretch, while they have failed to sufficiently exercise their muscles. They sacrifice all for a knowledge of the sciences, and pass to their graves.

Young ladies frequently give themselves up to study, to the neglect of other branches of education even more essential for practical life than the study of books. And after having obtained their education, they are often invalids for life. They neglected their health by remaining too much indoors, deprived of the pure air of heaven and of the God-given sunlight. These young ladies might have come from their schools in health had they combined with their studies household labor and exercise in the open air.

Health is a great treasure. It is the richest possession mortals can have. Wealth, honor, or learning is dearly purchased if it be at the loss of the vigor of health. None of these attainments can secure happiness, if health is wanting. It is a terrible sin to abuse the health that God has given us; for every abuse of health enfeebles us for life and makes us losers, even if we gain any amount of education.

In many cases parents who are wealthy do not feel the importance of giving their children an education in the practical duties of life as well as in the sciences. They do not see the necessity, for the good of their children's minds and morals, and for their future usefulness, of giving them a thorough understanding of useful labor. This is due their children, that, should misfortune come, they could stand forth in noble independence, knowing how to use their hands. If they have a capital of strength, they cannot be poor, even if they have not a dollar. Many who in youth were in affluent circumstances may be robbed of all their riches and be left with parents and brothers and sisters dependent upon them for sustenance. Then how important that every youth be educated to labor, that they may be prepared for any emergency! Riches are indeed a curse when their possessors let them stand in the way of their sons and daughters' obtaining a knowledge of useful labor, that they may be qualified for practical life.

Those who are not compelled to labor, frequently do not have sufficient active exercise for physical health. Young men, for want of having their minds and hands employed in active labor, acquire habits of indolence and frequently obtain what is most to be dreaded, a street education, lounging about stores, smoking, drinking, and playing cards. . . .

Poverty, in many cases, is a blessing; for it prevents youth and children from being ruined by inaction. The physical as well as the mental powers should be cultivated and properly developed. The first and constant care of parents should be to see that their children have firm constitutions, that they may be sound men and women. It is impossible to attain this object without physical exercise. For their own physical health and moral good, children should be taught to work, even if there is no necessity so far as want is concerned. If they would have pure and virtuous characters, they must have the discipline of well-regulated labor, which will bring into exercise all the muscles. The satisfaction that children will have in being useful, and in denying themselves to help others, will be the most healthful pleasure they ever enjoyed. Why should the wealthy rob themselves and their dear children of this great blessing?

Indolence Accursed

Parents, inaction is the greatest curse that ever came upon youth. Your daughters should not be allowed to lie in bed late in the morning, sleeping away the precious hours lent them of God to be used for the best purpose, and for which they will have to give an account to Him. The mother does her daughters great injury by bearing the burdens that they should share with her for their own present and future good. The course that many parents pursue in allowing their children to be indolent and to gratify their desire for reading romance, is unfitting them for real life. Novel and storybook reading are the greatest evils in which youth can indulge. Novel and lovestory readers always fail to make good, practical mothers. They are air-castle builders, living in an unreal, an imaginary world. They become sentimental and have sick fancies. Their artificial life spoils them for anything useful. They are dwarfed in intellect, although they may flatter themselves that they are superior in mind and manners. Exercise in household labor is of the greatest advantage to young girls.

Physical labor will not prevent the cultivation of the intellect. Far from it. The advantages gained by physical labor will balance a person and prevent the mind from being overworked. The toil will come upon the muscles and relieve the wearied brain. There are many listless, useless girls who consider it unladylike to engage in active labor. But their characters are too transparent to deceive sensible persons in regard to their real worthlessness. They simper and giggle and are all affectation. They appear as though they could not speak their words fairly and squarely, but torture all they say with lisping and simpering. Are these ladies? They were not born fools, but were educated such. It does not require a frail, helpless, overdressed, simpering thing to make a lady. A sound body is required for a sound intellect. Physical soundness and a practical knowledge of all the necessary household duties will never be hindrances to a welldeveloped intellect; both are highly important for a lady.

Physical Culture

The question of suitable recreation for their pupils is one that teachers often find perplexing. Gymnastic exercises fill a useful place in many schools, but without careful supervision they are often carried to excess. In the gymnasium many youth, by their attempted feats of strength, have done themselves lifelong injury.

Exercise in a gymnasium, however well conducted, cannot supply the place of recreation in the open air, and for this our schools should offer better opportunity. Vigorous exercise the pupils must have. Few evils are more to be dreaded than indolence and aimlessness. Yet the tendency of most athletic sports is a subject of anxious thought to those who have at heart the well-being of the youth. Teachers are troubled as they consider the influence of these sports both on the student's progress in school and on his success in afterlife. The games that occupy so much of his time are diverting the mind from study. They are not helping to prepare the youth for practical, earnest work in life. Their influence does not tend toward refinement, generosity, or real manliness.

Some of the most popular amusements, such as football and boxing, have become schools of brutality. They are developing the same characteristics as did the games of ancient Rome. The love of domination, the pride in mere brute force, the reckless disregard of life, are exerting upon the youth a power to demoralize that is appalling.

Other athletic games, though not so brutalizing, are scarcely less objectionable, because of the excess to which they are carried. They stimulate the love of pleasure and excitement, thus fostering a distaste for useful labor, a

---

Education, pages 210-213 (1903).

disposition to shun practical duties and responsibilities. They tend to destroy a relish for life's sober realities and its tranquil enjoyments. Thus the door is opened to dissipation and lawlessness, with their terrible results.

Parties of Pleasure

As ordinarily conducted, parties of pleasure also are a hindrance to real growth, either of mind or of character. Frivolous associations, habits of extravagance, of pleasure seeking, and too often of dissipation, are formed, that shape the whole life for evil. In place of such amusements, parents and teachers can do much to supply diversions wholesome and life-giving.

In this, as in all things else that concern our well-being, Inspiration has pointed the way. In early ages, with the people who were under God's direction, life was simple. They lived close to the heart of nature. Their children shared in the labor of the parents and studied the beauties and mysteries of nature's treasure house. And in the quiet of field and wood they pondered those mighty truths handed down as a sacred trust from generation to generation. Such training produced strong men.

Outdoor Occupations

In this age, life has become artificial and men have degenerated. While we may not return fully to the simple habits of those early times, we may learn from them lessons that will make our seasons of recreation what the name implies—seasons of true upbuilding for body and mind and soul.

With the question of recreation the surroundings of the home and the school have much to do. In the choice of a home or the location of a school these things should be considered. Those with whom mental and physical well-being is of greater moment than money or the claims and customs of society should seek for their children the benefit of nature's teaching, and recreation amidst her surroundings. It would be a great aid in educational work could every school be so situated as to afford the pupils land for cultivation and access to the fields and woods.

In lines of recreation for the student, the best results will be attained through the personal co-operation of the teacher. The true teacher can impart to his pupils few gifts so valuable as the gift of his own companionship. It is true of men and women, and how much more of youth and children, that only as we come in touch through sympathy can we understand them; and we need to understand in order most effectively to benefit. To strengthen the tie of sympathy between teacher and student there are few means that count so much as pleasant association together outside the schoolroom. In some schools the teacher is always with his pupils in their hours of recreation. He unites in their pursuits, accompanies them in their excursions, and seems to make himself one with them. Well would it be for our schools were this practice more generally followed. The sacrifice demanded of the teacher would be great, but he would reap a rich reward.

No recreation helpful only to themselves will prove so great a blessing to the children and youth as that which makes them helpful to others. Naturally enthusiastic and impressible, the young are quick to respond to suggestions. In planning for the culture of plants, let the teacher seek to awaken an interest in beautifying the school grounds and the schoolroom. A double benefit will result. That which the pupils seek to beautify they will be unwilling to have marred or defaced. A refined taste, a love of order, and a habit of caretaking will be encouraged; and the spirit of fellowship and co-operation developed will prove to the pupils a lifelong blessing.

So also a new interest may be given to the work of the garden or the excursion in field and wood, as the pupils are encouraged to remember those shut in from these pleasant places and to share with them the beautiful things of nature.

The watchful teacher will find many opportunities for directing pupils to acts of helpfulness. By little children especially the teacher is regarded with almost unbounded confidence and respect. Whatever he may suggest as to ways of helping in the home, faithfulness in the daily tasks, ministry to the sick or the poor, can hardly fail of bringing forth fruit. And thus again a double gain will be secured. The kindly suggestion will react upon its author. Gratitude and co-operation on the part of the parents will lighten the teacher's burden and brighten his path.

A Safeguard Against Evil

Attention to recreation and physical culture will at times, no doubt, interrupt the regular routine of schoolwork; but the interruption will prove no real hindrance. In the invigoration of mind and body, the fostering of an unselfish spirit and the binding together of pupil and teacher by the ties of common interest and friendly association, the expenditure of time and effort will be repaid a hundredfold. A blessed outlet will be afforded for that restless energy which is so often a source of danger to the young. As a safeguard against evil, the preoccupation of the mind with good is worth more than unnumbered barriers of law and discipline.

Health and Efficiency

It is necessary, in order to pursue this great and arduous work, that the ministers of Christ should possess physical health. To attain this end they must become regular in their habits and adopt a healthful system of living. Many are continually complaining and suffering from various indispositions. This is almost always because they do not labor wisely nor observe the laws of health. They frequently remain too much indoors, occupying heated rooms filled with impure air. Here they apply themselves closely to study or writing, taking little physical exercise and having little change of employment. As a consequence, the blood becomes sluggish, and the powers of the mind are enfeebled.

The whole system needs the invigorating influence of exercise in the open air. A few hours of manual labor each day would tend to renew the bodily vigor and rest and relax the mind. In this way the general health would be promoted and a greater amount of pastoral labor could be performed. The incessant reading and writing of many ministers unfit them for pastoral work. They consume valuable time in abstract study, which should be expended in helping the needy at the right moment. . . .

Our ministers who have reached the age of forty or fifty years should not feel that their labor is less efficient than formerly. Men of years and experience are just the ones to put forth strong and well-directed efforts. They are especially needed at this time; the churches cannot afford to part with them. Such ones should not talk of physical and mental feebleness, nor feel that their day of usefulness is over.

Testimonies for the Church, vol. 4, pp. 264-270 (1876).

Many of them have suffered from severe mental taxation, unrelieved by physical exercise. The result is a deterioration of their powers and a tendency to shirk responsibility. What they need is more active labor. This is not alone confined to those whose heads are white with the frost of time, but men young in years have fallen into the same state and have become mentally feeble. They have a list of set discourses; but if they get beyond the boundaries of these, they lose their soundings.

The old-fashioned pastor, who traveled on horseback, and spent much time in visiting his flock, enjoyed much better health, notwithstanding his hardships and exposures, than our ministers of today, who avoid all physical exertion as far as possible and confine themselves to their books.

Ministers of age and experience should feel it their duty, as God's hired servants, to go forward, progressing every day, continually becoming more efficient in their work and constantly gathering fresh matter to set before the people. Each effort to expound the gospel should be an improvement upon that which preceded it. Each year they should develop a deeper piety, a tenderer spirit, a greater spirituality, and a more thorough knowledge of Bible truth. The greater their age and experience, the nearer should they be able to approach the hearts of the people, having a more perfect knowledge of them.

Periods of Relaxation

I was shown that Sabbathkeepers as a people labor too hard, without allowing themselves change or periods of rest. Recreation is needful to those who are engaged in physical labor, and is still more essential for those whose labor is principally mental. It is not essential to our salvation, nor for the glory of God, to keep the mind laboring constantly and excessively, even upon religious themes. There are amusements, such as dancing, card playing, chess, checkers, etc., which we cannot approve, because Heaven condemns them. These amusements open the door for great evil. They are not beneficial in their tendency, but have an exciting influence, producing in some minds a passion for those plays which lead to gambling and dissipation. All such plays should be condemned by Christians, and something perfectly harmless should be substituted in their place.

I saw that our holidays should not be spent in patterning after the world, yet they should not be passed by unnoticed, for this will bring dissatisfaction to our children. On these days when there is danger that our children will be exposed to evil influences and become corrupted by the pleasures and excitement of the world, let the parents study to get up something to take the place of more dangerous amusements. Give your children to understand that you have their good and happiness in view.

Let several families living in a city or village unite and leave the occupations which have taxed them physically and mentally and make an excursion into the country to the side of a fine lake or to a nice grove, where the scenery of nature is beautiful. They should provide themselves

Testimonies for the Church, vol. 1, pp. 514, 515 (1867).

with plain, hygienic food, the very best fruits and grains, and spread their table under the shade of some tree or under the canopy of heaven. The ride, the exercise, and the scenery will quicken the appetite, and they can enjoy a repast which kings might envy.

On such occasions parents and children should feel free from care, labor, and perplexity. Parents should become children with their children, making everything as pleasant for them as possible. Let the whole day be given to recreation. Exercise in the open air, for those whose employment has been within doors and sedentary, will be beneficial to health. All who can should feel it a duty to pursue this course. Nothing will be lost, but much gained. They can return to their occupations with new life and new courage to engage in their labor with zeal, and they are better prepared to resist disease.

Sunlight in the Home

If you would have your homes sweet and inviting, make them bright with air and sunshine. Remove your heavy curtains, open the windows, throw back the blinds, and enjoy the rich sunlight, even if it be at the expense of the colors of your carpets. The precious sunlight may fade your carpets, but it will give a healthful color to the cheeks of your children. If you have God's presence and possess earnest, loving hearts, a humble home, made bright with air and sunlight, and cheerful with the welcome of unselfish hospitality, will be to your family and to the weary traveler a heaven below.—*Testimonies for the Church,* vol. 2, p. 527 (1870).

Reference for further study: *Testimonies for the Church,* vol. 2, pp. 585-594, "Christian Recreation."

Prohibited Amusements

Those who are engaged in study should have relaxation. The mind must not be constantly confined to close thought, for the delicate mental machinery becomes worn. The body as well as the mind must have exercise. But there is great need of temperance in amusements, as in every other pursuit. And the character of these amusements should be carefully and thoroughly considered. Every youth should ask himself, What influence will these amusements have on physical, mental, and moral health? Will my mind become so infatuated as to forget God? Shall I cease to have His glory before me?

Card playing should be prohibited. The associations and tendencies are dangerous. The prince of the powers of darkness presides in the gaming room and wherever there is card playing. Evil angels are familiar guests in these places. There is nothing in such amusements beneficial to soul or body. There is nothing to strengthen the intellect, nothing to store it with valuable ideas for future use. The conversation is upon trivial and degrading subjects. There is heard the unseemly jest, the low, vile talk, which lowers and destroys the true dignity of manhood. These games are the most senseless, useless, unprofitable, and dangerous employments the youth can have. Those who engage in card playing become intensely excited, and soon lose all relish for useful and elevating occupations. Expertness in handling cards will soon lead to a desire to put this knowledge and tact to some use for personal benefit. A small sum is staked, and then a larger, until a thirst for gaming is acquired, which leads to certain ruin. How many has this pernicious amusement led

Testimonies for the Church, vol. 4, pp. 652, 653 (1831).

to every sinful practice, to poverty, to prison, to murder, and to the gallows! And yet many parents do not see the terrible gulf of ruin that is yawning for our youth.

Among the most dangerous resorts for pleasure is the theater. Instead of being a school of morality and virtue, as is so often claimed, it is the very hotbed of immorality. Vicious habits and sinful propensities are strengthened and confirmed by these entertainments. Low songs, lewd gestures, expressions, and attitudes, deprave the imagination and debase the morals. Every youth who habitually attends such exhibitions will be corrupted in principle. There is no influence in our land more powerful to poison the imagination, to destroy religious impressions, and to blunt the relish for the tranquil pleasures and sober realities of life, than theatrical amusements. The love for these scenes increases with every indulgence, as the desire for intoxicating drink strengthens with its use. The only safe course is to shun the theater, the circus, and every other questionable place of amusement.

There are modes of recreation which are highly beneficial to both mind and body. An enlightened, discriminating mind will find abundant means for entertainment and diversion, from sources not only innocent, but instructive. Recreation in the open air, the contemplation of the works of God in nature, will be of the highest benefit.

Exercise as a Restorer

The idea that those who have overtaxed their mental and physical powers, or who have been broken down in body or mind, must suspend activity in order to regain health is a great error. In a few cases, entire rest for a time may be necessary, but such instances are rare. In most cases the change would be too great to be beneficial.

Those who have broken down by intense mental labor should have rest from wearing thought; yet to teach them that it is wrong, or even dangerous, for them to exercise their mental powers at all, leads them to view their condition as worse than it really is. They are nervous and finally become a burden to themselves as well as to those who care for them. In this state of mind their recovery is doubtful indeed.

Those who have overtaxed their physical powers should not be advised to forgo labor entirely. To shut them away from all exercise would in many cases prevent their restoration to health. The will goes with the labor of the hands; and when the will power is dormant, the imagination becomes abnormal, so that it is impossible for the sufferer to resist disease. Inactivity is the greatest curse that could come upon one in such a condition.

Nature's fine and wonderful mechanism needs to be constantly exercised in order to be in a condition to accomplish the object for which it was designed. The do-nothing system is a dangerous one in any case. Physical exercise in the direction of useful labor has a happy influence upon the mind, strengthens the muscles, improves the circulation, and gives the invalid the satisfaction of knowing how much he can endure, and that he is not

Christian Temperance, pages 100, 101 (1890).

wholly useless in this busy world; whereas, if this is restricted, his attention is turned to himself and he is in constant danger of exaggerating his difficulties. If invalids
would engage in some well-directed physical exercise,
using their strength but not abusing it, they would find
it an effective agent in their recovery.

Walking for Exercise

Those who are feeble and indolent should not yield to
their inclination to be inactive, thus depriving themselves
of air and sunlight, but should practice exercising out of
doors in walking or working in the garden. They will
become very much fatigued, but this will not injure them.
. . . It is not good policy to give up the use of certain
muscles because pain is felt when they are exercised. The
pain is frequently caused by the effort of nature to give
life and vigor to those parts that have become partially
lifeless through inaction. The motion of these long-dis-
used muscles will cause pain, because nature is awakening them to life.

Walking, in all cases where it is possible, is the best
remedy for diseased bodies, because in this exercise all
the organs of the body are brought into use. Many who
depend upon the movement cure could accomplish more
for themselves by muscular exercise than the movements
can do for them. In some cases, want of exercise causes
the bowels and muscles to become enfeebled and
shrunken, and these organs that have become enfeebled
for want of use will be strengthened by exercise. There
is no exercise that can take the place of walking. By
it the circulation of the blood is greatly improved.—*Testimonies for the Church,* vol. 3, p. 78 (1871).

The Evils of Inactivity

Physical exercise and labor combined have a happy influence upon the mind, strengthen the muscles, improve the circulation, and give the invalid the satisfaction of knowing his own power of endurance; whereas, if he is restricted from healthful exercise and physical labor, his attention is turned to himself. He is in constant danger of thinking himself worse than he really is, and of having established within him a diseased imagination which causes him to continually fear that he is overtaxing his powers of endurance. As a general thing, if he should engage in some well-directed labor, using his strength and not abusing it, he would find that physical exercise would prove a more powerful and effective agent in his recovery than even the water treatment he is receiving.

The inactivity of the mental and physical powers, as far as useful labor is concerned, is that which keeps many invalids in a condition of feebleness which they feel powerless to rise above. It also gives them a greater opportunity to indulge an impure imagination—an indulgence which has brought many of them into their present condition of feebleness. They are told that they have expended too much vitality in hard labor, when, in nine cases out of ten, the labor they performed was the only redeeming thing in their lives and was the means of saving them from utter ruin. While their minds were thus engaged they could not have as favorable an opportunity to debase their bodies and to complete the work of destroying themselves. To have all such persons cease to labor with brain and muscle is to give them ample opportunity to be taken captive by the temptations of Satan.—*Testimonies for the Church,* vol. 4, pp. 94, 95 (1876).

Open the Windows of the Soul

The burden of sin, with its unrest and unsatisfied desires, lies at the very foundation of a large share of the maladies the sinner suffers. Christ is the Mighty Healer of the sin-sick soul. These poor, afflicted ones need to have a clearer knowledge of Him whom to know aright is life eternal. They need to be patiently and kindly yet earnestly taught how to throw open the windows of the soul and let the sunlight of God's love come in to illuminate the darkened chambers of the mind. The most exalted spiritual truths may be brought home to the heart by the things of nature. The birds of the air, the flowers of the field in their glowing beauty, the springing grain, the fruitful branches of the vine, the trees putting forth their tender buds, the glorious sunset, the crimson clouds predicting a fair morrow, the recurring seasons—all these may teach us precious lessons of trust and faith. The imagination has here a fruitful field in which to range. The intelligent mind may contemplate with the greatest satisfaction those lessons of divine truth which the world's Redeemer has associated with the things of nature.

Christ sharply reproved the men of His time because they had not learned from nature the spiritual lessons which they might have learned. All things, animate and inanimate, express to man the knowledge of God. The same divine mind that is working upon the things of nature is speaking to the minds and hearts of men and creating an inexpressible craving for something they have not. The things of the world cannot satisfy their longing. —*Testimonies for the Church,* vol. 4, pp. 579, 580 (1881).

SANITARIUMS—THEIR OBJECTS AND AIMS

God's Design in Our Sanitariums

Every institution established by Seventh-day Adventists is to be to the world what Joseph was in Egypt and what Daniel and his fellows were in Babylon. As in the providence of God these chosen ones were taken captive, it was to carry to heathen nations the blessings that come to humanity through a knowledge of God. They were to be representatives of Jehovah. They were never to compromise with idolaters; their religious faith and their name as worshipers of the living God they were to bear as a special honor.

And this they did. In prosperity and adversity they honored God, and God honored them. . . .

So the institutions established by God's people today are to glorify His name. The only way in which we can fulfill His expectation is by being representatives of the truth for this time. God is to be recognized in the institutions established by Seventh-day Adventists. By them the truth for this time is to be represented before the world with convincing power.

We are called to represent to the world the character of God as it was revealed to Moses. In answer to the prayer of Moses, "Show me Thy glory," the Lord promised, "I will make all My goodness pass before thee." "And the Lord passed by before him, and proclaimed, The

Testimonies for the Church, vol. 6, pp. 219-228 (1900).

(203)

Lord, The Lord God, merciful and gracious, long-suffering, and abundant in goodness and truth, keeping mercy for thousands, forgiving iniquity and transgression and sin." Exodus 33:18, 19; 34:6, 7. This is the fruit that God desires from His people. In the purity of their characters, in the holiness of their lives, in their mercy and loving-kindness and compassion, they are to demonstrate that "the law of the Lord is perfect, converting the soul." Psalm 19:7.

God's purpose for His institutions today may also be read in the purpose which He sought to accomplish through the Jewish nation. Through Israel it was His design to impart rich blessings to all peoples. Through them the way was to be prepared for the diffusion of His light to the whole world. . . .

God desired to make of His people Israel a praise and a glory. Every spiritual advantage was given them. God withheld from them nothing favorable to the formation of character that would make them representatives of Himself.

Their obedience to the laws of God would make them marvels of prosperity before the nations of the world. He who could give them wisdom and skill in all cunning work would continue to be their teacher, and would ennoble and elevate them through obedience to His laws. If obedient, they would be preserved from the diseases that afflicted other nations and would be blessed with vigor of intellect. The glory of God, His majesty and power, were to be revealed in all their prosperity. They were to be a kingdom of priests and princes. God furnished them with every facility for becoming the greatest nation on the earth. . . .

The Lord years ago gave me special light in regard

to the establishment of a health institution where the sick could be treated on altogether different lines from those followed in any other institution in our world. It was to be founded and conducted upon Bible principles, as the Lord's instrumentality, and it was to be in His hands one of the most effective agencies for giving light to the world. It was God's purpose that it should stand forth with scientific ability, with moral and spiritual power, and as a faithful sentinel of reform in all its bearings. All who should act a part in it were to be reformers, having respect to its principles and heeding the light of health reform shining upon us as a people.

A Beacon Light

God designed that the institution which He should establish should stand forth as a beacon of light, of warning and reproof. He would prove to the world that an institution conducted on religious principles, as an asylum for the sick, could be sustained without sacrificing its peculiar, holy character; that it could be kept free from the objectionable features found in other health institutions. It was to be an instrumentality for bringing about great reforms.

The Lord revealed that the prosperity of the sanitarium was not to be dependent alone upon the knowledge and skill of its physicians, but upon the favor of God. It was to be known as an institution where God was acknowledged as the Monarch of the universe, an institution that was under His special supervision. Its managers were to make God first and last and best in everything. And in this was to be its strength. If conducted in a manner that God could approve, it would be highly successful and would stand in advance of all other institutions of the kind in the world. Great light, great knowledge, and superior privileges were given. And in accordance with the light received would be the responsibility of those to whom the carrying forward of the institution was entrusted.

As our work has extended and institutions have multiplied, God's purpose in their establishment remains the same. The conditions of prosperity are unchanged.

The human family is suffering because of transgression of the laws of God. The Lord desires that men shall be led to understand the cause of their suffering and the only way to find relief. He desires them to see that their well-being, physical, mental, and moral, depends upon their obedience to His law. It is His purpose that our institutions shall be as object lessons showing the results of obedience to right principles.

To Promulgate Health Principles

In the preparation of a people for the Lord's second coming, a great work is to be accomplished through the promulgation of health principles. The people are to be instructed in regard to the needs of the physical organism and the value of healthful living as taught in the Scriptures, that the bodies which God has created may be presented to Him a living sacrifice, fitted to render Him acceptable service. There is a great work to be done for suffering humanity in relieving their sufferings by the use of the natural agencies that God has provided, and in teaching them how to prevent sickness by the regulation of the appetites and passions. The people should be taught that transgression of the laws of nature is transgression of the laws of God. They should be taught the truth in physical as well as in spiritual lines, that "the fear of the

Lord tendeth to life." Proverbs 19:23. "If thou wilt enter into life," Christ says, "keep the commandments." Matthew 19:17. Live out My law "as the apple of thine eye." God's commandments, obeyed, are "life unto those that find them, and health to all their flesh." Proverbs 4:22.

Our sanitariums are an educating power to teach the people in these lines. Those who are taught can in turn impart to others a knowledge of health-restoring and health-preserving principles. Thus our sanitariums are to be an instrumentality for reaching the people, an agency for showing them the evil of disregarding the laws of life and health, and for teaching them how to preserve the body in the best condition. Sanitariums are to be established in different countries that are entered by our missionaries, and are to be centers from which a work of healing, restoring, and educating shall be carried on.

We are to labor both for the health of the body and for the saving of the soul. Our mission is the same as that of our Master, of whom it is written that He went about doing good and healing all who were oppressed by Satan. Acts 10:38. Of His own work He says: "The Spirit of the Lord God is upon Me; because the Lord hath anointed Me to preach good tidings unto the meek." "He hath sent Me to heal the brokenhearted, to preach deliverance to the captives, and recovering of sight to the blind, to set at liberty them that are bruised." Isaiah 61:1; Luke 4:18. As we follow Christ's example of labor for the good of others, we shall awaken their interest in the God whom we love and serve.

Memorials for God

Our sanitariums in all their departments should be memorials for God, His instrumentalities for sowing the seeds of truth in human hearts. This they will be if rightly conducted.

The living truth of God is to be made known in our medical institutions. Many persons who come to them are hungering and thirsting for truth, and when it is rightly presented they will receive it with gladness. Our sanitariums have been the means of elevating the truth for this time and bringing it before thousands. The religious influence that pervades these institutions inspires the guests with confidence. The assurance that the Lord presides there, and the many prayers offered for the sick, make an impression upon their hearts. Many who have never before thought of the value of the soul are convicted by the Spirit of God, and not a few are led to change their whole course of life. Impressions that will never be effaced are made upon many who have been self-satisfied, who have thought their own standard of character to be sufficient, and have felt no need of the righteousness of Christ. When the future test comes, when enlightenment comes to them, not a few of these will take their stand with God's remnant people.

God is honored by institutions conducted in this way. In His mercy He has made the sanitariums such a power in the relief of physical suffering that thousands have been drawn to them to be cured of their maladies. And with many, physical healing is accompanied by the healing of the soul. From the Saviour they receive the forgiveness of their sins. They receive the grace of Christ and identify themselves with Him, with His interests, His honor. Many go away from our sanitariums with new hearts. The change is decided. These, returning to their homes, are as lights in the world. The Lord makes them His witnesses. Their testimony is, "I have seen His greatness,

I have tasted His goodness. 'Come and hear, all ye that fear God, and I will declare what He hath done for my soul.'" Psalm 66:16.

Thus through the prospering hand of God upon them, our sanitariums have been the means of accomplishing great good. And they are to rise still higher. God will work with the people who will honor Him.

Fountains of Life

Wonderful is the work which God designs to accomplish through His servants, that His name may be glorified. God made Joseph a fountain of life to the Egyptian nation. Through Joseph the life of that whole people was preserved. Through Daniel God saved the life of all the wise men of Babylon. And these deliverances were as object lessons; they illustrated to the people the spiritual blessings offered them through connection with the God whom Joseph and Daniel worshiped. So through His people today God desires to bring blessings to the world. Every worker in whose heart Christ abides, everyone who will show forth His love to the world, is a worker together with God for the blessing of humanity. As he receives from the Saviour grace to impart to others, from his whole being flows forth the tide of spiritual life. Christ came as the Great Physician to heal the wounds that sin has made in the human family, and His Spirit, working through His servants, imparts to sin-sick, suffering human beings a mighty healing power that is efficacious for the body and the soul. "In that day," says the Scripture, "there shall be a fountain opened to the house of David and to the inhabitants of Jerusalem for sin and for uncleanness." Zechariah 13:1. The waters of this fountain contain medicinal properties that will heal both physical and spiritual infirmities.

From this fountain flows the mighty river seen in Ezekiel's vision. "These waters issue out toward the east country, and go down into the desert, and go into the sea: which being brought forth into the sea, the waters shall be healed. And it shall come to pass, that everything that liveth, which moveth, whithersoever the rivers shall come, shall live. . . . And by the river upon the bank thereof, on this side and on that side, shall grow all trees for meat, whose leaf shall not fade, neither shall the fruit thereof be consumed: it shall bring forth new fruit according to his months, because their waters they issued out of the sanctuary: and the fruit thereof shall be for meat, and the leaf thereof for medicine." Ezekiel 47:8-12.

Such a river of life and healing God designs that, by His power working through them, our sanitariums shall be.

The Church Qualified for Service

Christ has empowered His church to do the same work that He did during His ministry. Today He is the same compassionate physician that He was while on this earth. We should let the afflicted understand that in Him there is healing balm for every disease, restoring power for every infirmity. His disciples in this time are to pray for the sick as verily as His disciples of old prayed. And recoveries will follow, for "the prayer of faith shall save the sick." James 5:15. We need the Holy Spirit's power, the calm assurance of faith that can claim God's promises.—*Review and Herald,* June 9, 1904.

Reference for further study: *Testimonies for the Church,* vol. 8, pp. 181-191, "God's Purpose in Establishing the Sanitarium."

Living Waters for Thirsty Souls

The Lord wants wise men and women, acting in the capacity of nurses, to comfort and help the sick and the suffering. . . .

It is for the object of soul saving that our sanitariums are established. In our daily ministrations we see many careworn, sorrowful faces. What does the sorrow on these faces show? The need of the soul for the peace of Christ. Poor, sad human beings go to broken cisterns, which can hold no water, thinking to quench their thirst. Let them hear a voice saying, "Ho, everyone that thirsteth, come ye to the waters." "Come to Me, that ye might have life." Isaiah 55:1; John 5:40.

It is that thirsting souls may be led to the living water that we plead for sanitariums—not expensive, mammoth sanitariums, but homelike institutions in pleasant places.

The sick are to be reached, not by massive buildings, but by the establishment of many small sanitariums, which are to be as lights shining in a dark place. Those who are engaged in this work are to reflect the sunlight of Christ's face. They are to be as salt that has not lost its savor. By sanitarium work, properly conducted, the influence of true, pure religion will be extended to many souls.

From our sanitariums, trained workers are to go forth into places where the truth has never been proclaimed, and do missionary work for the Master, claiming the promise, "Lo, I am with you alway, even unto the end of the world." Matthew 28:20.—*Special Testimonies,* Series B, No. 8, pp. 13, 14 (1907).

Sanitariums and Gospel Work

Our sanitariums are one of the most successful means of reaching all classes of people. Christ is no longer in this world in person, to go through our cities and towns and villages healing the sick. He has commissioned us to carry forward the medical missionary work that He began, and in this work we are to do our very best. Institutions for the care of the sick are to be established, where men and women may be placed under the care of God-fearing medical missionaries and be treated without drugs. To these institutions will come those who have brought disease on themselves by improper habits of eating and drinking. These are to be taught the principles of healthful living. They are to be taught the value of self-denial and self-restraint. They are to be provided with a simple, wholesome, palatable diet and are to be cared for by wise physicians and nurses.

Our sanitariums are the right hand of the gospel, opening doors whereby suffering humanity may be reached with the glad tidings of healing through Christ. In these institutions the sick may be taught to commit their cases to the Great Physician, who will co-operate with their earnest efforts to regain health, bringing to them healing of soul as well as healing of body.

There is most precious missionary work to be done in our sanitariums. In them Christ and the angels work to relieve suffering caused by bodily disease. And the work is by no means to stop there. The prayers offered for the sick and the opening of the Scriptures to them give them a knowledge of the great Medical Missionary. Their attention is called to Him as the One who can heal all

Review and Herald, March 23, 1906.

disease. They learn about the great gift of eternal life, which the Lord Jesus is longing to bestow on those who receive Him. They learn how to prepare for the mansions that Christ has gone to prepare for those that love Him. If I go away, He said, "I will come again, and receive you unto Myself; that where I am, there ye may be also." John 14:3. In the word of God there are gracious promises, from which those who are suffering, whether in body or in mind, may receive comfort and hope and encouragement.

The plan to provide institutions for the proper care of the sick originated with the Lord. He has instructed His people that these institutions should be established. With them are to be connected intelligent, God-fearing physicians, who know how to treat the sick from the standpoint of the skillful Christian physician. These physicians are to be earnest and active, serving the Lord in their activity. They are to remember that they are working in the place and under the oversight of the Great Physician. They stand as guardians of the beings that Christ has purchased with His own blood, and it is therefore essential that they be governed by high, noble principles, carrying out the will of the divine Medical Missionary, who is ever watching over the sick and suffering.

He who is set as a guardian of the health of the sick should understand by experience the soothing power of the grace of Christ, so that to those who come to him for treatment he can impart in words the uplifting, health-giving power of God's own truth. A physician is not fit for medical missionary work until he has gained a knowledge of Him who came to save perishing, sin-sick souls. If Christ is his teacher, if he has an experimental knowledge of the truth, he can hold up the Saviour before the sick and dying.

The sick note carefully the looks and words and acts of their physician, and as the Christian physician kneels beside the bedside of the sufferer, asking the Great Physician to take the case into His own hands, an impression is made upon the mind of the sick one that may result in the saving of his soul.

Plants Needed in Many Places

Christ embraced the world in His missionary work, and the Lord has shown me by revelation that it is not His plan for large centers to be made, for large institutions to be established, and for the funds of our people in all parts of the world to be exhausted in the support of a few large institutions, when the necessities of the times call for something to be done, as Providence opens the way, in many places. Plants should be established in various places all over the world. First one, and then another part of the vineyard is to be entered, until all has been cultivated. Efforts are to be put forth wherever the need is greatest. But we cannot carry on this aggressive warfare and at the same time make an extravagant outlay of means in a few places.

The Battle Creek Sanitarium is too large. A great many workers will be required to care for the patients who come. A tenth of the number of patients who come to that institution is as many as can be cared for with the best results in one medical missionary center. Centers should be made in all the cities that are unacquainted with the great work that the Lord would have done to warn the world that the end of all things is at hand. "There is too much," said the Great Teacher, "in one place."—*Testimonies for the Church,* vol. 8, pp. 204, 205 (1903).

In All the World

God has qualified His people to enlighten the world. He has entrusted them with faculties by which they are to extend His work until it shall encircle the globe. In all parts of the earth they are to establish sanitariums, schools, publishing houses, and kindred facilities for the accomplishment of His work.

The closing message of the gospel is to be carried to "every nation, and kindred, and tongue, and people." Revelation 14:6. In foreign countries many enterprises for the advancement of this message must yet be begun and carried forward. The opening of hygienic restaurants and treatment rooms, and the establishment of sanitariums for the care of the sick and the suffering, is just as necessary in Europe as in America. In many lands medical missions are to be established to act as God's helping hand in ministering to the afflicted.

Christ co-operates with those who engage in medical missionary work. Men and women who unselfishly do what they can to establish sanitariums and treatment rooms in many lands will be richly rewarded. Those who visit these institutions will be benefited physically, mentally, and spiritually—the weary will be refreshed, the sick restored to health, the sin-burdened relieved. In far-off countries, from those whose hearts are by these agencies turned from the service of sin unto righteousness, will be heard thanksgiving and the voice of melody. By their songs of grateful praise a testimony will be borne that will win others to allegiance and to fellowship with Christ.

The conversion of souls to God is the greatest, the noblest work in which human beings can have a part.

Testimonies for the Church, vol. 7, pp. 51-60 (1902).

In this work are revealed God's power, His holiness, His forbearance, and His unbounded love. Every true conversion glorifies Him and causes the angels to break forth into singing.

We are nearing the end of this earth's history, and the different lines of God's work are to be carried forward with much more self-sacrifice than is at present manifest. The work for these last days is in a special sense a missionary work. The presentation of present truth, from the first letter of its alphabet to the last, means missionary effort. The work to be done calls for sacrifice at every advance step. From this unselfish service the workers will come forth purified and refined as gold tried in the fire.

The sight of souls perishing in sin should arouse us to put forth greater effort to give the light of present truth to those who are in darkness, and especially to those in fields where as yet very little has been done to establish memorials for God. In all parts of the world a work that should have been done long ago is now to be entered upon and carried forward to completion.

In European Countries

Our brethren generally have not taken the interest that they ought in the establishment of sanitariums in the European countries. In the work in these countries the most perplexing questions will arise, because of the circumstances peculiar to the various fields. But from the light given me, institutions will be established which, though at first small, will, by God's blessing, become larger and stronger.

Our institutions for any land are not to be crowded together in one locality. God never designed that the light of truth should be thus restricted. For a time the

Jewish nation was required to worship at Jerusalem. But Jesus said to the Samaritan woman: "Believe Me, the hour cometh, when ye shall neither in this mountain, nor yet at Jerusalem, worship the Father." "The hour cometh, and now is, when the true worshipers shall worship the Father in spirit and in truth: for the Father seeketh such to worship Him. God is a Spirit: and they that worship Him must worship Him in spirit and in truth." John 4:21, 23, 24. Truth is to be planted in every place to which we can possibly gain access. It is to be carried to regions that are barren of the knowledge of God. Men will be blessed in receiving the One in whom their hopes of eternal life are centered. The acceptance of the truth as it is in Jesus will fill their hearts with melody to God.

To absorb a large amount of means in a few places is contrary to Christian principles. Every building is to be erected with reference to the need for similar buildings in other places. God calls upon men in positions of trust in His work not to block the way of advance by selfishly using in a few favored places, or in one or two lines of work, all the means that can be secured.

In the early days of the message, very many of our people possessed the spirit of self-denial and self-sacrifice. Thus a right beginning was made, and success attended the efforts put forth. But the work has not developed as it should have developed. Too much has been centered in Battle Creek and in Oakland and in a few other places. Our brethren should never have built so largely in any one place as they have in Battle Creek.

The Lord has signified that His work should be carried forward in the same spirit in which it was begun. The world is to be warned. Field after field is to be entered. The command given us is, "Add new territory."

Shall we not as a people, by our business arrangements, by our attitude toward a world unsaved, bear a testimony even more clear and decisive than that borne by us twenty or thirty years ago?

Upon us has shone great light in regard to the last days of this earth's history. Let not our lack of wisdom and energy give evidence of spiritual blindness. God's messengers must be clothed with power. They must have for the truth an elevating reverence that they do not now possess. The Lord's solemn, sacred message of warning must be proclaimed in the most difficult fields and in the most sinful cities—in every place where the light of the third angel's message has not yet dawned. To everyone is to be given the last call to the marriage supper of the Lamb.

In proclaiming the message, God's servants will be called upon to wrestle with numerous perplexities and to surmount many obstacles. Sometimes the work will go hard, as it did when the pioneers were establishing the institutions in Battle Creek, in Oakland, and in other places. But let all do their best, making the Lord their strength, avoiding all selfishness, and blessing others by their good works. . . .

In All Lands

The Lord is calling upon us to awake to a realization of our responsibilities. God has given to every man his work. Each one may live a life of usefulness. Let us learn all that we can and then be a blessing to others by imparting a knowledge of truth. Let every one do according to his several ability, willingly helping to bear the burdens.

Everywhere there is a work to be done for all classes of society. We are to come close to the poor and depraved, those who have fallen through intemperance. And, at the same time, we are not to forget the higher classes—the lawyers, ministers, senators, and judges, many of whom are slaves to intemperate habits. We are to leave no effort untried to show them that their souls are worth saving, that eternal life is worth striving for. To those in high positions we are to present the total-abstinence pledge, asking them to give the money they would otherwise spend for the harmful indulgences of liquor and tobacco to the establishment of institutions where children and youth may be prepared to fill positions of usefulness in the world.

Angels Waiting to Co-operate

Great light has been shining upon us, but how little of this light we reflect to the world? Heavenly angels are waiting for human beings to co-operate with them in the practical carrying out of the principles of truth. It is through the agency of our sanitariums and kindred enterprises that much of this work is to be done. These institutions are to be God's memorials, where His healing power can reach all classes, high and low, rich and poor. Every dollar invested in them for Christ's sake will bring blessings both to the giver and to suffering humanity.

Medical missionary work is the right hand of the gospel. It is necessary to the advancement of the cause of God. As through it men and women are led to see the importance of right habits of living, the saving power of the truth will be made known. Every city is to be entered by workers trained to do medical missionary work. As the right hand of the third angel's message, God's methods of treating disease will open doors for the entrance of present truth. Health literature must be circulated in many lands. Our physicians in Europe and other countries should awake to the necessity of having health works prepared by men who are on the ground and who can meet the people where they are with the most essential instruction.

Co-operation of Sanitariums

The Lord will give to our sanitariums whose work is already established an opportunity to co-operate with Him in assisting newly established plants. Every new institution is to be regarded as a sister helper in the great work of proclaiming the third angel's message. God has given our sanitariums an opportunity to set in operation a work that will be as a stone instinct with life, growing as it is rolled by an invisible hand. Let this mystic stone be set in motion.

The Lord has instructed me to warn those who in the future establish sanitariums in new places, to begin their work in humility, consecrating their abilities to His service. The buildings erected are not to be large or expensive. Small local sanitariums are to be established in connection with our training schools. In these sanitariums young men and young women of ability and consecration are to be gathered—those who will conduct themselves in the love and fear of God, those who, when prepared for graduation, will not feel that they know all that they need to know, but will diligently study and carefully practice the lessons given by Christ. The righteousness of Christ will go before such ones, and the glory of God will be their rearward.

The Sydney Sanitarium to Be Educational

The Lord has repeatedly given instruction regarding the importance of this institution and the necessity for its establishment. He desires the sanitarium to be built that we may co-operate with His instrumentalities in relieving the sufferings of humanity.

In the work in the sanitarium, physicians, matron, and nurses are to co-operate with God in restoring the sick to health. In doing this, they co-operate with Him in restoring His image in the soul. Let us not limit the Holy One of Israel. Is not Christ officiating for us in the sanctuary above, at the right hand of God? Is He not making intercession for those who are suffering physically and those who are suffering spiritually? He invites them to come to Him who was dead, but is alive forevermore.

God desires suffering human beings to be taught how to avoid sickness by the practice of correct habits of eating, drinking, and dressing. Many are suffering under the oppressive power of sinful practices, who might be restored to health by an intelligent observance of the laws of life and health, by co-operating with Him who died that they might have eternal life. This is the knowledge that men and women need. They need to be taught how to study the divine laws given by Christ for the good of all mankind. This is the work that is to be done in our sanitarium.

God's instrumentalities should seek to follow in the footsteps of the divine Healer. Those who come to the sanitarium should be taught how to take care of the body, remembering the words, "Ye are not your own; for ye are bought with a price: therefore glorify God in your

---

A Systematic Offering for the Sydney Sanitarium, pages 3-6 (1899).

body, and in your spirit, which are God's." 1 Corinthians
6:19, 20. Yes, we are God's property, and the path of
obedience to nature's laws is the direct path to heaven.
He who is converted from errors in eating, drinking, and
dressing is being prepared to hear and receive the truth
into a good and willing heart. Many, by practicing the
laws of nature and by receiving the renovating grace of
God into the soul, obtain a new lease of physical and spiritual life. "The fear of the Lord is the beginning of wisdom." Proverbs 9:10. Let wisdom's voice be heard, for
"her ways are ways of pleasantness, and all her paths are
peace." Proverbs 3:17. . . .

The Glory of the Gospel

It is the glory of the gospel that it is founded upon
the principle of restoring in the fallen race the divine
image by a constant manifestation of benevolence. This
work began in the heavenly courts. There God decided
to give human beings unmistakable evidence of the love
with which He regarded them. He "so loved the world,
that He gave His only-begotten Son, that whosoever believeth in Him should not perish, but have everlasting
life." John 3:16.

The Godhead was stirred with pity for the race, and
the Father, the Son, and the Holy Spirit gave Themselves
to the working out of the plan of redemption. In order
fully to carry out this plan, it was decided that Christ, the
only-begotten Son of God, should give Himself an offering for sin. What line can measure the depth of this love?
God would make it impossible for man to say that He
could have done more. With Christ He gave all the resources of heaven, that nothing might be wanting in the
plan for man's uplifting. Here is love—the contemplation

of which should fill the soul with inexpressible gratitude! Oh, what love, what matchless love! The contemplation of this love will cleanse the soul from all selfishness. It will lead the disciple to deny self, take up the cross, and follow the Redeemer.

All Should Have a Part

The establishment of churches and sanitariums is only a further manifestation of the love of God, and in this work all God's people should have a part. Christ formed His church here below for the express purpose of showing forth through the members the grace of God. Throughout the world His people are to raise memorials of His Sabbath—the sign between Him and them that He is the One who sanctifies them. Thus they are to show that they have returned to their loyalty and stand firmly for the principles of His law.

Agricultural Advantages

The Lord permitted fire to consume the principal buildings of the Review and Herald and the sanitarium, and thus removed the greatest objection urged against moving out of Battle Creek. It was His design that instead of rebuilding the one large sanitarium, our people should make plants in several places. These smaller sanitariums should have been established where land could be secured for agricultural purposes. It is God's plan that agriculture shall be connected with the work of our sanitariums and schools. Our youth need the education to be gained from this line of work. It is well, and more than well,—it is essential,—that efforts be made to carry out the Lord's plan in this respect.—*Testimonies for the Church*, vol. 8, pp. 227, 228 (1903).

A Warning Against Centralization

Saint Helena, California, Sept. 4, 1902.

To the Leaders in Our Medical Work—

DEAR BRETHREN: The Lord is working impartially for every part of His vineyard. It is men who disorganize His work. He does not give to His people the privilege of gathering in so much means to establish institutions in a few places, that nothing will be left for the establishment of similar institutions in other places.

Many plants are to be established in the cities of America, and especially in the Southern cities, where as yet little has been done. And in foreign lands many medical missionary enterprises are to be started, and carried forward to success. The establishment of sanitariums is as essential in Europe, and other foreign countries, as in America.

The Lord desires His people to have a right understanding of the work to be done, and, as faithful stewards, to move forward wisely in the investment of means. In the erection of buildings, He desires them to count the cost to see whether they have enough with which to finish. He also desires them to remember that they should not selfishly gather all the means possible to invest in a few places, but that they should work with reference to the many other places where institutions must be established.

Economy and Benevolence

From the light given me, the managers of all our institutions, and especially of newly established sanitariums, are to be careful to economize in the expenditure of means, that they may be in a position to help similar institutions

---

Testimonies for the Church, vol. 7, pp. 99-102 (1902).

that are to be established in other parts of the world. Even if they have a large amount of money in the treasury, they should make every plan with reference to the needs of God's great missionary field.

It is not the Lord's will for His people to erect mammoth sanitariums anywhere. Many sanitariums are to be established. They are not to be large, but sufficiently complete to do a good and successful work.

Cautions have been given me in reference to the work of training nurses and medical missionary evangelists. We are not to centralize this work in any one place. In every sanitarium established, young men and young women should be trained to be medical missionaries. The Lord will open the way before them as they go forth to work for Him.

The evidences before us of the fulfillment of prophecy declare that the end of all things is at hand. Much important work is to be done out of and away from the places where in the past our work has been largely centered.

When we bring a stream of water into a garden to irrigate it, we do not provide for the watering of one place only, leaving the other parts dry and barren, to cry, "Give us water." And yet this represents the way in which the work has been carried forward in a few places, to the neglect of the great field. Shall the desolate places remain desolate? No. Let the stream flow through every place, carrying with it gladness and fertility.

Lowliness and Unselfishness

Never are we to rely upon worldly recognition and rank. Never are we, in the establishment of institutions, to try to compete with worldly institutions in size or splendor. We shall gain the victory, not by erecting massive buildings, in rivalry with our enemies, but by cherishing a Christlike spirit—a spirit of meekness and lowliness. Better far the cross and disappointed hopes, with eternal life at last, than to live with princes and forfeit heaven.

The Saviour of mankind was born of humble parentage, in a sin-cursed, wicked world. He was brought up in obscurity at Nazareth, a small town in Galilee. He began His work in poverty and without worldly rank. Thus God introduced the gospel, in a way altogether different from the way in which many in our day deem it wise to proclaim the same gospel.

At the very beginning of the gospel dispensation He taught His church to rely, not on worldly rank and splendor, but on the power of faith and obedience. The favor of God is of greater value than gold and silver. The power of His Spirit is of inestimable worth.

Thus saith the Lord: "Buildings will give character to My work only when those who erect them follow My instruction in regard to the establishment of institutions. Had those who have managed and sustained the work in the past always been controlled by pure, unselfish principles, there never would have been the selfish gathering of a large share of My means into one or two places. Institutions would have been established in many localities. The seeds of truth, sown in many more fields, would have sprung up and borne fruit to My glory.

"Places that have been neglected are now to receive attention. My people are to do a sharp, quick work. Those who with purity of purpose fully consecrate themselves to Me, body, soul, and spirit, shall work in My way and in My name. Everyone shall stand in his lot, looking to Me, his Guide and Counselor.

"I will instruct the ignorant and anoint with heavenly eyesalve the eyes of many who are now in spiritual darkness. I will raise up agents who will carry out My will to prepare a people to stand before Me in the time of the end. In many places that before this ought to have been provided with sanitariums and schools, I will establish My institutions, and these institutions will become educational centers for the training of workers."

Providential Opportunities

The Lord will work upon human minds in unexpected quarters. Some who apparently are enemies of the truth will, in God's providence, invest their means to develop properties and erect buildings. In time, these properties will be offered for sale at a price far below their cost. Our people will recognize the hand of Providence in these offers and will secure valuable property for use in educational work. They will plan and manage with humility, self-denial, and self-sacrifice. Thus men of means are unconsciously preparing auxiliaries that will enable the Lord's people to advance His work rapidly.

In various places, properties are to be purchased to be used for sanitarium purposes. Our people should be looking for opportunities to purchase properties away from the cities, on which are buildings already erected and orchards already in bearing. Land is a valuable possession. Connected with our sanitariums there should be lands, small portions of which can be used for the homes of the helpers and others who are receiving a training for medical missionary work.

Duty to the Poor

The managers of the sanitarium should not be governed by the principles which control other institutions of this kind, in which the leaders, acting from policy, too often pay deference to the wealthy, while the poor are neglected. The latter are frequently in great need of sympathy and counsel, which they do not always receive, although for moral worth they may stand far higher in the estimation of God than the more wealthy. The apostle James has given definite counsel with regard to the manner in which we should treat the rich and the poor:

"For if there come unto your assembly a man with a gold ring, in goodly apparel, and there come in also a poor man in vile raiment; and ye have respect to him that weareth the gay clothing, and say unto him, Sit thou here in a good place; and say to the poor, Stand thou there, or sit here under my footstool: are ye not then partial in yourselves, and are become judges of evil thoughts? Hearken, my beloved brethren, Hath not God chosen the poor of this world rich in faith, and heirs of the kingdom which He hath promised to them that love Him?" James 2:2-5.

Although Christ was rich in the heavenly courts, yet He became poor that we through His poverty might be made rich. Jesus honored the poor by sharing their humble condition. From the history of His life we are to learn how to treat the poor. Some carry the duty of beneficence to extremes, and really hurt the needy by doing too much for them. The poor do not always exert themselves as they should. While they are not to be neglected and left to suffer, they must be taught to help themselves.

Testimonies for the Church, vol. 4, pp. 550-552 (1881).

The cause of God should not be overlooked that the poor may receive our first attention. Christ once gave His disciples a very important lesson on this point. When Mary poured the ointment on the head of Jesus, covetous Judas made a plea in behalf of the poor, murmuring at what he considered a waste of money. But Jesus vindicated the act, saying, "Why trouble ye her? she hath wrought a good work on Me." "Wheresoever this gospel shall be preached throughout the whole world, this also that she hath done shall be spoken of for a memorial of her." Mark 14:6, 9. By this we are taught that Christ is to be honored in the consecration of the best of our substance. Should our whole attention be directed to relieving the wants of the poor, God's cause would be neglected. Neither will suffer if His stewards do their duty, but the cause of Christ should come first.

The poor should be treated with as much interest and attention as the rich. The practice of honoring the rich, and slighting and neglecting the poor, is a crime in the sight of God. Those who are surrounded with all the comforts of life, or who are petted and pampered by the world because they are rich, do not feel the need of sympathy and tender consideration as do persons whose lives have been one long struggle with poverty. The latter have but little in this life to make them happy or cheerful, and they will appreciate sympathy and love. Physicians and helpers should in no case neglect this class, for by doing so they may neglect Christ in the person of His saints.

Responsibilities of the Church

Our sanitarium was erected to benefit suffering humanity, rich and poor, the world over. Many of our churches have but little interest in this institution, notwithstanding they have sufficient evidence that it is one of the instrumentalities designed of God to bring men and women under the influence of truth and to save many souls. The churches that have the poor among them should not neglect their stewardship and throw the burden of the poor and sick upon the sanitarium. All the members of the several churches are responsible before God for their afflicted ones. They should bear their own burdens. If they have sick persons among them, whom they wish to be benefited by treatment, they should, if able, send them to the sanitarium. In doing this, they will not only be patronizing the institution which God has established, but will be helping those who need help, caring for the poor as God requires us to do.

It was not the purpose of God that poverty should ever leave the world. The ranks of society were never to be equalized; for the diversity of conditions which characterizes our race is one of the means by which God has designed to prove and develop character. Many have urged with great enthusiasm that all men should have an equal share in the temporal blessings of God; but this was not the purpose of the Creator. Christ has said that we shall have the poor always with us. The poor, as well as the rich, are the purchase of His blood; and among His professed followers, in most cases, the former serve Him with singleness of purpose, while the latter are constantly fastening their affections on their earthly treasures, and Christ is forgotten. The cares of this life and the greed for riches eclipse the glory of the eternal world. It would be the greatest misfortune that has ever befallen mankind if all were to be placed upon an equality in worldly possessions.

Our Southern California Sanitariums

Physicians and ministers are to unite in an effort to lead men and women to obey God's commandments. They need to study the intimate relationship existing between obedience and health. Solemn is the responsibility resting upon medical missionaries. They are to be missionaries in the true sense of the term. The sick and the suffering who entrust themselves to the care of the helpers in our medical institutions must not be disappointed. They are to be taught how to live in harmony with heaven. As they learn to obey God's law, they will be richly blessed in body and in spirit.

Value of Outdoor Life

The advantage of outdoor life must never be lost sight of. How thankful we should be that God has given us beautiful sanitarium properties at Paradise Valley and Glendale and Loma Linda! "Out of the cities! out of the cities!"—this has been my message for years. We cannot expect the sick to recover rapidly when they are shut in within four walls, in some city, with no outside view but houses, houses, houses—nothing to animate, nothing to enliven. And yet how slow some are to realize that the crowded cities are not favorable places for sanitarium work!

Even in Southern California not many years ago, there were some who favored the erection of a large sanitarium building in the heart of Los Angeles. In the light of the instruction God had given, we could not consent to the carrying out of any such plan. In the visions of the night the Lord had shown me unoccupied properties in the

Review and Herald, June 21, 1906.

country, suitable for sanitarium purposes, and for sale at a price far below the original cost.

Finding Suitable Places

It was some time before we found these places. First, we secured the Paradise Valley Sanitarium, near San Diego. A few months later, in the good providence of God, the Glendale property came to the notice of our people and was purchased and fitted up for service. But light came that our work of establishing sanitariums in Southern California was not complete, and on several different occasions testimonies were given that medical missionary work must be done somewhere in the vicinity of Redlands.

In an article published in the *Review* of April 6, 1905, I wrote:

"On our way back to Redlands, as our train passed through miles of orange groves, I thought of the efforts that should be made in this beautiful valley to proclaim the truth for this time. I recognized this section of Southern California as one of the places that had been presented to me with the word that it should have a fully equipped sanitarium.

"Why have such fields as Redlands and Riverside been left almost unworked? As I looked from the car window and saw the trees laden with fruit, I thought, Would not earnest, Christlike efforts have brought forth just as abundant a harvest in spiritual lines? In a few years these towns have been built up and developed, and as I looked upon their beauty and the fertility of the country surrounding them, there rose before me a vision of what the spiritual harvest might have been had earnest, Christlike efforts been put forth for the salvation of souls.

"The Lord would have brave, earnest men and women take up His work in these places. The cause of God is to make more rapid advancement in Southern California than it has in the past. Every year thousands of people visit Southern California in search of health, and by various methods we should seek to reach them with the truth. They must hear the warning to prepare for the great day of the Lord, which is right upon us. . . .

"We are called upon by God to present the truth for this time to those who year by year come to Southern California from all parts of America. Workers who can speak to the multitudes are to be located where they can meet the people and give them the warning message. Ministers and canvassers should be on the ground, watching their opportunity to present the truth and to hold meetings. Let them be quick to seize opportunities to place present truth before those who know it not. Let them give the message with clearness and power, that those who have ears to hear may hear." . . .

Let us remember that one most important agency is our medical missionary work. Never are we to lose sight of the great object for which our sanitariums are established—the advancement of God's closing work in the earth.

Loma Linda is to be not only a sanitarium, but an educational center. With the possession of this place comes the weighty responsibility of making the work of the institution educational in character. A school is to be established here for the training of gospel medical missionary evangelists.

The Sabbath in Our Sanitariums

I have been instructed that our medical institutions are to stand as witnesses for God. They are established to relieve the sick and the afflicted, to awaken a spirit of inquiry, to disseminate light, and to advance reform. These institutions, rightly conducted, will be the means of bringing a knowledge of the reforms essential to prepare a people for the coming of the Lord, before many that otherwise it would be impossible for us to reach.

Many of the patrons of our medical institutions have high ideas in regard to the presence of God abiding in the institution they visit, and they are very susceptible to the spiritual influences that prevail. If all the physicians, nurses, and helpers are walking circumspectly before God, they have more than human power in dealing with these men and women. Every institution whose helpers are consecrated is pervaded by divine power; and the patrons not only obtain relief from bodily infirmities, but find a healing balm for their sin-sick souls.

Let the leaders among our people emphasize the necessity of a strong religious influence being maintained in our medical institutions. The Lord designs that these shall be places where He will be honored in word and in deed, places where His law will be magnified and the truths of the Bible made prominent. Medical missionaries are to do a great work for God. They are to be wide-awake and vigilant, having on every piece of the Christian armor, and fighting manfully. They are to be loyal to their Leader, obeying His commandments, including the one by which they reveal the sign of their order.

Testimonies for the Church, vol. 7, pp. 104-109 (1902).

The Sign of Our Order

The observance of the Sabbath is the sign between God and His people. Let us not be ashamed to bear the sign that distinguishes us from the world. As I considered this matter in the night season recently, One of authority counseled us to study the instruction given the Israelites in regard to the Sabbath. "Verily My Sabbaths ye shall keep," the Lord declared to them; "for it is a *sign* between Me and you throughout your generations; that ye may know that I am the Lord that doth sanctify you. Ye shall keep the Sabbath therefore; for it is holy unto you. . . . Six days may work be done; but in the seventh is the Sabbath of rest, holy to the Lord: whosoever doeth any work in the Sabbath day, he shall surely be put to death. Wherefore the children of Israel shall keep the Sabbath, to observe the Sabbath throughout their generations, for a perpetual covenant. It is a *sign* between Me and the children of Israel forever." Exodus 31:13-17.

The Sabbath is ever the sign that distinguishes the obedient from the disobedient. With masterly power Satan has worked to make null and void the fourth commandment, that the sign of God may be lost sight of. The Christian world have trodden underfoot the Sabbath of the Lord and observe a sabbath instituted by the enemy. But God has a people who are loyal to Him. His work is to be carried forward in right lines. The people who bear His sign are to establish churches and institutions as memorials to Him. These memorials, however humble in appearance, will constantly bear witness against the false sabbath instituted by Satan, and in favor of the Sabbath instituted by the Lord in Eden, when the morning stars sang together and all the sons of God shouted for joy.

A spirit of irreverence and carelessness in the observance of the Sabbath is liable to come into our sanitariums. Upon the men of responsibility in the medical missionary work rests the duty of giving instruction to physicians, nurses, and helpers in regard to the sanctity of God's holy day. Especially should every physician endeavor to set a right example. The nature of his duties naturally leads him to feel justified in doing on the Sabbath many things that he should refrain from doing. So far as possible, he should so plan his work that he can lay aside his ordinary duties.

The Suffering Never to Be Neglected

Often physicians and nurses are called upon during the Sabbath to minister to the sick, and sometimes it is impossible for them to take time for rest and for attending devotional services. The needs of suffering humanity are never to be neglected. The Saviour by His example has shown us that it is right to relieve suffering on the Sabbath. But unnecessary work, such as ordinary treatments and operations that can be postponed, should be deferred. Let the patients understand that physicians and helpers should have one day for rest. Let them understand that the workers fear God and desire to keep holy the day that He has set apart for His followers to observe as a sign between Him and them.

The educators and those being educated in our medical institutions should remember that to keep the Sabbath aright means much to them and to the patrons. In keeping the Sabbath, which God declares shall be kept holy, they give the sign of their order, showing plainly that they are on the Lord's side.

Free From Worldly Entanglements

Now and ever we are to stand as a distinct and peculiar people, free from all worldly policy, unembarrassed by confederating with those who have not wisdom to discern God's claims so plainly set forth in His law. All our medical institutions are established as Seventh-day Adventist institutions, to represent the various features of gospel medical missionary work, and thus to prepare the way for the coming of the Lord. We are to show that we are seeking to work in harmony with Heaven. We are to bear witness to all nations, kindreds, and tongues that we are a people who love and fear God, a people who keep holy His memorial of creation, the sign between Him and His obedient children that He sanctifies them. And we are plainly to show our faith in the soon coming of our Lord in the clouds of heaven.

As a people we have been greatly humiliated by the course that some of our brethren in responsible positions have taken in departing from the old landmarks. There are those who, in order to carry out their plans, have by their words denied their faith. This shows how little dependence can be placed on human wisdom and human judgment. Now, as never before, we need to see the danger of being led unguardedly away from loyalty to God's commandments. We need to realize that God has given us a decided message of warning for the world, even as He gave Noah a message of warning for the antediluvians. Let our people beware of belittling the importance of the Sabbath, in order to link up with unbelievers. Let them beware of departing from the principles of our faith, making it appear that it is not wrong to conform to the world. Let them be afraid of heeding the counsel of any man, whatever his position may be, who works counter to that which God has wrought in order to keep His people separate from the world.

The Lord is testing His people to see who will be loyal to the principles of His truth. Our work is to proclaim to the world the first, second, and third angels' messages. In the discharge of our duties we are neither to despise nor to fear our enemies. To bind ourselves up by contracts with those not of our faith is not in the order of God. We are to treat with kindness and courtesy those who refuse to be loyal to God, but we are never, never to unite with them in counsel regarding the vital interests of His work. Putting our trust in God, we are to move steadily forward, doing His work with unselfishness, in humble dependence upon Him, committing to His providence ourselves and all that concerns our present and future, holding the beginning of our confidence firm unto the end, remembering that we receive the blessings of Heaven, not because of our worthiness, but because of Christ's worthiness and our acceptance, through faith in Him, of God's abounding grace.

Called to Be a Holy People

I pray that my brethren may realize that the third angel's message means much to us, and that the observance of the true Sabbath is to be the sign that distinguishes those who serve God from those who serve Him not. Let those who have become sleepy and indifferent awake. We are called to be holy, and we should carefully avoid giving the impression that it is of little consequence whether or not we retain the peculiar features of our faith. Upon us rests the solemn obligation of taking a more decided stand for truth and righteousness than we have taken in the past. The line of demarcation between those who keep the commandments of God and those who do not is to be revealed with unmistakable clearness. We are conscientiously to honor God, diligently using every means of keeping in covenant relation with Him, that we may receive His blessings—the blessings so essential for the people who are to be so severely tried. To give the impression that our faith, our religion, is not a dominating power in our lives is greatly to dishonor God. Thus we turn from His commandments, which are our life, denying that He is our God and that we are His people.

Mammoth Sanitariums Not a Necessity

I have been repeatedly shown that it is not wise to erect mammoth institutions. It is not by the largeness of an institution that the greatest work for souls is to be accomplished. A mammoth sanitarium requires many workers. And where so many are brought together, it is exceedingly difficult to maintain a high standard of spirituality. In a large institution it often happens that responsible places are filled by workers who are not spiritual-minded, who do not exercise wisdom in dealing with those who, if wisely treated, would be awakened, convicted, and converted.

Not one quarter of the work has been done in opening the Scriptures to the sick that might have been done, and that would have been done, in our sanitariums, if the workers had themselves received thorough instruction in religious lines.

Where many workers are gathered together in one place, management of a much higher spiritual tone is required than has been maintained in our large sanitariums. —*Testimonies for the Church,* vol. 7, pp. 102, 103 (1902).

Amusements in Our Sanitariums

Those who bear the responsibility at the sanitarium should be exceedingly guarded that the amusements shall not be of a character to lower the standard of Christianity, bringing this institution down upon a level with others and weakening the power of true godliness in the minds of those who are connected with it. Worldly or theatrical entertainments are not essential for the prosperity of the sanitarium or for the health of the patients. The more they have of this kind of amusements, the less will they be pleased unless something of the kind shall be continually carried on. The mind is in a fever of unrest for something new and exciting, the very thing it ought not to have. And if these amusements are once allowed, they are expected again, and the patients lose their relish for any simple arrangement to occupy the time. But repose, rather than excitement, is what many of the patients need.

As soon as these entertainments are introduced, the objections to theatergoing are removed from many minds, and the plea that moral and high-toned scenes are to be acted at the theater breaks down the last barrier. Those who would permit this class of amusements at the sanitarium would better be seeking wisdom from God to lead these poor, hungry, thirsting souls to the Fountain of joy and peace and happiness.

When there has been a departure from the right path, it is difficult to return. Barriers have been removed, safeguards broken down. One step in the wrong direction prepares the way for another. A single glass of wine may open the door of temptation which will lead to habits of drunkenness. A single vindictive feeling indulged may open the way to a train of feelings which will end in murder. The least deviation from right and principle will lead to separation from God and may end in apostasy. . . . It takes less time and labor to corrupt our ways before God than to ingraft upon the character habits of righteousness and truth. Whatever a man becomes accustomed to, be its influence good or evil, he finds it difficult to abandon.

The managers of the sanitarium may as well conclude at once that they will never be able to satisfy that class of minds that can find happiness only in something new and exciting. To many persons this has been the intellectual diet during their lifetime; there are mental as well as physical dyspeptics. Many are suffering from maladies of the soul far more than from diseases of the body, and they will find no relief until they shall come to Christ, the wellspring of life. Complaints of weariness, loneliness, and dissatisfaction will then cease. Satisfying joys will give vigor to the mind and health and vital energy to the body.

If physicians and workers flatter themselves that they are to find a panacea for the varied ills of their patients by supplying them with a round of amusements similar to those which have been the curse of their lives, they will be disappointed. Let not these entertainments be placed in the position which the living Fountain should occupy. The hungry, thirsty soul will continue to hunger and thirst as long as it partakes of these unsatisfying pleasures. But those who drink of the living water will thirst no more for frivolous, sensual, exciting amusements. The ennobling principles of religion will strengthen the mental powers and will destroy a taste for these gratifications.

Encourage One Another

In the building of our sanitariums we must guard carefully against any unnecessary extravagance in our outlay of means. It is our duty to study simplicity. Yet there are a few places of special importance and influence where better accommodations and more room are needed than for sanitarium work in other places. The impression that we desire to be left upon the minds of the patients is that of the truths we teach rather than of the grandeur of the buildings.

We have none too many sanitariums. There is in our world a great field for true medical missionary work. Our sanitariums are to be as lights shining amid the moral darkness. In them the sick and suffering are to behold the miracle-working power of Christ as revealed in the lives of the workers. "Let your light so shine before men," says Christ, "that they may see your good works, and glorify your Father which is in heaven." Matthew 5:16. Let the lamp of light from the word of God shine forth unmistakably.

Let everything connected with the sanitarium and its surroundings be kept orderly and neat, that the work may stand high in the esteem of the people, and may exert constantly an uplifting influence. . . .

Schools Near Sanitariums

An educational work should be carried on in connection with all our sanitariums. There is a close relation between the work of our schools and our sanitariums, and wherever it is practicable, there are decided advantages in having a school in close connection with a sanitarium.

Review and Herald, August 8, 1907.

There would be in such an arrangement decided advantages to both lines of work.

Speak Words of Encouragement

Let us not discourage one another. Let us take hold unitedly to make every line of the Lord's work a success. If someone comes to you and talks discouragingly about the work in one or another of our institutions, telling you that they are extravagant beyond measure, say to them, "I am sorry if that is so, but let us help them out if they are in difficulty." If you will speak thus you may avoid much of the evil that might result were you to withdraw your sympathy, and should you refuse to help those who, possibly, may have been misrepresented. Let us never discourage even those who have done wrong, by treating them as if they had committed against us an unpardonable sin. Let us rather encourage them in every way possible, and if we see that they are lifting hard in a worthy enterprise, let us lift with them. . . .

We need to be instant in prayer. It is our great privilege to hang our helpless souls upon Jesus Christ, and to rest for our salvation upon His merits. Let us speak words that will elevate and ennoble, and that will make pleasant impressions on the minds of those with whom we converse. The Lord wants us to be sanctified and to walk in humility of mind before Him. If we are obedient to His commandments, not a reproach can fall on us justly. Others may talk about us, they may spread evil reports concerning us, but these reports need not be true.

Christlike Deportment

In our institutions, where many persons of varied temperaments are brought together, it is necessary that each should cultivate a spirit of unselfishness. Let no one feel that it is his place to mold others to his individual mind or opinions. While each will manifest an individuality, yet it should be an individuality that is under the control of the Holy Spirit. If we are kind and Christlike, there will be a blending of hearts and of interests that will be beneficial to all alike.

Our sanitariums are to be agencies for imparting to the sick a health that is maintained in happiness and peace of soul. Every worker is to co-operate with the physician, for by the manifestation of kindness and tenderness he may bring to the suffering ones a healing balm.

Everyone is responsible to God for the use he makes of his abilities. He is responsible for making a daily growth in grace. Let no one feel, even though he may theoretically be established in the present truth, that he makes no mistakes. But if mistakes are made, let there be a readiness to correct them. And let us avoid everything that is likely to create dissension and strife, for there is a heaven before us, and among its inhabitants there will be no strife.

We are to live, not to elevate ourselves, but that we may, as God's little children, do to the very best of our ability the work that He has committed to us. It is our business to give a right impression to others. We are preparing for eternity, for the sanitarium above, where the Great Physician shall wipe away the tears from every eye, and where the leaves of the tree of life are for the healing of the nation.

Denominational Views Not to Be Urged Upon Patients

The religion of Christ is not to be placed in the background and its holy principles laid down to meet the approval of any class, however popular. If the standard of truth and holiness is lowered, the design of God will not then be carried out in this institution.

But our peculiar faith should not be discussed with patients. Their minds should not be unnecessarily excited upon subjects wherein we differ, unless they themselves desire it; and then great caution should be observed not to agitate the mind by urging upon them our peculiar faith. The Health Institute[1] is not the place to be forward to enter into discussion upon points of our faith wherein we differ with the religious world generally. Prayer meetings are held at the Institute, in which all may take part if they choose; but there is an abundance to dwell upon in regard to Bible religion without touching objectionable points of difference. Silent influence will do more than open controversy.

In exhortation in the prayer meetings, some Sabbath-keepers have felt that they must bring in the Sabbath and the third angel's message, or they could not have freedom. This is characteristic of narrow minds. Patients not acquainted with our faith do not know what is meant by the third angel's message. The introduction of these terms without a clear explanation of them does only harm. We must meet the people where they are, and yet we need not sacrifice one principle of the truth. The prayer meeting will prove a blessing to patients, helpers, and physi-

Testimonies for the Church, vol. 3, pp. 166, 167 (1872).
[1] The name of the Battle Creek Sanitarium in its early days.

cians. Brief and interesting seasons of prayer and social worship will increase the confidence of patients in their physicians and helpers. The helpers should not be deprived of these meetings by work, unless it is positively necessary. They need them and should enjoy them.

By thus establishing regular meetings, the patients gain confidence in the Institute and feel more at home. And thus the way is prepared for the seed of truth to take root in some hearts. These meetings especially interest some who profess to be Christians and make a favorable impression upon those who do not. Mutual confidence is increased in one another, and prejudice is weakened and in many cases entirely removed. Then there is an anxiety to attend the Sabbath meeting. There, in the house of God, is the place to speak our denominational sentiments. There the minister can dwell with clearness upon the essential points of present truth, and with the spirit of Christ, in love and tenderness, urge home upon all the necessity of obedience to all the requirements of God, and let the truth convict hearts.

For All Sects and Classes

We are to invite everyone—the high and the low, the rich and the poor, all sects and classes—to share the benefits of our medical institutions. We receive into our institutions people of all denominations. But as for ourselves, we are strictly denominational; we are sacredly denominated by God and are under His theocracy. But we are not unwisely to press upon anyone the peculiar points of our faith.—*Testimonies for the Church,* vol. 7, p. 109 (1902).

Medical Treatment, Right Living, and Prayer

I saw that the reason why God did not hear the prayers of His servants for the sick among us more fully was that He could not be glorified in so doing while they were violating the laws of health. And I also saw that He designed the health reform and Health Institute to prepare the way for the prayer of faith to be fully answered. Faith and good work should go hand in hand in relieving the afflicted among us, and in fitting them to glorify God here and to be saved at the coming of Christ. God forbid that these afflicted ones should ever be disappointed and grieved in finding the managers of the Institute working only from a worldly standpoint, instead of adding to the hygienic practice the blessings and virtues of nursing fathers and mothers in Israel.

Let no one obtain the idea that the Institute is the place for them to come to be raised up by the prayer of faith. This is the place to find relief from disease by treatment and right habits of living, and to learn how to avoid sickness. But if there is one place under the heavens more than another where soothing, sympathizing prayer should be offered by men and women of devotion and faith, it is at such an institute. Those who treat the sick should move forward in their important work with strong reliance upon God for His blessing to attend the means which He has graciously provided, and to which He has in mercy called our attention as a people, such as pure air, cleanliness, healthful diet, proper periods of labor and repose, and the use of water. They should have no selfish interest outside of this important and solemn work.—*Testimonies for the Church,* vol. 1, p. 561 (1865).

Centers of Influence and Training

The Lord has ordained that sanitariums be established in many places to stand as memorials for Him. This is one of His chosen ways of proclaiming the third angel's message. By this means the truth will reach many who, but for these agencies, would never be lightened by the brightness of the gospel message. In the presentation of truth some will be attracted by one phase of the gospel message and some by another. We are instructed by the Lord to work in such a way that all classes will be reached. The message must go to the whole world. Our sanitarium work is to help make up the number of God's people. Through this line of missionary effort infidels will be converted. By the wonderful restorations taking place in our sanitariums many will be led to look to Christ as the healer of soul and body.

Self-sacrificing workers, who have full faith in God, should be chosen to take charge of these institutions. Wise men and women, acting in the capacity of nurses, are to comfort and help the sick and suffering. Our sanitariums are to be as lights shining in a dark place, because physicians, nurses, and helpers reflect the sunlight of Christ's righteousness. . . .

Sanitariums are to be so established and conducted that they will be educational in character. They are to show to the world the benevolence of Heaven. Though Christ's visible presence is not discerned, yet the workers may claim the promise, "Lo, I am with you alway, even unto the end of the world." Matthew 28:20. He has assured His followers that to those who love and fear Him He will give power to continue the work that He began.

Review and Herald, May 2, 1912.

He went about doing good, teaching the ignorant and healing the sick. His work did not stop with an exhibition of His power over disease. He made each work of healing an occasion of implanting in the heart the divine principles of His love and benevolence. Thus His followers are to work. Christ is no longer in this world in person, but He has commissioned us to carry forward the medical missionary work that He began; and in this work we are to do our very best. For the furtherance of this work institutions for the care of the sick are to be established, where men and women suffering from disease may be placed under the care of God-fearing physicians and nurses.

In our sanitariums truth is to be cherished, not banished nor hidden from sight; and from them the light of present truth is to shine forth in clear, distinct rays. These institutions are the Lord's agencies for the revival of a pure, elevated morality. We do not establish them as a speculative business, but to help men and women to follow right habits of living. Those who are now ignorant are to become wise. Suffering is to be relieved, and health restored. People are to be taught how, by exercising care in their habits, they may keep well. Christ died to save men from ruin. Our sanitariums are to be His helping hand, teaching men and women how to live in such a way as to honor and glorify God. If this work is not carried on in our sanitariums, those who are conducting them will make a great mistake.

The High Calling of Our Sanitarium Workers

The workers in our sanitariums have a high and holy calling. They need to awake to a realization of the sacredness of their work. The character of this work and the extent of its influence call for earnest effort and unreserved consecration.

In our sanitariums the sick and suffering are to be led to realize that they need spiritual help as well as physical restoration. They are to be given every advantage for the restoration of physical health; and they should be shown also what it means to be blessed with the light and life of Christ, what it means to be bound up with Him. They are to be led to see that the grace of Christ in the soul uplifts the whole being. And in no better way can they learn of Christ's life than by seeing it revealed in the lives of His followers.

The faithful worker keeps his eyes fixed on Christ. Remembering that his hope of eternal life is due to the cross of Christ, he is determined never to dishonor Him who gave His life for him. He takes a deep interest in suffering humanity. He prays and works, watching for souls as one that must give an account, knowing that the souls whom God brings in contact with truth and righteousness are worth saving.

Our sanitarium workers are engaged in a holy warfare. To the sick and the afflicted they are to present the truth as it is in Jesus; they are to present it in all its solemnity, yet with such simplicity and tenderness that souls will be drawn to the Saviour. Ever, in word and deed, they are to keep Him uplifted as the hope of eternal life. Not a harsh word is to be spoken, not a selfish act done. The workers are to treat all with kindness. Their words are to be gentle and loving. Those who show true modesty and Christian courtesy will win souls to Christ.

The Atmosphere of Peace

We should strive to restore to physical and spiritual health those who come to our sanitariums. Let us therefore make preparation to draw them for a season away from those surroundings that lead away from God, into a purer atmosphere. Out of doors, surrounded by the beautiful things that God has made, breathing the fresh, health-giving air, the sick can best be told of the new life in Christ. Here God's words can be taught. Here the sunshine of Christ's righteousness can shine into hearts darkened by sin. Patiently, sympathetically, lead the sick to see their need of the Saviour. Tell them that He gives power to the faint, and that to those who have no might He increases strength.

We need to appreciate more fully the meaning of the words, "I sat down under His shadow with great delight." Song of Solomon 2:3. These words do not bring to our minds the picture of hasty transit, but of quiet rest. There are many professing Christians who are anxious and depressed, many who are so full of busy activity that they cannot find time to rest quietly in the promises of God, who act as if they could not afford to have peace and quietness. To all such Christ's invitation is, "Come unto Me, . . . and I will give you rest." Matthew 11:28.

Let us turn from the dusty, heated thoroughfares of life to rest in the shadow of Christ's love. Here we gain strength for conflict. Here we learn how to lessen toil and worry, and how to speak and sing to the praise of

God. Let the weary and the heavy-laden learn from Christ the lesson of quiet trust. They must sit under His shadow if they would be possessors of His peace and rest.

A Treasure House of Experience

Those who engage in sanitarium work should have a treasure house full of rich experience, because the truth is implanted in the heart, and as a holy thing is tended and fed by the grace of God. Rooted and grounded in the truth, they should have a faith that works by love and purifies the soul. Constantly asking for blessings, they should keep the windows of the soul closed earthward against the malarious atmosphere of the world, and opened heavenward to receive the bright beams of the Sun of Righteousness.

Who is preparing to take hold understandingly of medical missionary work? By this work the minds of those who come to our sanitariums for treatment are to be led to Christ and taught to unite their weakness with His strength. Every worker should be understandingly efficient. Then in a high, broad sense he can present the truth as it is in Jesus.

The workers in our sanitariums are continually exposed to temptation. They are brought in contact with unbelievers, and those who are not sound in the faith will be harmed by the contact. But those who are abiding in Christ will meet unbelievers as He met them, refusing to be drawn from their allegiance, but always ready to speak a word in season, always ready to sow the seeds of truth. They will watch unto prayer, firmly maintaining their integrity, and daily showing the consistency of their religion. The influence of such workers is a blessing to many. By a well-ordered life they draw souls to the cross. A true Christian constantly acknowledges Christ. He is always cheerful, always ready to speak words of hope and comfort to the suffering.

"The fear of the Lord is the beginning of knowledge." Proverbs 1:7. One sentence of Scripture is of more value than ten thousand of man's ideas or arguments. Those who refuse to follow God's way will finally receive the sentence, "Depart from Me." But when we submit to God's way, the Lord Jesus guides our minds and fills our lips with assurance. We may be strong in the Lord and in the power of His might. Receiving Christ, we are clothed with power. An indwelling Saviour makes His power our property. The truth becomes our stock in trade. No unrighteousness is seen in the life. We are able to speak words in season to those who know not the truth. Christ's presence in the heart is a vitalizing power, strengthening the entire being.

Self-Sufficiency a Peril

I am instructed to say to our sanitarium workers that unbelief and self-sufficiency are the dangers against which they must constantly guard. They are to carry forward the warfare against evil with such earnestness and devotion that the sick will feel the uplifting influence of their unselfish efforts.

No taint of self-seeking is to mar our service. "Ye cannot serve God and mammon." Matthew 6:24. Lift Him up, the Man of Calvary. Lift Him up by living faith in God, that your prayers may prevail. Do we realize how near Jesus will come to us? He is speaking to us individually. He will reveal Himself to everyone who is willing to be clothed with the robe of His righteousness. He declares, "I the Lord thy God will hold thy right hand."

Isaiah 41:13. Let us place ourselves where He can hold us by the hand, where we can hear Him saying with assurance and authority, "I am He that liveth, and was dead; and, behold, I am alive forevermore." Revelation 1:18.

Wholesome Substitutes

When flesh food is discarded, its place should be supplied with a variety of grains, nuts, vegetables, and fruits, that will be both nourishing and appetizing. This is especially necessary in the case of those who are weak or who are taxed with continuous labor. In some countries, where poverty abounds, flesh is the cheapest food. Under these circumstances the change will be made with greater difficulty; but it can be effected. We should, however, consider the situation of the people and the power of lifelong habit, and should be careful not to urge even right ideas unduly. None should be urged to make the change abruptly. The place of meat should be supplied with wholesome foods that are inexpensive. In this matter very much depends on the cook. With care and skill, dishes may be prepared that will be both nutritious and appetizing, and will, to a great degree, take the place of flesh food. —*The Ministry of Healing,* pages 316, 317 (1905).

SUCCESSFUL INSTITUTIONAL WORK

The Secret of Success

The success of the sanitarium depends upon its maintaining the simplicity of godliness and shunning the world's follies in eating, drinking, dressing, and amusements. It must be reformatory in all its principles. Let nothing be invented to satisfy the wants of the soul and take the room and time which Christ and His service demand, for this will destroy the power of the institution as God's instrumentality to convert poor, sin-sick souls, who, ignorant of the way of life and peace, have sought for happiness in pride and vain folly.

"Standing by a purpose true" should be the position of all connected with the sanitarium. While none should urge our faith upon the patients or engage in religious controversy with them, our papers and publications, carefully selected, should be in sight almost everywhere. The religious element must predominate. This has been and ever will be the power of that institution. Let not our health asylum be perverted to the service of worldliness and fashion. There are hygienic institutions enough in our land that are more like an accommodating hotel than a place where the sick and suffering can obtain relief for their bodily infirmities, and the sin-sick soul can find that peace and rest in Jesus to be found nowhere else. Let religious principles be made prominent and kept so; let pride and popularity be discarded; let simplicity and plainness, kindness and faithfulness, be seen everywhere; then the sanitarium will be just what God intended it should be; then the Lord will favor it.—*Testimonies for the Church*, vol. 4, pp. 586, 587 (1881).

Moral and Intellectual Culture

In the view given me October 9, 1878, I was shown the position which our sanitarium at Battle Creek should occupy, and the character and influence which should be maintained by all connected with it. This important institution has been established by the providence of God, and His blessing is indispensable to its success. The physicians are not quacks nor infidels, but men who understand the human system and the best methods of treating disease, men who fear God and who have an earnest interest for the moral and spiritual welfare of their patients. This interest for spiritual as well as physical good the managers of the institution should make no effort to conceal. By a life of true Christian integrity they can give to the world an example worthy of imitation; and they should not hesitate to let it be seen that in addition to their skill in treating disease, they are continually gaining wisdom and knowledge from Christ, the greatest teacher the world has ever known. They must have this connection with the Source of all wisdom to make their labor successful.

The Power of Truth

Truth has a power to elevate the receiver. If Bible truth exerts its sanctifying influence upon the heart and character, it will make believers more intelligent. A Christian will understand his responsibility to God and to his fellow men, if he is truly connected with the Lamb of God, who gave His life for the world. Only by a continual improvement of the intellectual as well as the moral powers can we hope to answer the purpose of our Creator.

Testimonies for the Church, vol. 4, pp. 545-549 (1878).

Inefficiency Displeasing to God

God is displeased with those who are too careless or indolent to become efficient, well-informed workers. The Christian should possess more intelligence and keener discernment than the worldling. The study of God's word is continually expanding the mind and strengthening the intellect. There is nothing that will so refine and elevate the character and give vigor to every faculty as the continual exercise of the mind to grasp and comprehend weighty and important truths.

The human mind becomes dwarfed and enfeebled when dealing with commonplace matters only, never rising above the level of the things of time and sense to grasp the mysteries of the unseen. The understanding is gradually brought to the level of the subjects with which it is constantly familiar. The mind will contract its powers and lose its ability if it is not exercised to acquire additional knowledge and put to the stretch to comprehend the revelations of divine power in nature and in the Sacred Word.

But an acquaintance with facts and theories, however important they may be in themselves, is of little real value unless put to a practical use. There is danger that those who have obtained their education principally from books will fail to realize that they are novices, so far as experimental knowledge is concerned. This is especially true of those connected with the sanitarium. This institution needs men of thought and ability. The physicians, superintendent, matron, and helpers should be persons of culture and experience. But some fail to comprehend what is needed at such an establishment, and they plod on, year after year, making no marked improvement. They seem to be stereotyped; each succeeding day is but a repetition of the past one.

The minds and hearts of these mechanical workers are impoverished. Opportunities are before them; if studious, they might obtain an education of the highest value, but they do not appreciate their privileges. None should rest satisfied with their present education. All may be daily qualifying themselves to fill some office of trust. ...

Influence of God-Fearing Workers

Intelligent, God-fearing workers can do a vast amount of good in the way of reforming those who come as invalids to be treated at the sanitarium. These persons are diseased, not only physically, but mentally and morally. The education, the habits, and the entire life of many have been erroneous. They cannot in a few days make the great changes necessary for the adoption of correct habits. They must have time to consider the matter and to learn the right way. If all connected with the sanitarium are correct representatives of the truth of health reform and of our holy faith, they are exerting an influence to mold the minds of their patients. The contrast of erroneous habits with those which are in harmony with the truth of God has a convicting power.

Man is not what he might be and what it is God's will that he should be. The strong power of Satan upon the human race keeps them upon a low level; but this need not be so, else Enoch could not have become so elevated and ennobled as to walk with God. Man need not cease to grow intellectually and spiritually during his lifetime. But the minds of many are so occupied with themselves and their own selfish interests as to leave no room for higher and nobler thoughts. And the standard of intellectual as well as spiritual attainments is far too low. With many, the more responsible the position they occupy, the better pleased are they with themselves; and they cherish the idea that the position gives character to the man. Few realize that they have a constant work before them to develop forbearance, sympathy, charity, conscientiousness, and fidelity—traits of character indispensable to those who occupy positions of responsibility. All connected with the sanitarium should have a sacred regard for the rights of others, which is but obeying the principles of the law of God.

Some at this institution are sadly deficient in the qualities so essential to the happiness of all connected with them. The physicians and the helpers in the various branches of the work should carefully guard against a selfish coldness, a distant, unsocial disposition, for this will alienate the affection and confidence of the patients. Many who come to the sanitarium are refined, sensitive people, of ready tact and keen discernment. These persons discover such defects at once and comment upon them. Men cannot love God supremely and their neighbor as themselves and be as cold as icebergs. Not only do they rob God of the love due Him, but they rob their neighbor as well. Love is a plant of heavenly growth and it must be fostered and nourished. Affectionate hearts, truthful, loving words, will make happy families and exert an elevating influence upon all who come within the sphere of their influence.

Those who make the most of their privileges and opportunities will be, in the Bible sense, talented and educated men; not learned merely, but educated, in mind, in manners, in deportment. They will be refined, tender, pitiful, affectionate. . . .

Both Learners and Teachers

We should ever bear in mind that we are not only learners but teachers in this world, fitting ourselves and others for a higher sphere of action in the future life. The measure of man's usefulness is in knowing the will of God and doing it. It is within our power to so improve in mind and manners that God will not be ashamed to own us. There must be a high standard at the sanitarium. If there are men of culture, of intellectual and moral power, to be found in our ranks, they must be called to the front to fill places in our institutions.

The physicians should not be deficient in any respect. A wide field of usefulness is open before them, and if they do not become skillful in their profession they have only themselves to blame. They must be diligent students; and, by close application and faithful attention to details, they should become caretakers. It should be necessary for no one to follow them to see that their work is done without mistakes.

Those who occupy responsible positions should so educate and discipline themselves that all within the sphere of their influence may see what man can be, and what he can do, when connected with the God of wisdom and power. And why should not a man thus privileged become intellectually strong? Again and again have worldlings sneeringly asserted that those who believe present truth are weak-minded, deficient in education, without position or influence. This we know to be untrue; but is there not some reason for these assertions? Many have considered it a mark of humility to be ignorant and uncultivated. Such persons are deceived as to what constitutes true humility and Christian meekness.

Health Reform at the Sanitarium

Among the greatest dangers to our health institutions is the influence of physicians, superintendents, and helpers who profess to believe the present truth, but who have never taken their stand fully upon health reform. Some have no conscientious scruples in regard to their eating, drinking, and dressing. How can the physician or anyone else present the matter as it is when he himself is indulging in the use of harmful things? God's blessing will rest upon every effort made to awaken an interest in health reform, for it is needed everywhere. There must be a revival in regard to this matter, for God purposes to accomplish much through this agency.

Drug medication, as it is generally practiced, is a curse. Educate away from drugs. Use them less and less, and depend more upon hygienic agencies; then nature will respond to God's physicians—pure air, pure water, proper exercise, a clear conscience. Those who persist in the use of tea, coffee, and flesh meats will feel the need of drugs, but many might recover without one grain of medicine if they would obey the laws of health. Drugs need seldom be used.

If the heart is purified through obedience to the truth, there will be no selfish preferences, no corrupt motives; there will be no partiality. Lovesick sentimentalism, whose blighting influence has been felt in all our institutions, will not be developed. Strict guard should be kept that this curse shall not poison or corrupt our health institutions.—*Health, Philanthropic, and Medical Missionary Work*, pages 42, 43 (1890).

Results of Faithful Effort

I saw that there was a large amount of surplus means among our people, a portion of which should be put into the Health Institute. I also saw that there are many worthy poor among our people, who are sick and suffering, and who have been looking toward the Institute for help, but who are not able to pay the regular prices for board, treatment, etc. The Institute has struggled hard with debts the last three years, and could not treat patients, to any considerable extent, without full pay. It would please God for all our people who are able to do so, to take stock liberally in the Institute, to place it in a condition where it can help God's humble, worthy poor. In connection with this, I saw that Christ identifies Himself with suffering humanity, and that what we have the privilege of doing for even the least of His children, whom He calls His brethren, we do to the Son of God. . . .

To raise the Health Institute from its low state in the autumn of 1869 to its present prosperous, hopeful condition has demanded sacrifices and exertions of which its friends abroad know but little. Then it had a debt of thirteen thousand dollars, and had but eight paying patients. And what was worse still, the course of former managers had been such as to so far discourage its friends that they had no heart to furnish means to lift the debt, or to recommend the sick to patronize the Institute. It was at this discouraging point that my husband decided in his mind that the Institute property must be sold to pay the debts, and the balance, after the payment of debts, be refunded to stockholders in proportion to the amount

Testimonies for the Church, vol. 3, pp. 173-176 (1872).

of stock each held. But one morning, in prayer at the family altar, the Spirit of God came upon him as he was praying for divine guidance in matters pertaining to the Institute, and he exclaimed, while bowed upon his knees, "The Lord will vindicate every word He has spoken through vision relative to the Health Institute, and it will be raised from its low estate and prosper gloriously."

From that point of time we took hold of the work in earnest and have labored side by side for the Institute, to counteract the influence of selfish men who had brought embarrassment upon it. We have given of our means, thus setting an example to others. We have encouraged economy and industry on the part of all connected with the Institute and have urged that physicians and helpers work hard for small pay, until the Institute should again be fully established in the confidence of our people. We have borne a plain testimony against the manifestation of selfishness in anyone connected with the Institute and have counseled and reproved wrongs. We knew that the Health Institute would not succeed unless the blessing of the Lord rested upon it. If His blessing attended it, the friends of the cause would have confidence that it was the work of God and would feel safe to donate means to make it a living enterprise, that it might be able to accomplish the design of God.

The physicians and some of the helpers went to work earnestly. They worked hard, under great discouragement. Doctors Ginley, Chamberlain, and Lamson worked with earnestness and energy, for small pay, to build up this sinking institution. And, thank God, the original debt has been removed and large additions for the accommodation of patients have been made and paid for. The circulation of the *Health Reformer,* which lies at the very foundation of the success of the Institute, has been doubled, and it has become a live journal. Confidence in the Institute has been fully restored in the minds of most of our people, and there have been as many patients at the Institute, nearly the year round, as could well be accommodated and properly treated by our physicians.

Maintain a High Standard

It is far easier to allow matters in our important institutions to go in a lax, loose way than to weed out that which is offensive, which will corrupt and destroy confidence and faith. But it would be far better to have a smaller number of workers, to accomplish less, and as far as possible to have these who are engaged in the work truehearted, firm as rock in principle, loving the whole truth, obedient to all the commandments of God.

The white-robed ones who surround the throne of God are not composed of that company who were lovers of pleasure more than lovers of God, and who choose to drift with the current rather than to breast the waves of opposition. All who remain pure and uncorrupted from the spirit and influence prevailing at this time will have stern conflicts. They will come through great tribulations; they will wash their robes of character, and make them white in the blood of the Lamb. These will sing the song of triumph in the kingdom of glory. Those who suffer with Christ will be partakers of His glory.—*Review and Herald,* Oct. 16, 1883.

The Location of Sanitariums

Those who have to do with the locating of our sanitariums should prayerfully study the character and aim of sanitarium work. They should ever bear in mind that they are working for the restoration of the image of God in man. In one hand they are to carry remedies for the relief of physical suffering, and in the other the gospel for the relief of sin-burdened souls. Thus they are to work as true medical missionaries. In many hearts they are to sow the seeds of truth.

No selfishness, no personal ambition, is to be allowed to enter into the work of selecting locations for our sanitariums. Christ came to this world to show us how to live and labor. Let us learn from Him not to choose for our sanitariums the places most agreeable to our taste, but those places best suited to our work.

Out of the Cities

Light has been given me that in medical missionary work we have lost great advantages by failing to realize the need of a change in our plans in regard to the location of sanitariums. It is the Lord's will that these institutions shall be established outside the city. They should be situated in the country, in the midst of surroundings as attractive as possible. In nature—the Lord's garden—the sick will always find something to divert their attention from themselves and lift their thoughts to God.

I have been instructed that the sick should be cared for away from the bustle of the cities, away from the noise of streetcars and the continual rattling of carts and carriages. People who come to our sanitariums from country homes

Testimonies for the Church, vol. 7, pp. 80-83 (1902).

will appreciate a quiet place, and in retirement patients will be more readily influenced by the Spirit of God.

Amid the Scenes of Nature

The Garden of Eden, the home of our first parents, was exceedingly beautiful. Graceful shrubs and delicate flowers greeted the eye at every turn. In the garden were trees of every variety, many of them laden with fragrant and delicious fruit. On their branches the birds caroled their songs of praise. Adam and Eve, in their untainted purity, delighted in the sights and sounds of Eden. And today, although sin has cast its shadow over the earth, God desires His children to find delight in the works of His hands. To locate our sanitariums amidst the scenes of nature would be to follow God's plan, and the more closely this plan is followed, the more wonderfully will He work to restore suffering humanity. For our educational and medical institutions, places should be chosen where, away from the dark clouds of sin that hang over the great cities, the Sun of Righteousness can arise, "with healing in His wings." Malachi 4:2.

Let the leaders in our work instruct the people that sanitariums should be established in the midst of the most pleasant surroundings, in places not disturbed by the turmoil of the city—places where by wise instruction the thoughts of the patients can be bound up with the thoughts of God. Again and again I have described such places, but it seems that there has been no ear to hear. Recently, in a most clear and convincing manner, the advantage of establishing our institutions, especially our sanitariums and schools, outside the cities, was presented to me.

City Surroundings Unfavorable

Why are our physicians so eager to be located in the cities? The very atmosphere of the cities is polluted. In them, patients who have unnatural appetites to overcome cannot be properly guarded. To patients who are victims of strong drink, the saloons of a city are a continual temptation. To place our sanitariums where they are surrounded by ungodliness is to counterwork the efforts made to restore the patients to health.

In the future the condition of things in the cities will grow more and more objectionable, and the influence of city surroundings will be acknowledged as unfavorable to the accomplishment of the work that our sanitariums should do.

From the standpoint of health, the smoke and dust of the cities are very objectionable. And the patients who for a large part of their time are shut up within four walls, often feel that they are prisoners in their rooms. When they look out of a window, they see nothing but houses, houses, houses. Those who are thus confined to their rooms are liable to brood over their suffering and sorrow. Sometimes an invalid is poisoned by his own breath.

Many other evils follow the establishment of great medical institutions in the large cities.

Effects of Outdoor Life

Why deprive patients of the health-restoring blessing to be found in outdoor life? I have been instructed that as the sick are encouraged to leave their rooms and spend time in the open air, cultivating flowers, or doing some other light, pleasant work, their minds will be called from self to something more health-giving. Exercise in the open air should be prescribed as a beneficial, life-giving necessity. The longer patients can be kept out of doors the less care will they require. The more cheerful their surroundings, the more hopeful will they be. Surround them with the beautiful things of nature, place them where they can see the flowers growing and hear the birds singing, and their hearts will break into song in harmony with the song of the birds. Shut them in rooms and, be these rooms ever so elegantly furnished, they will grow fretful and gloomy. Give them the blessing of outdoor life; thus their souls will be uplifted. Relief will come to body and mind.

"Out of the cities," is my message. Our physicians ought to have been wide-awake on this point long ago. I hope and pray and believe that they will now arouse to the importance of getting out into the country.

The Perils of City Life

The time is near when the large cities will be visited by the judgments of God. In a little while these cities will be terribly shaken. No matter how large or how strong their buildings, no matter how many safeguards against fire may have been provided, let God touch these buildings, and in a few minutes or a few hours they are in ruins.

The ungodly cities of our world are to be swept away by the besom of destruction. In the calamities that are now befalling immense buildings and large portions of cities, God is showing us what will come upon the whole earth. He has told us, "Now learn a parable of the fig tree; When his branch is yet tender, and putteth forth leaves, ye know that summer is nigh: so likewise ye, when ye shall see all these things, know that it [the coming of the Son of man] is near, even at the doors." Matthew 24: 32, 33.

Not Among the Wealthy

It might seem to us that it would be best to select for our sanitariums places among the wealthy, that this would give character to our work and secure patronage for our institutions. But in this there is no light. "The Lord seeth not as man seeth." 1 Samuel 16:7. Man looks at the outward appearance; God looks at the heart. The fewer grand buildings there are around our institutions, the less vexation we shall experience. Many of the wealthy property owners are irreligious and irreverent. Worldly thoughts fill their minds. Worldly amusements, merriment, and hilarity occupy their time. Extravagance in dress and luxurious living absorb their means. The heavenly messengers are not welcomed to their homes. They want God afar off.

Humility is a difficult lesson for humanity to learn, and it is especially difficult for the rich and the self-indulgent. Those who do not regard themselves as accountable to God for all that they possess are tempted to exalt self, as if the riches comprehended by lands and bank stock made them independent of God. Full of pride and conceit, they place on themselves an estimate measured by their wealth.

There are many rich men who in God's sight are unfaithful stewards. In their acquirement and use of means, He has seen robbery. They have neglected the great Proprietor of all and have not used the means entrusted to them to relieve the suffering and the oppressed. They have been laying up for themselves wrath against the day of wrath, for God will reward every man according as his work shall be. These men do not worship God; self is their idol. They put justice and mercy out of the mind,

Testimonies for the Church, vol. 7, pp. 88, 89 (1902).

replacing them with avarice and strife. God says, "Shall I not visit them for these things?" Jeremiah 9:9.

God would not be pleased to have any of our institutions located in a community of this character, however great its apparent advantages. Selfish, wealthy men have a molding influence upon other minds, and the enemy would work through them to hedge up our way. Evil associations are always detrimental to piety and devotion, and principles that are approved by God may be undermined by such associations. God would have none of us like Lot, who chose a home in a place where he and his family were brought into constant contact with evil. Lot went into Sodom rich; he left with nothing, led by an angel's hand, while messengers of wrath waited to pour forth the fiery blasts that were to consume the inhabitants of that highly favored city and blot out its entrancing beauty making bleak and bare a place that God had once made very beautiful.

Our sanitariums should not be situated near the residences of rich men, where they would be looked upon as an innovation and an eyesore and unfavorably commented upon because they receive suffering humanity of all classes. Pure and undefiled religion makes those who are children of God one family, bound up with Christ in God. But the spirit of the world is proud, partial, exclusive, favoring only a few.

In erecting our buildings, we must keep away from the homes of the great men of the world and let them seek the help they need by withdrawing from their associates into more retired places. We shall not please God by building our sanitariums among people extravagant in dress and living, who are attracted to those who can make a great display.

Not for Pleasure Seekers

Why do we establish sanitariums? That the sick who come to them for treatment may receive relief from physical suffering and may also receive spiritual help. Because of their condition of health, they are susceptible to the sanctifying influence of the medical missionaries who labor for their restoration. Let us work wisely, for their best interests.

We are not building sanitariums for hotels. Receive into our sanitariums only those who desire to conform to right principles, those who will accept the foods that we can conscientiously place before them. Should we allow patients to have intoxicating liquor in their rooms, or should we serve them with meat, we could not give them the help they should receive in coming to our sanitariums. We must let it be known that from principle we exclude such articles from our sanitariums and our hygienic restaurants. Do we not desire to see our fellow beings freed from disease and infirmity, and in the enjoyment of health and strength? Then let us be as true to principle as the needle to the pole.

Those whose work it is to labor for the salvation of souls must keep themselves free from worldly policy plans. They must not, for the sake of obtaining the influence of someone who is wealthy, become entangled in plans dishonoring to their profession of faith. They must not sell their souls for financial advantage. They must do nothing that will retard the work of God and lower the standard of righteousness. We are God's servants, and we are to be workers together with Him, doing His work in His way, that all for whom we labor may see

Testimonies for the Church, vol. 7, pp. 95-97 (1902).

that our desire is to reach a higher standard of holiness. Those with whom we come in contact are to see that we not only talk of self-denial and sacrifice, but that we reveal it in our lives. Our example is to inspire those with whom we come in contact in our work, to become better acquainted with the things of God.

If we are to go to the expense of building sanitariums in order that we may work for the salvation of the sick and afflicted, we must plan our work in such a way that those we desire to help will receive the help they need. We are to do all in our power for the healing of the body; but we are to make the healing of the soul of far greater importance. Those who come to our sanitariums as patients are to be shown the way of salvation, that they may repent and hear the words, Thy sins are forgiven thee; go in peace, and sin no more. . . .

We are not to absorb the time and strength of men capable of carrying forward the Lord's work in the way He has outlined, in an enterprise for the accommodation and entertainment of pleasure seekers, whose greatest desire is to gratify self. To connect workers with such an enterprise would be perilous to their safety. Let us keep our young men and young women from all such dangerous influences. And should our brethren engage in such an enterprise, they would not advance the work of soul saving as they think they would.

Our sanitariums are to be established for one object —the advancement of present truth. And they are to be so conducted that a decided impression in favor of the truth will be made on the minds of those who come to them for treatment. The conduct of the workers, from the head manager to the worker occupying the humblest position, is to tell on the side of truth. The institution is to be pervaded by a spiritual atmosphere. We have a warning message to bear to the world, and our earnestness, our devotion to God's service, is to impress those who come to our sanitariums. . . .

We are living in the very close of this earth's history, and we are to move cautiously, understanding what the will of the Lord is, and, imbued with His Spirit, doing work that will mean much to His cause, work that will proclaim the warning message to a world infatuated, deceived, perishing in sin.

City Conditions

For years I have been given special light that we are not to center our work in the cities. The turmoil and confusion that fill these cities, the conditions brought about by the labor unions and the strikes, would prove a great hindrance to our work. Men are seeking to bring those engaged in the different trades under bondage to certain unions. This is not God's planning, but the planning of a power that we should in no wise acknowledge. God's word is fulfilling; the wicked are binding themselves up in bundles ready to be burned.

We are now to use all our entrusted capabilities in giving the last warning message to the world. In this work we are to preserve our individuality. We are not to unite with secret societies or with trades unions. We are to stand free in God, looking constantly to Christ for instruction. All our movements are to be made with a realization of the importance of the work to be accomplished for God.—*Testimonies for the Church,* vol. 7, p. 84 (1902).

Reference for further study: *The Ministry of Healing,* pages 261-268, "In Contact With Nature."

Economy in Establishing Sanitariums

As the chosen people of God, we cannot copy the habits, aims, practices, or fashions of the world. We are not left in darkness, to pattern after worldly models and to depend on outward appearance for success. The Lord has told us whence comes our strength. "This is the word of the Lord unto Zerubbabel, saying, Not by might, nor by power, but by My Spirit, saith the Lord of hosts." Zechariah 4:6. As the Lord sees fit He imparts, to those who keep His way, power that enables them to exert a strong influence for good. On God they are dependent, and to Him they must give an account of the way in which they use the talents He has entrusted to them. They are to realize that they are God's stewards and are to seek to magnify His name.

Outward Display Undesirable

Those whose affections are set on God will succeed. They will lose sight of self in Christ, and worldly attractions will have no power to allure them from their allegiance. They will realize that outward display does not give strength. It is not ostentation, outward show, that gives a correct representation of the work that we, as God's chosen people, are to do. Those who are connected with our sanitarium work should be adorned with the grace of Christ. This will give them the greatest influence for good.

The Lord is in earnest with us. His promises are given on condition that we faithfully do His will; therefore, in the building of sanitariums He is to be made first and last and best in everything.

Let all who are connected with the service of God be

guarded, lest by desire for display they lead others into indulgence and self-glorification. God does not want any of His servants to enter into unnecessary, expensive undertakings, which bring heavy burdens of debt upon the people, thus depriving them of means that would provide facilities for the work of the Lord. So long as those who claim to believe the truth for this time walk in the way of the Lord, to do justice and judgment, they may expect that the Lord will give them prosperity. But when they choose to wander from the narrow way, they bring ruin upon themselves and upon those who look to them for guidance.

Examples of Unselfishness

Those who lead out in the establishment of medical institutions must set a right example. Even if the money is in sight, they should not use more than is absolutely needed. The Lord's work should be conducted with reference to the necessities of every part of His vineyard. We are all members of one family, children of one Father, and the Lord's revenue must be used with reference to the interests of His cause throughout the world. The Lord looks upon all parts of the field, and His vineyard is to be cultivated as a whole.

We must not absorb in a few places all the money in the treasury, but must labor to build up the work in many places. New territory is to be added to the Lord's kingdom. Other parts of His vineyard are to be furnished with facilities that will give character to the work. The Lord forbids us to use selfish schemes in His service. He forbids us to adopt plans that will rob our neighbor of facilities that would enable him to act his part in representing the truth. We are to love our neighbor as ourselves.

Our Buildings to Represent Our Faith

We must also remember that our work is to correspond with our faith. We believe that the Lord is soon to come, and should not our faith be represented in the buildings we erect? Shall we put a large outlay of money into a building that will soon be consumed in the great conflagration? Our money means souls, and it is to be used to bring a knowledge of the truth to those who, because of sin, are under the condemnation of God. Then let us bind about our ambitious plans; let us guard against extravagance or improvidence, lest the Lord's treasury become empty and the builders have not means to do their appointed work.

Much more money than was necessary has been expended on our older institutions. Those who have done this have supposed that this outlay would give character to the work. But this plea is no excuse for unnecessary expenditure.

God desires that the humble, meek, and lowly spirit of the Master, who is the Majesty of heaven, the King of glory, shall ever be revealed in our institutions. Christ's first advent is not studied as it should be. He came to be our example in all things. His life was one of strict self-denial. If we follow His example, we shall never expend means unnecessarily. Never are we to seek for outward show. Let our showing be such that the light of truth can shine through our good works, so that God will be glorified by the use of the very best methods to restore the sick and to relieve the suffering. Character is given to the work, not by investing means in large buildings, but by maintaining the true standard of religious principles, with noble Christlikeness of character.

The mistakes that have been made in the erection of buildings in the past should be salutary admonitions to us in the future. We are to observe where others have failed and, instead of copying their mistakes, make improvements. In all our advance work we must regard the necessity of economy. There must be no needless expense. The Lord is soon to come, and our outlay in buildings is to be in harmony with our faith. Our means is to be used in providing cheerful rooms, healthful surroundings, and wholesome food.

Our ideas of building and furnishing our institutions are to be molded and fashioned by a true, practical knowledge of what it means to walk humbly with God. Never should it be thought necessary to give an appearance of wealth. Never should appearance be depended on as a means of success. This is a delusion. The desire to make an appearance that is not in every way appropriate to the work that God has given us to do, an appearance that could be kept up only by expending a large sum of money, is a merciless tyrant. It is like a canker that is ever eating into the vitals.

Comfort More Important Than Elegance

Men of common sense appreciate comfort above elegance and display. It is a mistake to suppose that by keeping up an appearance, more patients, and therefore more means, would be gained. But even if this course would bring an increase of patronage, we could not consent to have our sanitariums furnished according to the luxurious ideas of the age. Christian influence is too valuable to be sacrificed in this way. All the surroundings, inside and outside our institutions, must be in harmony with the teachings of Christ and the expression of our faith. Our work in all its departments should be an illustration, not of display and extravagance, but of sanctified judgment.

It is not large, expensive buildings, it is not rich furniture, it is not tables loaded with delicacies, that will give our work influence and success. It is the faith that works by love and purifies the soul; it is the atmosphere of grace that surrounds the believer, the Holy Spirit working upon the mind and heart, that makes him a savor of life unto life and enables God to bless his work.

God can communicate with His people today and give them wisdom to do His will, even as He communicated with His people of old and gave them wisdom in building the tabernacle. In the construction of this building He gave a representation of His power and majesty, and His name is to be honored in the buildings that are erected for Him today. Faithfulness, stability, and fitness are to be seen in every part.

Laborers Together With God

Those who have in hand the erecting of a sanitarium are to represent the truth by working in the spirit and love of God. As Noah in his day warned the world in the building of the ark, so, by the faithful work that is done today in erecting the Lord's institutions, sermons will be preached and the hearts of some will be convicted and converted. Then let the workers feel the greatest anxiety for the constant help of Christ, that the institutions which are established may not be in vain. While the work of building is going forward, let them remember that, as in the days of Noah and of Moses God arranged every detail of the ark and of the tabernacle, so in the building of His institutions today He Himself is watching the work done. Let them remember that the great Master

Builder, by His word, by His Spirit, and by His providence, designs to direct His work. They should take time to ask counsel of Him. The voice of prayer and the melody of holy song should ascend as sweet incense. All should realize their entire dependence upon God; they should remember that they are erecting an institution in which is to be carried forward a work of eternal consequence, and that, in doing this work, they are to be laborers together with God. "Looking unto Jesus" is ever to be our motto. And the assurance is, "I will instruct thee and teach thee in the way which thou shalt go: I will guide thee with Mine eye." Psalm 32:8.

Advantages of Wooden Structures

Brick and stone buildings are not the most desirable for a sanitarium, for they are generally cold and damp. It may be said that a brick building presents a much more attractive appearance, and that the building should be attractive. But we need roomy buildings; and if brick is too costly, we must build of wood. Economy must be our study. This is a necessity, because of the greatness of the work that must be done in many lines in God's moral vineyard.

It has been suggested that patients will not feel safe from fire in a wooden structure. But if we are in the country, and not in the cities where buildings are crowded together, a fire would originate from within, not from without; therefore brick would not be a safeguard. It should be presented to the patients that for health a wooden building is preferable to one of brick.—*Testimonies for the Church,* vol. 7, pp. 83, 84 (1902).

Economy in Operating

Economy in the outlay of means is an excellent branch of Christian wisdom. This matter is not sufficiently considered by those who occupy responsible positions in our institutions. Money is an excellent gift of God. In the hands of His children it is food for the hungry, drink for the thirsty, and raiment for the naked; it is a defense for the oppressed and a means of health to the sick. Means should not be needlessly or lavishly expended for the gratification of pride or ambition.

Principle Must Control

In order to meet the real wants of the people, the stern motives of religious principle must be a controlling power. When Christians and worldlings are brought together, the Christian element is not to assimilate with the unsanctified. The contrast between the two must be kept sharp and positive. They are servants of two masters. One class strive to keep the humble path of obedience to God's requirements,—the path of simplicity, meekness, and humility,—imitating the Pattern, Christ Jesus. The other class are in every way the opposite of the first. They are servants of the world, eager and ambitious to follow its fashions in extravagant dress and in the gratification of appetite. This is the field in which Christ has given those connected with the sanitarium their appointed work. We are not to lessen the distance between us and worldlings by coming to their standard, stepping down from the high path cast up for the ransomed of the Lord to walk in. But the charms exhibited in the Christian's life—the principles carried out in our daily work, in holding appetite under the control of reason, maintaining simplicity in dress, and engaging in holy conversation—will be a light continually shining upon the pathway of those whose habits are false. . . .

All who are connected with our institutions should have a jealous care that nothing be wasted, even if the matter does not come under the very part of the work assigned them. Everyone can do something toward economizing. All should perform their work, not to win praise of men, but in such a manner that it may bear the scrutiny of God.

Christ once gave His disciples a lesson upon economy, which is worthy of careful attention. He wrought a miracle to feed the hungry thousands who had listened to His teachings; yet after all had eaten and were satisfied, He did not permit the fragments to be wasted. He who could, in their necessity, feed the vast multitude by His divine power, bade His disciples gather up the fragments, that nothing might be lost. This lesson was given as much for our benefit as for those living in Christ's day. The Son of God has a care for the necessities of temporal life. He did not neglect the broken fragments after the feast, although He could make such a feast whenever He chose. The workers in our institutions would do well to heed this lesson: "Gather up the fragments that remain, that nothing be lost." John 6:12. This is the duty of all, and those who occupy a leading position should set the example.

Loyalty to Our Institutions

The sanitarium at Battle Creek has been built up under a pressure of difficulties. There have had to be decisive measures taken, contracts signed by those who were engaged as helpers that they would remain a certain number of years. This has been a positive necessity. After help has been secured, and by considerable painstaking efforts these have become efficient workers, wealthy patients have held out inducements of better wages to secure them as nurses for their own special benefit, at their own homes. And these helpers have often left the sanitarium and gone with them, without taking into consideration the labor that had been put forth to qualify them as efficient workers. This has not been the case in merely one or two instances, but in many cases.

Then people have come as patrons from other institutions that are not conducted on religious principles, and in a most artful manner have led away the help by promising to give them higher wages. Physicians have apostatized from the faith and from the institution, and have left because they could not have their own way in everything. Some have been discharged, and after obtaining the sympathy of others of the helpers and patients, have led these away; and after being at great expense and trying their own ways and methods to the best of their ability, they have made a failure and closed up, incurring debts that they could not meet. This has been tried again and again. Justice and righteousness have had no part in the movements of such. "The way of the Lord" has not been

---

Health, Philanthropic, and Medical Missionary Work, pages 29-33 (1888).

chosen, but their own way. They beguiled the unwary and made an easy conquest of those who love change. They were too much blinded to consider the right and wrong of this course, and too reckless to care.

Thus it has been necessary in the sanitarium at Battle Creek to make contracts binding those who connected with it as helpers, so that after they have been educated and trained as nurses and as bath hands, they shall not leave because others present inducements to them. Money has been advanced to some special ones that they might obtain a medical education and be useful to the institution. Dr.—— has placed hopes upon some of these, that they would relieve him of responsibilities that have rested most heavily upon him. Some have become uneasy and dissatisfied because those who have started institutions in other parts of the country have tried to flatter and induce them to come to their sanitariums, promising to do better by them. In this way the workers—some of them at least—have become uneasy, unsettled, self-sufficient, and unreliable, even if they did not disconnect with the sanitarium, because they felt there were openings for them elsewhere. Those who are just beginning to practice have felt ready to take large responsibilities which it would be unsafe to trust in their hands, because they have not proved faithful in that which is least.

Now we wish all to look at this matter from a Christian standpoint. These tests reveal the true material that goes to make up the character. There is in the Decalogue a commandment that says, "Thou shalt not steal." This commandment covers just such acts as these. Some have stolen the help that others have had the burden of bringing up and training for their own work. Any underhanded scheme, any influence brought to bear to try to secure help that others have engaged and trained, is nothing less than downright stealing.

There is another commandment that says, "Thou shalt not bear false witness against thy neighbor." There has been tampering with the help that has been secured and depended upon to do a certain kind of labor; efforts have been made to demerit the plans and find fault with the management of those who are conducting the institution. The course of the management has been questioned as regards those whose services they desired to secure. Their vanity has been flattered and insinuations made that they are not advanced as rapidly as they should be, they ought to be in more responsible positions.

The very gravest difficulty that the physicians and managers of our institutions have to meet is that men and women who have been led up step by step, educated and trained to fill positions of trust, have become self-inflated, self-sufficient, and placed altogether too high an estimate upon their own capabilities. If they have been entrusted with two talents, they feel perfectly capable of handling five. If they had wisely and judiciously used the two talents, coming up with faithfulness in the little things entrusted to them, thorough in everything they undertook, then they would be qualified to handle larger responsibilities. If they could climb every step of the ladder, round after round, showing faithfulness in that which is least, it would be an evidence that they were fitted to bear heavier burdens, and would be faithful in much. But many care only to skim the surface. They do not think deep, and become master of their duties. They feel ready to grasp the highest round of the ladder without the trouble of climbing up step after step. We are pained at heart as we compare the work coming forth from their hands with God's righteous standard of faithfulness which God alone can accept. There is a painful defect, a remissness, a superficial gloss, a wanting in solidity and in intelligent knowledge and carefulness and thoroughness. God cannot say to such, "Well done, thou good and faithful servant: thou hast been faithful over a few things, I will make thee ruler over many things." Matthew 25:21.

Men must get hold conscientiously and feel that they are doing the work of God. They must have the trust in their heart to correct all the sophistries and delusions of Satan that would throw them off the right track, so that they will not choose the way of the Lord, but follow the impulses of their own undisciplined characters. If the heart is sanctified and guided by the Holy Spirit, they will run no risks, but will be sure in all they undertake to do good work for Jesus; and in doing their work righteously they are standing securely in this life with a fast hold from above, and they will be guided into every good and holy way. They will be constant to principle. They will do their work, not to secure a great name or great wages, not for the purpose of weaving self into all their works, and of appearing to be somebody in the world, but to be right in everything in the sight of God. They will not be half as anxious to do a big work as to do whatever they have to do with fidelity and with an eye single to the glory of God. Such men are great in the sight of God. Such names are registered in the Lamb's book of life as the faithful servants of the most high God. These are the men who are more precious in the sight of God than fine gold, even more precious than the golden wedge of Ophir.

The Sanitarium as a Missionary Field

The sanitarium is to be a missionary institution in the fullest sense of the word, and its character in this respect must be preserved or it will not bear upon it the superscription of God. To keep it thus will require godliness of life and character in every worker. The success of this institution must be viewed in the light of God's word. True success will bear the heavenly credentials. The workers for God will rejoice in the Lord, and at the same time be dissatisfied with their own efforts. The moment of rejoicing in the Lord because of success will be the moment of self-abasement because of what has been left undone through neglect and unfaithfulness.

Men who accept a position in any of our health institutions should do so with as full a realization of its responsibilities as possible. The Lord has promised to be a present help in every time of need, and there is no excuse for not doing more real missionary work at the sanitarium. Far better attention should be paid to obtaining a fitness for every duty. Workers should seek to improve, that they may do their work in the best manner possible and with fidelity, so as to meet the approval of God. Opportunites for doing good have always been far in advance of the workers, for they have failed to see and improve them, because the enemy of right doing has had a controlling power over their minds.—*Health, Philanthropic, and Medical Missionary Work,* pages 46, 47 (1888).

Adherence to Principle

The temptations by which Christ was beset in the wilderness—appetite, love of the world, and presumption—are the three great leading allurements by which men are most frequently overcome. The managers of the sanitarium will often be tempted to depart from the principles which should govern such an institution. But they should not vary from the right course to gratify the inclinations or minister to the depraved appetites of wealthy patients or friends. The influence of such a course is only evil. Deviations from the teachings given in lectures or through the press have a most unfavorable effect upon the influence and morals of the institution and will, to a great extent, counteract all efforts to instruct and reform the victims of depraved appetites and passions and to lead them to Christ, the only safe refuge.

The evil will not end here. The influence affects not only the patients, but the workers as well. When the barriers are once broken down, step after step is taken in the wrong direction. Satan presents flattering worldly prospects to those who will depart from principle and sacrifice integrity and Christian honor to gain the approbation of the ungodly. His efforts are too often successful. He gains the victory where he should meet with repulse and defeat.

Christ resisted Satan in our behalf. We have the example of our Saviour to strengthen our weak purposes and resolves; but notwithstanding this, some will fall by Satan's temptations, and they will not fall alone. Every soul that fails to obtain the victory carries others down through his influence. Those who fail to connect with

Testimonies for the Church, vol. 4, pp. 576, 577 (1881).

God and to receive wisdom and grace to refine and elevate their own lives will be judged for the good they might have done, but failed to perform because they were content with earthliness of mind and friendship with the unsanctified.

All heaven is interested in the salvation of man, and is ready to pour upon him her beneficent gifts, if he will comply with the conditions Christ has made: "Come out from among them, and be ye separate, saith the Lord, and touch not the unclean." 2 Corinthians 6:17.

To the Glory of God

We are commanded, whether we eat or drink or whatever we do, to do all to the glory of God. How many have conscientiously moved from principle rather than impulse, and obeyed this command to the letter? How many of the youthful disciples in ——— have made God their trust and portion, and have earnestly sought to know and do His will? There are many who are servants of Christ in name, but who are not so in deed. Where religious principle governs, the danger of committing great errors is small; for selfishness, which always blinds and deceives, is subordinate. The sincere desire to do others good so predominates that self is forgotten. To have firm religious principles is an inestimable treasure. It is the purest, highest, and most elevated influence mortals can possess. Such have an anchor. Every act is well considered, lest its effect be injurious to another and lead away from Christ.—*Testimonies for the Church,* vol. 2, p. 129 (1868).

The Chaplain and His Work

It is of great importance that the one who is chosen to care for the spiritual interests of patients and helpers be a man of sound judgment and undeviating principle, a man who will have moral influence, who knows how to deal with minds. He should be a person of wisdom and culture, of affection as well as intelligence. He may not be thoroughly efficient in all respects at first; but he should, by earnest thought and the exercise of his abilities, qualify himself for this important work. The greatest wisdom and gentleness are needed to serve in this position acceptably, yet with unbending integrity, for prejudice, bigotry, and error of every form and description must be met.

This place should not be filled by a man who has an irritable temper, a sharp combativeness. Care must be taken that the religion of Christ be not made repulsive by harshness or impatience. The servant of God should seek, by meekness, gentleness, and love, rightly to represent our holy faith. While the cross must never be concealed, he should present also the Saviour's matchless love. The worker must be imbued with the spirit of Jesus, and then the treasures of the soul will be presented in words that will find their way to the hearts of those who hear. The religion of Christ, exemplified in the daily life of His followers, will exert a tenfold greater influence than the most eloquent sermons. . . . If all connected with the sanitarium are correct representatives of the truths of health reform and of our holy faith, they are exerting an influence to mold the minds of their patients. The contrast of erroneous habits with those which are in harmony with the truth of God, has a convicting power.—*Testimonies for the Church,* vol. 4, pp. 546, 547 (1878).

Hold the Truth in Its Purity

Those who are placed in charge of the Lord's institutions are in need of much of the strength and grace and keeping power of God, that they shall not walk contrary to the sacred principles of the truth. Many, many are very dull of comprehension in regard to their obligation to preserve the truth in its purity, uncontaminated by one vestige of error. Their danger is in holding the truth in light esteem, thus leaving upon minds the impression that it is of little consequence what we believe, if, by carrying out plans or human devising, we can exalt ourselves before the world as holding a superior position, as occupying the highest seat.

God calls for men whose hearts are as true as steel, and who will stand steadfast in integrity, undaunted by circumstances. He calls for men who will remain separate from the enemies of the truth. He calls for men who will not dare to resort to the arm of flesh by entering into partnership with worldlings in order to secure means for advancing His work—even for the building of institutions. Solomon, by his alliance with unbelievers, secured an abundance of gold and silver, but his prosperity proved his ruin. Men today are no wiser than he, and they are as prone to yield to the influences that caused his downfall. For thousands of years Satan has been gaining an experience in learning how to deceive; and to those who live in this age he comes with almost overwhelming power. Our only safety is found in obedience to God's word, which has been given us as a sure guide and counselor. God's people today are to keep themselves distinct and separate from the world, its spirit, and its influences.

Review and Herald, Feb. 1, 1906.

"Come out from among them, and be ye separate."
2 Corinthians 6:17. Shall we hear the voice of God and
obey, or shall we make halfway work of the matter and
try to serve God and mammon? There is earnest work
before each one of us. Right thoughts, pure and holy
purposes, do not come to us naturally. We shall have to
strive for them. In all our institutions, our publishing
houses and colleges and sanitariums, pure and holy principles must take root. If our institutions are what God
designs they should be, those connected with them will
not pattern after worldly institutions. They will stand as
peculiar, governed and controlled by the Bible standard.
They will not come into harmony with the principles of
the world in order to gain patronage. No motives will
have sufficient force to move them from the straight line
of duty. Those who are under the control of the Spirit
of God will not seek their own pleasure or amusement.
If Christ presides in the hearts of the members of His
church, they will answer to the call, "Come out from
among them, and be ye separate." "Be not partakers of
her sins." Revelation 18:4.

For the Welfare of Others

In their conduct toward the patients, all should be
actuated by higher motives than selfish interest. Everyone should feel that this institution is one of God's instrumentalities to relieve the disease of the body and
point the sin-sick soul to Him who can heal both soul
and body. In addition to the performance of the special
duties assigned them, all should have an interest for the
welfare of others. Selfishness is contrary to the spirit of
Christianity.—*Testimonies for the Church,* vol. 4, p. 564
(1881).

The Workers Needed

We should be careful that we connect with all our sanitariums those who will give a right mold to the work. Characters are to be formed here after the divine similitude. It is not the expensive dress that will give us influence, but it is by true Christian humility that we shall exalt our Saviour. Our only hope for success in doing good to the people of the world who come to our sanitariums as guests, is for the workers, each and every one, to maintain a living connection with God. The dress of sanitarium helpers is to be modest and neat, but the dress is not so important as the deportment. The matter of greatest consequence is that the truth be lived out in our lives, that our words be in harmony with the faith we profess to hold. If the workers in our sanitariums will surrender to God, and take a high position as believers in the truth, the Lord will recognize this, and we shall see a great work done in these institutions.

Experienced Helpers

It is not the wisest course to connect with our sanitariums too many who are inexperienced, who come as learners, while there is a lack of experienced, efficient workers. We need more matronly women, and men who are sound and solid in principle—substantial men who fear God and who can carry responsibilities wisely. Some may come and offer to work for small wages, because they enjoy being at a sanitarium, or because they wish to learn; but it is not true economy to supply an institution largely with inexperienced helpers.

If the right persons are connected with the work, and

Review and Herald, Dec. 30, 1909.

if all will humble their hearts before God, although there may now be a heavy debt resting upon the institution, the Lord will work in such a way that the debt will be lessened, and souls will be converted to the truth, because they see that the workers are following in the way of the Lord, and keeping His commandments. This is the only hope for the prosperity of our sanitariums. It is useless to think of any other way. We cannot expect the blessing of God to rest upon us, if we serve God at will, and let Him alone at pleasure.

It is not necessary that we should cater to the world's demands for pleasure. There are other places in the world where people may find amusement. We need at our sanitariums substantial men and women; we need those who will reveal the simplicity of true godliness. When the sick come to our institutions, they should be made to realize that there is a divine power at work, that angels of God are present.

Tact Essential

The spiritual work of our sanitariums is not to be under the control of physicians. This work requires thought and tact, and a broad knowledge of the Bible. Ministers possessing these qualifications should be connected with our sanitariums. They should uplift the standard of temperance from a Christian point of view, showing that the body is the temple of the Holy Spirit, and bringing to the minds of the people the responsibility resting upon them as God's purchased possession to make mind and body a holy temple, fit for the indwelling of the Holy Spirit.—*Testimonies for the Church,* vol. 7, p. 75 (1902).

Dealing With Sentimentalism

The guardians of the institution must ever maintain a high standard and carefully watch over the youth entrusted to them by parents as learners or helpers in the various departments. When young men and women work together a sympathy is created among them which frequently grows into sentimentalism. If the guardians are indifferent to this, lasting injury may be done to these souls and the high moral tone of the institution will be compromised. If any, patients or helpers, continue their familiarity by deception after having had judicious instruction, they should not be retained in the institution, for their influence will affect those who are innocent and unsuspecting. Young girls will lose their maidenly modesty and be led to act deceptively because their affections have become entangled. . . .

The young should be taught to be frank, yet modest, in their associations. They should be taught to respect just rules and authority. If they refuse to do this, let them be dismissed, no matter what position they occupy, for they will demoralize others. The forwardness of young girls in placing themselves in the company of young men, lingering around where they are at work, entering into conversation with them, talking common, idle talk, is belittling to womanhood. It lowers them, even in the estimation of those who themselves indulge in such things. . . .

Let not those who profess the religion of Christ descend to trifling conversation, to unbecoming familiarity with women of any class, whether married of single. Let them keep their proper places with all dignity. At the same

Health, Philanthropic, and Medical Missionary Work, pages 26-28 (1885).

(294)

time they should be sociable, kind, and courteous to all. Young ladies should be reserved and modest. They should give no occasion for their good to be evil spoken of. . . . Those who give evidence that their thoughts run in a low channel, whose conversation tends to corrupt rather than to elevate, should be removed at once from any connection with the institution, for they will surely demoralize others.

Ever bear in mind that our health institutions are missionary fields. . . . Will you excuse levity and careless acts by saying that it was the result of thoughtlessness on your part? Is it not the duty of the Christian to think soberly? If Jesus is enthroned in the heart, will the thoughts be running riot? . . .

Moral purity, self-respect, a strong power of resistance, must be firmly and constantly cherished. There should not be one departure from reserve. One act of familiarity, one indiscretion, may jeopardize the soul, by opening the door to temptation and thus weakening the power of resistance.

The Ennobling Power of Pure Thoughts

We need a constant sense of the ennobling power of pure thoughts. The only security for any soul is right thinking. As a man "thinketh in his heart, so is he." The power of self-restraint strengthens by exercise. That which at first seems difficult, by constant repetition grows easy, until right thoughts and actions become habitual. If we will, we may turn away from all that is cheap and inferior, and rise to a higher standard; we may be respected by men, and beloved of God.—*The Ministry of Healing,* page 491 (1905).

Criticizing and Faultfinding

Those visiting our institutions and seeing where work is not done to the best advantage, should, if they have had larger experience, and know of a more successful way to manage, counsel with those who are in trust and seek to help them to see the right way of action. Those who fail to do this neglect their duty, and are unfaithful to their God-given responsibility. Such an one, if he goes from that institution without saying anything to the proper persons and states to parties not connected with it that he saw failures in the management there, that he saw places where expense was incurred without benefiting the institution, has failed to manifest a Christian spirit and has been unfaithful to his brethren and to God. The Lord would have him diffuse light, if he has it to give; and if he has not a well-regulated plan to suggest, he does wrong to tell others of the mistakes which he has seen. If he fails to give the workers the benefit of his supposed superior wisdom, if he only finds fault without telling, in a right spirit, how to improve, he not only injures the reputation of the institution, but of the workers, who may be acting according to the very best light they have.

These things need to be carefully considered. Let every man and woman inquire, "On whose side am I? Am I working to build up or to tear down one of God's instrumentalities?"

One thing makes me feel very sad, and that is that there is not always harmony among the workers in our institutions. I have thought, Is it possible that there is anyone who will find fault with those connected with

Health, Philanthropic, and Medical Missionary Work, pages 23-26 (1885).

them in the work? Is there anyone who will suggest to patients or to visitors or fellow workers that there are many things which ought to be done that are not done, and many other things which are not done right? If they do this, they are not doing the work of Christians.

Men who have been appointed to different positions of trust are to be respected. We do not expect to find men who are perfect in every respect. They may be seeking for perfection of character, but they are finite and liable to err. Those who are engaged in our institutions should feel it their duty jealously to guard both the work and the workers from unjust criticism. They should not readily accept or speak words of censure against any who are connected with the work of God, for in thus doing God Himself may be reproached and the work that He is doing through instrumentalities may be greatly hindered. The wheels of progress may be blocked when God says "Go forward."

It is a great evil, and one which exists among our people to a great extent, to give loose rein to the thoughts, to question and criticize everything another does, making mountains out of molehills, and thinking their own ways are right, whereas, if they were in the same place as their brother, they might not do half as well as he does. It is just as natural for some to find fault with what another does as it is for them to breathe. They have formed the habit of criticizing others, when they themselves are the ones who should be brought severely to task and their wicked speeches and hard feelings be burned out of their souls by the purifying fire of God's love. . . .

A person who will allow any degree of suspicion or censure to rest upon his fellow workers, while he neither rebukes the complainers nor faithfully presents the matter before the one condemned, is doing the work of the enemy. He is watering the seeds of discord and of strife, the fruit of which he will have to meet in the day of God. . . .

This disrespect for others, this disregard for right and justice, is not a rare thing. It is found to a greater or less extent in all our institutions. If one makes a mistake, there are some who make it their business to talk about it until it grows to large proportions. Instead of this, there should be in all engaged in our institutions a sacred principle to guard the interest and reputation of everyone with whom they are associated, even as they would wish their own reputation guarded.

Results of Fostered Sin

The strongest bulwark of vice in our world is not the iniquitous life of the abandoned sinner or the degraded outcast; it is that life which otherwise appears virtuous, honorable, and noble, but in which one sin is fostered, one vice indulged. To the soul that is struggling in secret against some giant temptation, trembling upon the very verge of the precipice, such an example is one of the most powerful enticements to sin. He who, endowed with high conceptions of life and truth and honor, does yet willfully transgress one precept of God's holy law, has perverted his noble gifts into a lure to sin. Genius, talent, sympathy, even generous and kindly deeds, may become decoys of Satan to entice other souls over the precipice of ruin for this life and the life to come.—*Mount of Blessing,* pp. 94, 95 (1896).

Looking Unto Jesus

Last night I had a wonderful experience. I was in an assembly where questions were being asked and answered. I awoke at one o'clock and arose. For a time I walked the room, praying most earnestly for clearness of mind, for strength of eyesight, and for strength to write the things that must be written. I entreated the Lord to help me to bear a testimony that would awake His people before it is forever too late. . . .

My soul was drawn out in the consideration of matters relating to the future carrying forward of God's work. Those who have had little experience in the beginning of the work often err in judgment in regard to how it should be advanced. They are tempted on many points. They think that it would be better if the talented workers had higher wages, according to the importance of the work they do.

But one of authority stood among us in the assembly in which I was present last night and spoke words that must decide the question. He said: "Looking unto Jesus, the Author and Finisher of your faith, trace His work after He assumed humanity, and remember that He is your pattern. In the work of soul saving, His divine-human life in our world is to be your guide. He made the world, yet when He lived on this earth He had not where to lay His head."

Were the most talented workers given higher wages, those who do the more laborious part of the work would desire larger wages also, and would say that their work is just as essential as any work that is done.

Work is to be carried forward in many lines. New ter-

Special Testimonies, Series B, No. 19, pp. 29-31 (1902).

ritory is to be annexed. But no Jerusalem-centers are to be made. If such centers are made, there will be a scattering of the people out of them, by the Lord God of heaven.

The work of God is to be carried on without outward display. In establishing institutions, we are never to compete with the institutions of the world in size or splendor. We are to enter into no confederacy with those who do not love or fear God. Those who have not the light of present truth, who are unable to endure the seeing of Him who is invisible, are surrounded by spiritual darkness that is as the darkness of midnight. Within, all is dreariness. They know not the meaning of joy in the Lord. They take no interest in eternal realities. Their attention is engrossed by the trifling things of earth. They make haste unto vanity, striving by unfair means to obtain advantages. Having forsaken God, the fountain of living waters, they hew out for themselves broken cisterns that can hold no water. Let it not be thus with those who have tasted the power of the world to come.

Economy and Self-Denial

Sow the seeds of truth wherever you have opportunity. In establishing the work in new places, economize in every possible way. Gather up the fragments; let nothing be lost. . . .

We are nearing the end of this earth's history, and the different lines of God's work are to be carried forward with much more self-sacrifice than they have yet been. The work for these last days is a missionary work. Present truth, from the first letter of its alphabet to the last, means missionary effort. The work to be done calls for sacrifice at every step of advance. The workers are to come forth from trial purified and refined, as gold tried in the fire.

Co-operation Between Schools and Sanitariums

It is well that our training schools for Christian workers should be established near to our health institutions, that the students may be educated in the principles of healthful living. Institutions that send forth workers who are able to give a reason for their faith, and who have a faith which works by love and purifies the soul, are of great value. I have clear instruction that, wherever it is possible, schools should be established near to our sanitariums, that each institution may be a help and strength to the other. He who created man has an interest in those who suffer. He has directed in the establishment of our sanitariums and in the building up of our schools close to our sanitariums, that they may become efficient mediums in training men and women for the work of ministering to suffering humanity.

Let Seventh-day Adventist medical workers remember that the Lord God omnipotent reigneth. Christ was the greatest Physician that ever trod this sin-cursed earth. The Lord would have His people come to Him for their power of healing. He will baptize them with His Holy Spirit and fit them for service that will make them a blessing in restoring the spiritual and physical health of those who need healing. . . .

The Lord would have the workers make special efforts to point the sick and suffering to the Great Physician who made the human body.—*Testimonies for the Church,* vol. 9, p. 178 (1909).

Equity in the Matter of Wages

DEAR BROTHER:

I did not suppose that it would be so long before I fulfilled my promise to write to you. I have been thinking of the question that was agitating your mind in regard to wages. You suggest that if we paid higher wages, we could secure men of ability to fill important positions of trust. This might be so, but I should very much regret to see our workers held to our work by the wages they receive. There are needed in the cause of God workers who will make a covenant with Him by sacrifice, who will labor for the love of souls, not for the wages they receive.

Your sentiment regarding wages, my much-respected brother, is the language of the world. Service is service, and one kind of work is as essential as the other. To every man is given his work. There is stern, taxing labor to be performed, labor involving disagreeable taxation and requiring skill and tact. In the work of God, the physical as well as the mental powers are drawn upon, and both are essential. One is as necessary as the other. Should we attempt to draw a line between mental and physical work, we would place ourselves in very difficult positions.

The experiment of giving men high wages has been tried in the publishing institutions. Some men have grasped high wages, while others, doing work just as severe and taxing, have had barely enough to sustain their families. Yet their taxation was just as great, and often men have been overworked and overwearied, while others, bearing not half the burdens, received double the wages. The Lord sees all these things, and He will surely call

Special Testimonies, Series B, No. 19, pp. 32, 33 (1902).

men to account; for He is a God of justice and equity.

Those who have a knowledge of the truth for this time should be pure and clean and noble in all their business transactions. None among God's servants should hunger and thirst for the highest place as director or manager. Such positions are fraught with great temptation.

Our nurses are encouraged to pledge themselves to work for certain parties for a certain sum. They bind themselves to serve thus and so, and afterward they are dissatisfied. It is necessary that more equality be shown in dealing with our nurses. There are among us intelligent, conscientious nurses, who work faithfully and at all times. It is nurses such as these that we need, and they should receive better wages, so that should they fall sick, they would have money enough laid by to enable them to have a rest and a change. Then again, often the parents of these nurses practice great self-denial to make it possible for their children to take the nurses' course. It is only right that when these children have received their education, they should be given sufficient remuneration to enable them to help their parents, should they need help.

Economical From Principle

Those whose hands are open to respond to the calls for means to sustain the cause of God and to relieve the suffering and the needy, are not the ones who are found loose and lax and dilatory in their business management. They are always careful to keep their outgoes within their income. They are economical from principle; they feel it their duty to save, that they may have something to give. —*Testimonies for the Church,* vol. 4, p. 573 (1881).

Compensation

God does not want His work to be continually embarrassed with debt. When it seems desirable to add to the buildings or other facilities of an institution, beware of going beyond your means. Better to defer the improvements until Providence shall open the way for them to be made without contracting heavy debts and having to pay interest.

The publishing houses have been made places of deposit by our people and have thus been enabled to furnish means to support branches of the work in different fields and have aided in carrying other enterprises. This is well. None too much has been done in these lines. The Lord sees it all. But, from the light He has given me, every effort should be made to stand free from debt.

The publishing work was founded in self-denial and should be conducted upon strictly economical principles. The question of finance can be managed, if, when there is a pressure for means, the workers will consent to a reduction in wages. This was the principle the Lord revealed to me to be brought into our institutions. When money is scarce, we should be willing to restrict our wants.

Let the proper estimate be placed upon the publications, and then let all in our publishing houses study to economize in every possible way, even though considerable inconvenience is thus caused. Watch the little outgoes. Stop every leak. It is the little losses that tell heavily in the end. Gather up the fragments; let nothing be lost. Waste not the minutes in talking; wasted minutes mar

Testimonies for the Church, vol. 7, pp. 206-209 (1902).

This article, addressed to managers and workers in our publishing houses, is included here because the principles apply to sanitarium workers.

the hours. Persevering diligence, working in faith, will always be crowned with success.

Some think it beneath their dignity to look after small things. They think it the evidence of a narrow mind and a niggardly spirit. But small leaks have sunk many a ship. Nothing that would serve the purpose of any should be allowed to waste. A lack of economy will surely bring debt upon our institutions. Although much money may be received, it will be lost in the little wastes of every branch of the work. Economy is not stinginess.

Every man or woman employed in the publishing house should be a faithful sentinel, watching that nothing be wasted. All should guard against supposed wants that require an expenditure of means. Some men live better on four hundred dollars a year than others do on eight hundred. Just so it is with our institutions; some persons can manage them with far less capital than others can. God desires all the workers to practice economy, and especially to be faithful accountants.

Every worker in our institutions should receive fair compensation. If the workers receive suitable wages, they have the gratification of making donations to the cause. It is not right that some should receive a large amount, and others, who are doing essential and faithful work, very little.

Yet there are cases where a difference must be made. There are men connected with the publishing houses who carry heavy responsibilities, and whose work is of great value to the institution. In many other positions they would have far less care, and, financially, much greater profit. All can see the injustice of paying such men no higher wages than are paid to mere mechanical workers.

If a woman is appointed by the Lord to do a certain

work, her work should be estimated according to its value. Some may think it good policy to allow persons to devote their time and labor to the work without compensation. But God does not sanction such arrangements. When self-denial is required because of a dearth of means, the burden is not to rest wholly upon a few persons. Let all unite in the sacrifice.

The Lord desires those entrusted with His goods to show kindness and liberality, not niggardliness. Let them not, in their deal, try to exact every cent possible. God looks with contempt on such methods. . . .

The Lord wants men who see the work in its greatness, and who understand the principles that have been interwoven with it from its rise. He will not have a worldly order of things come in to fashion the work in altogether different lines from those He has marked out for His people. The work must bear the character of its Originator.

In the sacrifice of Christ for fallen men, mercy and truth have met together, righteousness and peace have kissed each other. When these attributes are separated from the most wonderful and apparently successful work, there is nothing to it.

God has not singled out a few men for His favor, and left others uncared for. He will not lift up one, and cast down and oppress another. All who are truly converted will manifest the same spirit. They will treat their fellow men as they would treat Christ. No one will ignore the rights of another.

God's servants should have so great respect for the sacred work they are handling that they will not bring into it one vestige of selfishness.

No Exorbitant Salaries

No man should be granted an exorbitant salary, even though he may possess special capabilities and qualifications. The work done for God and His cause is not to be placed on a mercenary basis. The workers in the publishing house have no more taxing labor, no greater expense, no more weighty responsibilities, than have the workers in other lines. Their labor is no more wearing than is that of the faithful minister. On the contrary, ministers, as a rule, make greater sacrifices than are made by the laborers in our institutions. Ministers go where they are sent; they are minutemen, ready to move at any moment, to meet any emergency. They are necessarily separated, to a great degree, from their families. The workers in the publishing houses, as a rule, have a permanent home and can live with their families. This is a great saving of expense and should be considered in its bearing on the relative compensation of laborers in the ministry and in publishing houses.

Those who labor wholeheartedly in the Lord's vineyard, working to the utmost of their ability, are not the ones to set the highest estimate on their own services. Instead of swelling with pride and self-importance, and measuring with exactness every hour's work, they compare their efforts with the Saviour's work and account themselves unprofitable servants.

Brethren, do not study how little you may do, in order to reach the very lowest standard, but arouse to grasp the fullness of Christ, that you may do much for Him.—*Testimonies for the Church,* vol. 7, pp. 208, 209 (1902).

Helping Those Who Need Help

As God's agencies we are to have hearts of flesh, full of the charity that prompts us to be helpful to those more needy than ourselves. If we see our brethren and sisters struggling under poverty and debt, if we see churches that are in need of financial aid, we should manifest an unselfish interest in them and help them in proportion as God has prospered us. If you who have charge of an institution see other institutions bravely struggling for standing room, so that they may do a work similar to the work of the institutions with which you are connected, do not be jealous.

Do not seek to push a working force out of existence and to exalt yourself in conscious superiority. Rather curtail some of your large plans and help those who are struggling. Aid them in carrying out some of their plans to increase their facilities. Do not use every dollar in enlarging your facilities and increasing your responsibilities. Reserve part of your means for establishing in other places health institutions and schools. You will need great wisdom to know just where to place these institutions, so that the people will be the most benefited. All these matters must receive candid consideration.

Those in positions of responsibility will need wisdom from on high in order to deal justly, to love mercy, and to show mercy, not only to a few, but to everyone with whom they come in contact. Christ identifies His interests with those of His people, no matter how poor and needy they may be. Missions must be opened for the colored people, and everyone should seek to do something and to do it now.

Testimonies for the Church, vol. 8, pp. 136-144 (1890).

There is need that institutions be established in different places, that men and women may be set at work to do their best in the fear of God. No one should lose sight of his mission and work. Everyone should aim to carry forward to a successful issue the work placed in his hands. All our institutions should keep this in mind and strive for success; but at the same time let them remember that their success will increase in proportion as they exercise disinterested liberality, sharing their abundance with institutions that are struggling for a foothold. Our prosperous institutions should help those institutions that God has said should live and prosper, but which are still struggling for an existence. There is among us a very limited amount of real, unselfish love. The Lord says: "Everyone that loveth is born of God, and knoweth God. He that loveth not knoweth not God; for God is love." "If we love one another, God dwelleth in us, and His love is perfected in us." 1 John 4:7, 8, 12. It is not pleasing to God to see man looking only upon his own things, closing his eyes to the interests of others.

What One Institution Can Do for Another

In the providence of God the Battle Creek Sanitarium has been greatly prospered, and during this coming year those in charge should restrict their wants. Instead of doing all that they desire to do in enlarging their facilities, they should do unselfish work for God, reaching out the hand of charity to interests centered in other places. What benefit they could confer upon the Rural Health Retreat, at Saint Helena, by giving a few thousand dollars to this enterprise! Such a donation would give courage to those in charge, inspiring them to move forward and upward.

Donations were made to the Battle Creek Sanitarium

in its earlier history, and should not this sanitarium consider carefully what it can do for its sister institution on the Pacific Coast? My brethren in Battle Creek, does it not seem in accordance with God's order to restrict your wants, to curtail your building operations, not enlarging our institutions in that center? Why should you not feel that it is your privilege and duty to help those who need help?

A Reformation Needed

I have been instructed that a reformation is needed along these lines, that more liberality should prevail among us. There is constant danger that even Seventh-day Adventists will be overcome with selfish ambition and will desire to center all the means and power in the interests over which they especially preside. There is danger that men will permit a jealous feeling to arise in their hearts and that they will become envious of interests that are as important as those which they are handling. Those who cherish the grace of pure Christianity cannot look with indifference upon any part of the work in the Lord's great vineyard. Those who are truly converted will have an equal interest in the work in all parts of the vineyard and will be ready to help wherever help is needed.

It is selfishness that hinders men from sending help to those places where the work of God is not as prosperous as it is in the institution over which they have supervision. Those who bear responsibilities should carefully seek for the good of every branch of the cause and work of God. They should encourage and sustain the interests in other fields, as well as the interests in their own. Thus the bonds of brotherhood would be strengthened between members of God's family on earth and the door would be closed to the petty jealousies and heartburnings that position and prosperity are sure to arouse unless the grace of God controls the heart.

"This I say," Paul wrote: "He which soweth sparingly shall reap also sparingly; and he which soweth bountifully shall reap also bountifully. Every man according as he purposeth in his heart, so let him give; not grudgingly, or of necessity: for God loveth a cheerful giver. And God is able to make all grace abound toward you; that ye, always having all sufficiency in all things, may abound to every good work;" "being enriched in everything to all bountifulness, which causeth through us thanksgiving to God. For the administration of this service not only supplieth the want of the saints, but is abundant also by many thanksgivings unto God; whiles by the experiment of this ministration they glorify God for your professed subjection unto the gospel of Christ, and for your liberal distribution unto them, and unto all men; and by their prayer for you, which long after you for the exceeding grace of God in you. Thanks be unto God for His unspeakable gift." 2 Corinthians 9:6-8, 11-15. . . .

The Question of Wages

The institution is now in a prosperous condition, and its managers should not insist upon the low rate of wages that was necessary in its earlier years. Worthy, efficient workers should receive reasonable wages for their labor, and they should be left to exercise their own judgment as to the use they make of their wages. In no case should they be overworked. The physician in chief himself should have larger wages.

To the physician in chief I wish to say: Although you have not the matter of wages under your personal supervision, it is best for you to look carefully into this matter; for you are responsible, as the head of the institution. Do not call upon the workers to do so much of the sacrificing. Restrict your ambition to enlarge the institution and to accumulate responsibilities. Let some of the means flowing into the sanitarium be given to the institutions needing help. This is certainly right. It is in accordance with God's will and way, and it will bring the blessing of God upon the sanitarium.

I wish to say particularly to the board of directors: "Remember that the workers should be paid according to their faithfulness. God requires us to deal with one another in the strictest faithfulness. Some of you are overburdened with cares and responsibilities, and I have been instructed that there is danger of your becoming selfish and wronging those whom you employ."

Each business transaction, whether it has to do with a worker occupying a position of responsibility, or with the lowliest worker connected with the sanitarium, should be such as God can approve. Walk in the light while you have the light, lest darkness come upon you. It would be far better to expend less in building and give your workers wages that are in accordance with the value of their work, exercising toward them mercy and justice.

From the light that the Lord has been pleased to give me, I know that He is not pleased with many things which have taken place in reference to the workers. God has not laid every particular open to me, but warnings have come that in many things decided reformation is needed. I have been shown that there is need of fathers and mothers in Israel being united with the institution. Devoted men and women should be employed who, because they are not continually pressed with cares and responsibilities, can look after the spiritual interests of the employees. It is necessary that such men and women should be constantly at work in missionary lines in this large institution. Not half is being done that should be done in this respect. It should be the part of these men and women to labor for the employees in spiritual lines, giving them instruction that will teach them how to win souls, showing them that this is to be done, not by much talking, but by a consistent, Christlike life. The workers are exposed to worldly influences, but instead of being molded by these influences, they should be consecrated missionaries, controlled by an influence that elevates and refines. Thus they will learn how to meet unbelievers, and how to exert an influence that will win them to Christ.

Channels of Blessing

Cooranbong, N.S.W., August 28, 1895.

God has a work for every believer who labors in the sanitarium. Every nurse is to be a channel of blessing, receiving light from above and letting it shine forth to others. The workers are not to conform to fashionable display of those who come to the sanitarium for treatment, but are to consecrate themselves to God. The atmosphere that surrounds their souls is to be a savor of life unto life. Temptations will beset them on every side, but let them ask God for His presence and guidance. The Lord said to Moses: "Certainly I will be with thee;" and to every faithful, consecrated worker the same assurance is given.

Reference for further study: *Testimonies for the Church,* vol. 7, pp. 292-294, "Our Sanitariums a Refuge for Workers."

Sanitarium Workers

Dear Brother:

Have you learned how much Dr. ——— proposes to charge for his services? If a physician does his work skillfully, his talent should be recognized, but there is danger of our being brought into perplexity. If we introduce a new system of paying our surgeons high wages, there may be a hard problem to settle after a time. Other physicians will demand high wages, and our ministers will require consideration, also. . . .

There is great necessity for decided reforms to be made in regard to our dealings with the workers in our sanitariums. Faithful, conscientious workers should be employed, and when they have performed a reasonable amount of work in a day they should be relieved that they may secure needed rest.

Only a reasonable amount of labor should be required, and for this the worker should receive a reasonable wage. If helpers are not given proper periods for rest from their taxing labor they will lose their strength and vitality. They cannot possibly do justice to the work, nor can they represent what a sanitarium employee should be. More helpers should be employed, if necessary, and the work should be so arranged that when one has performed a day's labor he may be freed to take the rest necessary to the maintenance of his strength.

Let no man consider it his place to judge of the amount of labor a woman should perform. A competent woman should be employed as matron, and if anyone does not perform her work faithfully, the matron should deal with the matter. Just wages should be paid, and every

Special Testimonies, Series B, No. 19, pp. 35-37 (1905).

woman should be treated kindly and courteously, without reproach.

And let those who have charge of the men's work be careful lest they be too exacting. The men should have regular hours for service, and when they have worked full time, they are not to be begrudged their periods of rest. A sanitarium is to be all that the name indicates.

Every worker should seek to educate himself to perform his work expeditiously. The matron should teach those under her charge how to make quick, careful movements. Train the young to perform the work with tact and thoroughness. Then when the hours of work are over, all will feel that the time has been faithfully spent and the workers are rightfully entitled to a period of rest.

Educational advantages should be provided for the workers in every sanitarium. The workers should be given every possible advantage consistent with the work assigned them.

Recognition of Honest Labor

Workers should receive compensation according to the hours they give in honest labor. The one who gives full time is to receive according to the time. If one enlists mind, soul, and strength in bearing the burdens, he is to be paid accordingly.—*Testimonies for the Church,* vol. 7, p. 208 (1902).

The Example of Christ

Dear Brother:

At one time you made the suggestion that if the managers of our institutions offered higher wages, they would secure a higher class of workmen and thus a higher grade of work. My brother, such reasoning is not in harmony with the Lord's plans. We are all His servants. We are not our own. We have been bought with a price and we are to glorify God in our body and in our spirit, which are His. This is a lesson that we need to learn. We need the discipline so essential to the development of completeness of Christian character.

Our institutions are to be entirely under the supervision of God. They were established in sacrifice, and only in sacrifice can their work be successfully carried forward.

A Broadening Work

Upon all who are engaged in the Lord's work rests the responsibility of fulfilling the commission: "Go ye therefore, and teach all nations, baptizing them in the name of the Father, and of the Son, and of the Holy Ghost: teaching them to observe all things whatsoever I have commanded you." Matthew 28:19, 20.

Christ Himself has given us an example of how we are to work. Read the fourth chapter of Matthew, and learn what methods Christ, the Prince of life, followed in His teaching. "Leaving Nazareth, He came and dwelt in Capernaum, which is upon the seacoast, in the borders of Zabulon and Nephthalim: that it might be fulfilled which was spoken by Esaias the prophet, saying, The land of Zabulon, and the land of Nephthalim, by the way

Special Testimonies, Series B, No. 19, pp. 37-40 (1903).

of the sea, beyond Jordan, Galilee of the Gentiles; the people which sat in darkness saw great light; and to them which sat in the region and shadow of death light is sprung up." Matthew 4:13-16.

"And Jesus, walking by the sea of Galilee, saw two brethren, Simon called Peter, and Andrew his brother, casting a net into the sea: for they were fishers. And He saith unto them, Follow Me, and I will make you fishers of men. And they straightway left their nets, and followed Him. And going on from thence, He saw other two brethren, James the son of Zebedee, and John his brother, in a ship with Zebedee their father, mending their nets; and He called them. And they immediately left the ship and their father, and followed Him." Matthew 4:18-22.

These humble fishermen were Christ's first disciples. He did not say that they were to receive a certain sum for their services. They were to share with Him His self-denial and sacrifices.

"And Jesus went about all Galilee, teaching in their synagogues, and preaching the gospel of the kingdom, and healing all manner of sickness and all manner of disease among the people. And His fame went throughout all Syria: and they brought unto Him all sick people that were taken with divers diseases and torments, and those which were possessed with devils, and those which were lunatic, and those that had the palsy; and He healed them." Matthew 4:23, 24.

In every sense of the word Christ was a medical missionary. He came to this world to preach the gospel and to heal the sick. He came as a healer of the bodies as well as the souls of human beings. His message was that obedience to the laws of the kingdom of God would bring men and women health and prosperity. . . .

Christ might have occupied the highest place among the highest teachers of the Jewish nation. But He chose rather to take the gospel to the poor. He went from place to place, that those in the highways and byways might catch the words of the gospel of truth. He labored in the way in which He desires His workers to labor today. By the sea, on the mountainside, in the streets of the city, His voice was heard, explaining the Old Testament Scriptures. So unlike the explanation of the scribes and Pharisees was His explanation that the attention of the people was arrested. He taught as one having authority, and not as the scribes. With clearness and power He proclaimed the gospel message.

Never was there such an evangelist as Christ. He was the Majesty of heaven, but He humbled Himself to take our nature that He might meet men where they were. To all people, rich and poor, free and bond, Christ, the Messenger of the Covenant, brought the tidings of salvation. How the people flocked to Him! From far and near they came for healing, and He healed them all. His fame as the Great Healer spread throughout Palestine, from Jerusalem to Syria. The sick came to the places through which they thought He would pass, that they might call on Him for help, and He healed them of their diseases. Hither, too, came the rich, anxious to hear His words and to receive a touch of His hand. Thus He went from city to city, from town to town, preaching the gospel and healing the sick—the King of glory in the lowly garb of humanity. "Though He was rich, yet for your sakes He became poor, that ye, through His poverty might be rich." 2 Corinthians 8:9.

Simplicity and Economy

In the establishment and carrying forward of the work, the strictest economy is ever to be shown. Workers are to be employed who will be producers as well as consumers. In no case is money to be invested for display. The gospel medical missionary work is to be carried forward in simplicity, as was the work of the Majesty of heaven, who, seeing the necessity of a lost, sinful world, laid aside His royal robe and kingly crown and clothed His divinity with humanity, that He might stand at the head of humanity. He so conducted His missionary work as to leave a perfect example for human beings to follow. "If any man will come after Me," He declared, "let him deny himself, and take up his cross, and follow Me." Matthew 16:24. Every true medical missionary will obey these words. He will not strain every nerve to follow worldly customs and make a display, thus thinking to win souls to the Saviour. No, no. If the Majesty of heaven could leave His glorious home to come to a world all seared and marred by the curse, to establish correct methods of doing medical missionary work, we His followers ought to practice the same self-denial and self-sacrifice.

Christ gives to all the invitation: "Come unto Me, all ye that labor and are heavy-laden, and I will give you rest. Take My yoke upon you, and learn of Me; for I am meek and lowly in heart: and ye shall find rest unto your souls. For My yoke is easy, and My burden is light." Matthew 11:28-30. If all will wear Christ's yoke, if all will learn in His school the lessons that He teaches, there will be sufficient means to establish gospel medical missionary work in many places.

Special Testimonies, Series B, No. 19, pp. 27-29 (1904).

Let none say, "I will engage in this work for a stipulated sum. If I do not receive this sum, I will not do the work." Those who say this show that they are not wearing Christ's yoke; they are not learning His meekness and lowliness. Christ might have come to this world with a retinue of angels, but instead He came as a babe and lived a life of lowliness and poverty. His glory was in His simplicity. He suffered for us the privations of poverty. Shall we refuse to deny ourselves for His sake? Shall we refuse to become medical missionary workers unless we can follow the customs of the world, making a display such as worldlings make? . . .

My brother, my sister, take up your work right where you are. Do your best, ever looking to Jesus, the Author and Finisher of our faith. In no other way can we do the work of God and magnify His truth than by following in the footsteps of Him who gave up His high command to come to our world, that through His humiliation and suffering, human beings might become partakers of the divine nature. For our sake He became poor, that through His poverty we might come into possession of the eternal riches. . . .

Intelligent, self-denying, self-sacrificing men are now needed—men who realize the solemnity and importance of God's work, and who as Christian philanthropists will fulfill the commission of Christ. The medical missionary work given us to do means something to every one of us. It is a work of soul saving; it is the proclamation of the gospel message.

THE CHRISTIAN PHYSICIAN

A Responsible Calling

"The fear of the Lord is the beginning of wisdom." Psalm 111:10. Professional men, whatever their calling, need divine wisdom. But the physician is in special need of this wisdom in dealing with all classes of minds and diseases. He occupies a position even more responsible than that of the minister of the gospel. He is called to be a colaborer with Christ, and he needs stanch religious principles and a firm connection with the God of wisdom. If he takes counsel of God, he will have the Great Healer to work with his efforts and he will move with the greatest caution, lest by his mismanagement he injure one of God's creatures. He will be firm as a rock to principle, yet kind and courteous to all. He will feel the responsibility of his position, and his practice will show that he is actuated by pure, unselfish motives and a desire to adorn the doctrine of Christ in all things. Such a physician will possess a heaven-born dignity and will be a powerful agent for good in the world. Although he may not be appreciated by those who have no connection with God, yet he will be honored of Heaven. In God's sight he will be more precious than gold, even the gold of Ophir.

An Example in Temperance

The physician should be a strictly temperate man. The physical ailments of humanity are numberless, and he has to deal with disease in all its varied forms. He

---

Testimonies for the Church, vol. 5, pp. 439-449 (1885).

knows that much of the suffering he seeks to relieve is the result of intemperance and other forms of selfish indulgence. He is called to attend young men and men in the prime of life and in mature age, who have brought disease upon themselves by the use of the narcotic tobacco. If he is an intelligent physician, he will be able to trace disease to its cause; but unless he is free from the use of tobacco himself, he will hesitate to put his finger upon the plague spot and faithfully unfold to his patients the cause of their sickness. He will fail to urge upon the young the necessity of overcoming the habit before it becomes fixed. If he uses the weed himself, how can he present to the inexperienced youth its injurious effects, not only upon themselves, but upon those around them? . . .

Of all men in the world, the physician and the minister should have strictly temperate habits. The welfare of society demands total abstinence of them, for their influence is constantly telling for or against moral reform and the improvement of society. It is willful sin in them to be ignorant of the laws of health or indifferent to them, for they are looked up to as wise above other men. This is especially true of the physician, who is entrusted with human life. He is expected to indulge in no habit that will weaken the life forces. . . .

The question is not, What is the world doing? but, What are professional men doing in regard to the widespread and prevailing curse of tobacco using? Will men to whom God has given intelligence, and who are in positions of sacred trust, be true to follow intelligent reason? Will these responsible men, having under their care persons whom their influence will lead in a right or a wrong direction, be pattern men? Will they, by precept and example, teach obedience to the laws which govern the physical system? If they do not put to a practical use the knowledge they have of the laws that govern their own being, if they prefer present gratification to soundness of mind and body, they are not fit to be entrusted with the lives of others. They are in duty bound to stand in the dignity of their God-given manhood, free from the bondage of any appetite or passion.

The man who chews and smokes is doing injury, not only to himself, but to all who come within the sphere of his influence. If a physician must be called, the tobacco devotee should be passed by. He will not be a safe counselor. If the disease has its origin in the use of tobacco, he will be tempted to prevaricate and assign some other than the true cause, for how can he condemn himself in his own daily practice?

There are many ways of practicing the healing art, but there is only one way that Heaven approves. God's remedies are the simple agencies of nature, that will not tax or debilitate the system through their powerful properties. Pure air and water, cleanliness, a proper diet, purity of life, and a firm trust in God, are remedies for the want of which thousands are dying, yet these remedies are going out of date because their skillful use requires work that the people do not appreciate. Fresh air, exercise, pure water, and clean, sweet premises, are within the reach of all with but little expense; but drugs are expensive, both in the outlay of means and the effect produced upon the system.

A Healer of Spiritual Maladies

The work of the Christian physician does not end with healing the maladies of the body; his efforts should extend to the diseases of the mind, to the saving of the soul. It may not be his duty, unless asked, to present any theoretical points of truth; but he may point his patients to Christ. The lessons of the divine Teacher are ever appropriate. He should call the attention of the repining to the ever-fresh tokens of the love and care of God, to His wisdom and goodness as manifested in His created works. The mind can then be led through nature up to nature's God, and centered on the heaven which He has prepared for those that love Him.

The physician should know how to pray. In many cases he must increase suffering in order to save life; and whether the patient is a Christian or not, he feels greater security if he knows that his physician fears God. Prayer will give the sick an abiding confidence; and many times if their cases are borne to the Great Physician in humble trust, it will do more for them than all the drugs that can be administered.

Satan is the originator of disease, and the physician is warring against his work and power. Sickness of the mind prevails everywhere. Nine tenths of the diseases from which men suffer have their foundation here. Perhaps some living home trouble is, like a canker, eating to the very soul and weakening the life forces. Remorse for sin sometimes undermines the constitution and unbalances the mind. There are erroneous doctrines also, as that of an eternally burning hell and the endless torment of the wicked, that, by giving exaggerated and distorted views of the character of God, have produced the same result upon sensitive minds. Infidels have made the most of these unfortunate cases, attributing insanity to religion, but this is a gross libel, and one which they will not be pleased to meet by and by. The religion of Christ, so far from being the cause of insanity, is one of its most effectual remedies; for it is a potent soother of the nerves.

The physician needs more than human wisdom and power that he may know how to minister to the many perplexing cases of disease of the mind and heart with which he is called to deal. If he is ignorant of the power of divine grace, he cannot help the afflicted one, but will aggravate the difficulty; but if he has a firm hold upon God, he will be able to help the diseased, distracted mind. He will be able to point his patients to Christ and teach them to carry all their cares and perplexities to the great Burden Bearer.

There is a divinely appointed connection between sin and disease. No physician can practice for a month without seeing this illustrated. He may ignore the fact; his mind may be so occupied with other matters that his attention will not be called to it; but if he will be observing and honest, he cannot help acknowledging that sin and disease bear to each other the relationship of cause and effect. The physician should be quick to see this and to act accordingly. When he has gained the confidence of the afflicted by relieving their sufferings and bringing them back from the verge of the grave, he may teach them that disease is the result of sin, and that it is the fallen foe who seeks to allure them to health-and-soul-destroying practices. He may impress their minds with the necessity of denying self and obeying the laws of life and health. In the minds of the young especially he may instill right principles. God loves His creatures with a love that is both tender and strong. He has established the laws of nature; but His laws are not arbitrary exactions. Every "Thou shalt not," whether in physical or moral law, contains or implies a promise. If it is obeyed, blessings will attend our steps; if it is disobeyed, the result is danger and unhappiness. The laws of God are designed to bring His people closer to Himself. He will save them from the evil and lead them to the good, if they will be led; but force them He never will. . . .

Physicians who love and fear God are few compared with those who are infidels or openly irreligious; and these should be patronized in preference to the latter class. We may well distrust the ungodly physician. A door of temptation is open to him, a wily devil will suggest base thoughts and actions, and it is only the power of divine grace that can quell tumultuous passion and fortify against sin. To those who are morally corrupt, opportunities to corrupt pure minds are not wanting. But how will the licentious physician appear in the day of God? While professing to care for the sick, he has betrayed sacred trusts. He has degraded both the soul and the body of God's creatures and has set their feet in the path that leads to perdition. How terrible to trust our loved ones in the hands of an impure man, who may poison the morals and ruin the soul! How out of place is the godless physician at the bedside of the dying!

Familiarity With Suffering

The physician is almost daily brought face to face with death. He is, as it were, treading upon the verge of the grave. In many instances familiarity with scenes of suffering and death results in carelessness and indifference to human woe and recklessness in the treatment of the sick. Such physicians seem to have no tender sympathy. They are harsh and abrupt, and the sick dread their approach. Such men, however great their knowledge and skill, can do the suffering little good; but if the love and sympathy that Jesus manifested for the sick is combined with the physician's knowledge, his very presence will be a blessing. He will not look upon his patient as a mere piece of human mechanism, but as a soul to be saved or lost.

The Physician's Need of Sympathy

The duties of the physician are arduous. Few realize the mental and physical strain to which he is subjected. Every energy and capability must be enlisted with the most intense anxiety in the battle with disease and death. Often he knows that one unskillful movement of the hand, even but a hair's breadth in the wrong direction, may send a soul unprepared into eternity. How much the faithful physician needs the sympathy and prayers of the people of God. His claims in this direction are not inferior to those of the most devoted minister or missionary worker. Deprived, as he often is, of needed rest and sleep, and even of religious privileges on the Sabbath, he needs a double portion of grace, a fresh supply daily, or he will lose his hold on God and will be in danger of sinking deeper in spiritual darkness than men of other callings. And yet often he is made to bear unmerited reproaches and is left to stand alone, the subject of Satan's fiercest temptations, feeling himself misunderstood, betrayed by his friends.

Many, knowing how trying are the duties of the physician, and how few opportunities physicians have for release from care, even upon the Sabbath, will not choose this for their lifework. But the great enemy is constantly seeking to destroy the workmanship of God's hands, and men of culture and intelligence are called upon to combat his cruel power. More of the right kind of men are needed to devote themselves to this profession. Painstaking effort should be made to induce suitable men to qualify themselves for this work. They should be men whose characters are based upon the broad principles of the word of God—men who possess a natural energy, force, and perseverance that will enable them to reach a high standard of excellence. It is not everyone who can make a successful physician. Many have entered upon the duties of this profession every way unprepared. They have not the requisite knowledge, neither have they the skill and tact, the carefulness and intelligence, necessary to ensure success.

A physician can do much better work if he has physical strength. If he is feeble, he cannot endure the wearing labor incident to his calling. A man who has a weak constitution, who is a dyspeptic, or who has not perfect self-control, cannot become qualified to deal with all classes of disease. Great care should be taken not to encourage persons who might be useful in some less responsible position, to study medicine at a great outlay of time and means, when there is no reasonable hope that they will succeed.

Unfaithfulness and Infidelity

Some have been singled out as men who might be useful as physicians, and they have been encouraged to take a medical course. But some who commenced their studies in the medical colleges as Christians, did not keep the divine law prominent; they sacrificed principle and lost their hold on God. They felt that singlehanded they could not keep the fourth commandment and meet the jeers and ridicule of the ambitious, the world-loving, the superficial, the skeptic, and the infidel. This kind of persecution they were not prepared to meet. They were ambitious to climb higher in the world, and they stumbled on the dark mountains of unbelief and became untrustworthy. Temptations of every kind opened before them and they had no strength to resist. Some of these have become dishonest, scheming policy men and are guilty of grave sins.

In this age there is danger for everyone who shall enter upon the study of medicine. Often his instructors are worldly-wise men and his fellow students infidels who have no thought of God, and he is in danger of being influenced by these irreligious associations. Nevertheless, some have gone through the medical course and have remained true to principle. They would not continue their studies on the Sabbath, and they have proved that men may become qualified for the duties of a physician and not disappoint the expectations of those who furnish them means to obtain an education. Like Daniel, they have honored God, and He has kept them. Daniel purposed in his heart that he would not adopt the customs of kingly courts; he would not eat of the king's meat nor drink of his wine. He looked to God for strength and grace, and God gave him wisdom and skill and knowledge above that of the astrologers, the soothsayers, and the magicians of the kingdom. To him the promise was verified, "Them that honor Me I will honor." Samuel 2:30.

The young physician has access to the God of Daniel. Through divine grace and power he may become as efficient in his calling as Daniel was in his exalted position. But it is a mistake to make a scientific preparation the all-important thing, while religious principles, that lie at the very foundation of a successful practice, are neglected. Many are lauded as skillful men in their profession, who scorn the thought that they need to rely upon Jesus for wisdom in their work. But if these men who trust in their knowledge of science were illuminated by the light of Heaven, to how much greater excellence might they attain! How much stronger would be their powers, with how much greater confidence could they undertake difficult cases! The man who is closely connected with the Great Physician of soul and body has the resources of heaven and earth at his command, and he can work with a wisdom, an unerring precision, that the godless man cannot possess.

Those to whom the care of the sick is entrusted, whether as physicians or nurses, should remember that their work must stand the scrutiny of the piercing eye of Jehovah. There is no missionary field more important than that occupied by the faithful, God-fearing physician. There is no field where a man may accomplish greater good or win more jewels to shine in the crown of his rejoicing. He may carry the grace of Christ, as a sweet perfume, into all the sickrooms he enters; he may carry the true healing balm to the sin-sick soul. He can point the sick and dying to the Lamb of God that taketh away the sin of the world. He should not listen to the suggestion that it is dangerous to speak of their eternal interests to those whose lives are in peril, lest it should make them worse, for in nine cases out of ten the knowledge of a sin-pardoning Saviour would make them better both in mind and body. Jesus can limit the power of Satan. He is the physician in whom the sin-sick soul may trust to heal the maladies of the body as well as of the soul.

References for further study: *Testimonies for the Church,* vol. 6, pp. 243-253, "Responsibilities of Medical Workers;" *The Ministry of Healing,* pages 111-124, "The Co-working of the Divine and the Human."

The Physician's Work for Souls

Every medical practitioner may through faith in Christ have in his possession a cure of the highest value—a remedy for the sin-sick soul. The physician who is converted and sanctified through the truth is registered in heaven as a laborer together with God, a follower of Jesus Christ. Through the sanctification of the truth, God gives to physicians and nurses wisdom and skill in treating the sick, and this work is opening the fast-closed door to many hearts. Men and women are led to understand the truth which is needed to save the soul as well as the body.

This is an element that gives character to the work for this time. The medical missionary work is as the right arm of the third angel's message which must be proclaimed to a fallen world; and physicians, managers, and workers in any line, in acting faithfully their part, are doing the work of the message. Thus the sound of the truth will go forth to every nation and kindred and tongue and people. In this work the heavenly angels bear a part. They awaken spiritual joy and melody in the hearts of those who have been freed from suffering, and thanksgiving to God arises from the lips of many who have received the precious truth.

Every physician in our ranks should be a Christian. Only those physicians who are genuine Bible Christians can discharge aright the high duties of their profession.

The physician who understands the responsibility and accountability of his position will feel the necessity of Christ's presence with him in his work for those for whom such a sacrifice has been made. He will subordinate everything to the higher interests which concern the life that

Testimonies for the Church, vol. 6, pp. 229-234 (1900).

may be saved unto life eternal. He will do all in his power to save both the body and the soul. He will try to do the very work that Christ would do were He in his place. The physician who loves Christ and the souls for whom Christ died will seek earnestly to bring into the sickroom a leaf from the tree of life. He will try to break the bread of life to the sufferer. Notwithstanding the obstacles and difficulties to be met, this is the solemn, sacred work of the medical profession.

Christ's Methods to Be Copied

True missionary work is that in which the Saviour's work is best represented, His methods most closely copied, His glory best promoted. Missionary work that falls short of this standard is recorded in heaven as defective. It is weighed in the balances of the sanctuary and found wanting.

Physicians should seek to direct the minds of their patients to Christ, the Physician of soul and body. That which physicians can only attempt to do, Christ accomplishes. The human agent strives to prolong life. Christ is life itself. He who passed through death to destroy him that had the power of death is the Source of all vitality. There is balm in Gilead, and a Physician there. Christ endured an agonizing death under the most humiliating circumstances that we might have life. He gave up His precious life that He might vanquish death. But He rose from the tomb, and the myriads of angels who came to behold Him take up the life He had laid down heard His words of triumphant joy as He stood above Joseph's rent sepulcher proclaiming, "I am the resurrection and the life."

The question, "If a man die, shall he live again?" has been answered. By bearing the penalty of sin, by going down into the grave, Christ has brightened the tomb for all who die in faith. God in human form has brought life and immortality to light through the gospel. In dying, Christ secured eternal life for all who believe in Him. In dying, He condemned the originator of sin and disloyalty to suffer the penalty of sin—eternal death.

The possessor and giver of eternal life, Christ was the only one who could conquer death. He is our Redeemer, and blessed is every physician who is in a true sense of the word a missionary, a savior of souls for whom Christ gave His life. Such a physician learns day by day from the Great Physician how to watch and work for the saving of the souls and bodies of men and women. The Saviour is present in the sickroom, in the operating room; and His power for His name's glory accomplishes great things.

The Physician Can Point to Jesus

The physician can do a noble work if he is connected with the Great Physician. To the relatives of the sick, whose hearts are full of sympathy for the sufferer, he may find opportunity to speak the words of life; and he can soothe and uplift the mind of the sufferer by leading him to look to the One who can save to the uttermost all who come to Him for salvation.

When the Spirit of God works on the mind of the afflicted one, leading him to inquire for truth, let the physician work for the precious soul as Christ would work for it. Do not urge upon him any special doctrine, but point him to Jesus as the sin-pardoning Saviour. Angels of God will impress the mind. Some will refuse to be illuminated by the light which God would let shine into the chambers of the mind and into the soul temple; but many will respond to the light, and from these minds deception and error in their various forms will be swept away.

Every opportunity of working as Christ worked should be carefully improved. The physician should talk of the works of healing wrought by Christ, of His tenderness and love. He should believe that Jesus is his companion, close by his side. "We are laborers together with God." 1 Corinthians 3:9. Never should the physician neglect to direct the minds of his patients to Christ, the Chief Physician. If he has the Saviour abiding in his own heart, his thoughts will ever be directed to the Healer of soul and body. He will lead the minds of sufferers to Him who can restore, who, when on earth, restored the sick to health and healed the soul as well as the body, saying, "Son, thy sins be forgiven thee." Mark 2:5.

Never should familiarity with suffering cause the physician to become careless or unsympathetic. In cases of dangerous illness, the afflicted one feels that he is at the mercy of the physician. He looks to that physician as his only earthly hope, and the physician should ever point the trembling soul to One who is greater than himself, even the Son of God, who gave His life to save him from death, who pities the sufferer, and who by His divine power will give skill and wisdom to all who ask Him.

When the patient knows not how his case will turn is the time for the physician to impress the mind. He should not do this with a desire to distinguish himself, but that he may point the soul to Christ as a personal Saviour. If the life is spared, there is a soul for that physician to watch for. The patient feels that the physician is the very life of his life. And to what purpose should this great confidence be employed? Always to win a soul to Christ and magnify the power of God.

Let Praise Be Given to God

When the crisis has passed and success is apparent, be the patient a believer or an unbeliever, let a few moments be spent with him in prayer. Give expression to your thankfulness for the life that has been spared. The physician who follows such a course carries his patient to the One upon whom he is dependent for life. Words of gratitude may flow from the patient to the physician, for through God he has bound this life up with his own; but let the praise and thanksgiving be given to God, as to One who is present though invisible.

On the sickbed Christ is often accepted and confessed; and this will be done oftener in the future than it has been in the past, for a quick work will the Lord do in our world. Words of wisdom are to be on the lips of the physician, and Christ will water the seed sown, causing it to bring forth fruit unto eternal life.

A Word in Season

We lose the most precious opportunities by neglecting to speak a word in season. Too often a precious talent that ought to produce a thousandfold is left unused. If the golden privilege is not watched for it will pass. Something was allowed to prevent the physician from doing his appointed work as a minister of righteousness.

There are none too many godly physicians to minister in their profession. There is much work to be done, and ministers and doctors are to work in perfect union. Luke, the writer of the Gospel that bears his name, is called the beloved physician, and those who do a work similar to that which he did are living out the gospel.

Countless are the opportunities of the physician for warning the impenitent, cheering the disconsolate and hopeless, and prescribing for the health of mind and body. As he thus instructs the people in the principles of true temperance, and as a guardian of souls gives advice to those who are mentally and physically diseased, the physician is acting his part in the great work of making ready a people prepared for the Lord. This is what medical missionary work is to accomplish in its relation to the third angel's message.

Ministers and physicians are to work harmoniously with earnestness to save souls that are becoming entangled in Satan's snares. They are to point men and women to Jesus, their righteousness, their strength, and the health of their countenance. Continually they are to watch for souls. There are those who are struggling with strong temptations, in danger of being overcome in the fight with satanic agencies. Will you pass these by without offering them assistance? If you see a soul in need of help, engage in conversation with him even though you do not know him. Pray with him. Point him to Jesus.

This work belongs just as surely to the doctor as to the minister. By public and private effort the physician should seek to win souls to Christ.

In all our enterprises and in all our institutions God is to be acknowledged as the Master Worker. The physicians are to stand as His representatives. The medical fraternity have made many reforms, and they are still to advance. Those who hold the lives of human beings in their hands should be educated, refined, sanctified. Then will the Lord work through them in mighty power to glorify His name.

References for further study: *The Ministry of Healing,* pages 17-28, "Our Example;" pages 29-50, "Days of Ministry;" pages 73-94, "Healing of the Soul."

The Sphere of Leading Physicians

Precious light has been given me concerning our sanitarium workers. These workers are to stand in moral dignity before God. Physicians make a mistake when they confine themselves exclusively to the routine of sanitarium work, because they consider their presence essential to the welfare of the institution. Every physician should see the necessity of exerting all the influence the Lord has given him in as wide a sphere as possible; he is required to let his light shine before men, that they may see his good works and glorify the Father who is in heaven.

The head physicians in our sanitariums are not to exclude themselves from the work of speaking the truth to others. Their light is not to be hidden under a bushel, but placed where it can benefit believers and unbelievers. The Saviour said of His representatives: "Ye are the salt of the earth: but if the salt have lost his savor, wherewith shall it be salted? it is thenceforth good for nothing, but to be cast out, and to be trodden underfoot of men. Ye are the light of the world. A city that is set on an hill cannot be hid. Neither do men light a candle, and put it under a bushel, but on a candlestick; and it giveth light unto all that are in the house. Let your light so shine before men, that they may see your good works, and glorify your Father which is in heaven." Matthew 5:13-16. This is a work that is strangely neglected, and because of this neglect, souls will be lost. Wake up, my brethren, wake up!

Their Light to Shine Abroad

Our leading physicians do not glorify God when they confine their talents and their influence to one institu-

Review and Herald, Aug. 13, 1914.

tion. It is their privilege to show to the world that health reformers carry a decided influence for righteousness and truth. They should make themselves known outside of the institutions where they labor. It is their duty to give the light to all whom they can possibly reach. While the sanitarium may be their special field of labor, yet there are other places of importance that need their influence. To physicians the instruction is given: Let your light shine forth among men. Let every talent be used to meet unbelievers with wise counsel and instruction. If our Christian physicians will consider that there must be no daubing with untempered mortar and will learn to handle wisely the subjects of Bible truth, seeking to present its importance on every possible occasion, much prejudice will be broken down and souls will be reached. . . .

We are not to be an obscure church, but we are to let the light shine forth, that the world may receive it. "I will rejoice in Jerusalem, and joy in My people," God declares through His servant Isaiah. Isaiah 65:19. These words will be proved true when those who are capable of standing in positions of responsibility let the light shine forth. Our leading physicians have a work to do outside the compass of our own people. Their influence is not to be limited. Christ's methods of labor are to become their methods, and they are to learn to practice the teachings of His word. Everyone who stands at the head of an institution is under sacred obligation to God to show forth the light of present truth in increasingly bright rays in every place where opportunity offers.

The workers in our sanitariums are not to think that the prosperity of the institution depends upon the influence of the head physician alone. There should be in every institution men and women who will exert a righteous, refining influence, and who are capable of carrying responsibilities. The chief responsibilities should be shared by several workers, in order that the leading physician may not be confined too closely to his practice. He should be given opportunity to go where there is need of words of counsel and encouragement to be spoken. As a representative of the Chief Physician, now in the heavenly courts, he is to speak to new congregations, to broaden his experience. He needs to be constantly receiving new ideas, constantly imparting of his store of knowledge, constantly receiving from the Source of all wisdom. We need ever to keep ourselves in a position where we can receive increased light, have new and deeper thoughts, and obtain clearer views of the close relation that must exist between God and His people. And we obtain these views and these ideas by association with those to whom we are called to speak words of mercy and pardoning grace.

In all our work there should be kept in view the value of the exchange of talents. Strenuous efforts are to be put forth to reach souls and win them to the truth. We are required to make known the principles of health reform in the large gatherings of our people at our camp meetings. A variety of gifts is needed on these occasions, not only for the work of speaking before those not of our faith, but to instruct our own people how to work in order to secure the best success. Let our physicians learn how to take part in this work—a work by which they give to the world bright rays of light.

_____

Reference for further study: *Testimonies for the Church*, vol. 8, pp. 231-235, "A Division of Responsibility."

Ready for Every Good Work

The Lord will hear and answer the prayer of the Christian physician, and he may reach an elevated standard if he will but lay hold upon the hand of Christ and determine that he will not let go. Golden opportunities are open to the Christian physician, for he may exert a precious influence upon those with whom he is brought in contact. He may guide and mold and fashion the lives of his patients by holding before them heavenly principles.

The physician should let men see that he does not regard his work as of a cheap order, but looks upon it as high, noble, elevated work, even that to which is attached the sacred accountability of dealing with both the souls and the bodies of those for whom Christ has paid the infinite price of His most precious blood. If the physician has the mind of Christ, he will be cheerful, hopeful, and happy, but not trifling. He will realize that heavenly angels accompany him to the sickroom and will find words to speak readily, truthfully, to his patients, that will cheer and bless them. His faith will be full of simplicity, of childlike confidence in the Lord. He will be able to repeat to the repenting soul the gracious promises of God and thus place the trembling hand of the afflicted ones in the hand of Christ, that they may find repose in God.

Thus, through the grace imparted to him, the physician will fulfill his heavenly Father's claims upon him. In delicate and perilous operations he may know that Jesus is by his side to counsel, to strengthen, to nerve him to act with precision and skill in his efforts to save human

Health, Philanthropic, and Medical Missionary Work, pages 36-40 (1892).

life. If the presence of God is not in the sickroom, Satan will be there to suggest perilous experiments and will seek to unbalance the nerves, so that life will be destroyed rather than saved.

A physician occupies a more important position, because of dealing with morbid souls, diseased minds, and afflicted bodies, than does the minister of the gospel. The physician can present an elevated standard of Christian character, if he will be instant in season and out of season. He is thus a missionary for the Lord, doing the Master's work with fidelity, and will receive a reward by and by.

Let the Christian keep his own counsel and divulge no secret to unbelievers. Let him communicate no secret that will disparage God's people. Guard your thoughts, close the door to temptation. Do your work as in the sight of the divine Watcher. Work patiently, expecting that, through the grace of Christ, you will make a success in your profession. Keep up the barriers which the Lord has erected for your safety. Keep your heart with all diligence, for out of it are the issues of life, or of death.

A physician should attend strictly to his professional work. He should not allow anything to come in to divert his mind from his business, or to take his attention from those who are looking to him for relief from suffering. An assuring and hopeful word spoken in season to the sufferer will often relieve his mind and win for the physician a place in his confidence. Kindness and courtesy should be manifested; but the common, cheap talk which is so customary even among some who claim to be Christians, should not be heard in our institutions. The only way for us to become truly courteous, without affectation, without undue familiarity, is to drink in the spirit of Christ, to heed the injunction, "Be ye holy; for I am holy."

1 Peter 1:16. If we act upon the principles laid down in the word of God, we shall have no inclination to indulge in undue familiarity.

The workers in our institutions should be living examples of what they desire those to be who are patients in the institution. A right spirit and a holy life are a constant instruction to others. The hollowhearted courtesy of the fashionable world is of no value in the sight of Him by whom actions are weighed. There should be no partiality and no hypocrisy. The physician should be ready for every good work. If his life is hid with Christ in God, he will be a missionary in the highest sense.

When they are together, Christian physicians will conduct themselves as sons of God. They will realize that they are engaged to work in the same vineyard, and selfish barriers will be broken down. For each other they will feel a deep interest, untainted with selfishness. He who is himself a reformer can accomplish good in seeking to reform others. By precept and example he can be a savor of life unto life. Would that the curtain could be rolled back, and we could see how interestedly the angels of God are looking upon the institutions for the treatment of the sick. The work in which the physician is engaged —standing between the living and the dead—is of special importance.

God has given a great work into the hand of physicians. The afflicted children of men are in a degree at their mercy. How the patient watches him who cares for his physical welfare. The actions and words, the very expressions of the physician's countenance, are matters of study. What gratitude springs up in the heart of the suffering one when his pain is relieved through the efforts of his faithful physician. The patient feels that his life is in the hands of him who thus ministers to him, and the physician or the nurse can then easily approach him on religious subjects. If the sufferer is under the control of divine influences, how gently can the Christian physician or nurse drop the precious seeds of truth into the garden of the heart. He can bring the promise of God before the soul of the helpless one. If the physician has religion, he can impart the fragrance of heavenly grace to the softened and subdued heart of the suffering one. He can direct the thoughts of his patient to the Great Physician. He can present Jesus to the sin-sick soul.

How often the physician is made a confidant, and griefs and trials are laid open before him by the sick. At such a time what precious opportunities are afforded to speak words of comfort and consolation in the fear and love of God, and to impart Christian counsel. Deep love for souls for whom Christ died should imbue the physician. In the fear of God I tell you that none but a Christian physician can rightly discharge the duties of this sacred profession.

Bearing Witness to the Truth

Our sanitariums are to be established for one object —the proclamation of the truth for this time. And they are to be so conducted that a decided impression in favor of the truth will be made on the minds of those who come to them for treatment. The conduct of each worker is to tell on the side of right. We have a warning message to bear to the world, and our earnestness, our devotion to God's service, are to bear witness to the truth.—*Testimonies for the Church,* vol. 8, p. 200 (1904).

Mind Cure

The relation that exists between the mind and the body is very intimate. When one is affected, the other sympathizes. The condition of the mind affects the health to a far greater degree than many realize. Many of the diseases from which men suffer are the result of mental depression. Grief, anxiety, discontent, remorse, guilt, distrust, all tend to break down the life forces and to invite decay and death.

Disease is sometimes produced, and is often greatly aggravated, by the imagination. Many are lifelong invalids who might be well if they only thought so. Many imagine that every slight exposure will cause illness, and the evil effect is produced because it is expected. Many die from disease, the cause of which is wholly imaginary.

Courage, hope, faith, sympathy, love, promote health and prolong life. A contented mind, a cheerful spirit, is health to the body and strength to the soul. "A merry [rejoicing] heart doeth good like a medicine." Proverbs 17:22.

In the treatment of the sick, the effect of mental influence should not be overlooked. Rightly used, this influence affords one of the most effective agencies for combating disease.

Control of Mind Over Mind

There is, however, a form of mind cure that is one of the most effective agencies for evil. Through this so-called science, one mind is brought under the control of another, so that the individuality of the weaker is merged in that of the stronger mind. One person acts out the will of another. Thus it is claimed that the tenor of the thoughts

The Ministry of Healing, pages 241-244 (1905).

may be changed, that health-giving impulses may be imparted and patients may be enabled to resist and overcome disease.

This method of cure has been employed by persons who were ignorant of its real nature and tendency, and who believed it to be a means of benefit to the sick. But the so-called science is based upon false principles. It is foreign to the nature and spirit of Christ. It does not lead to Him who is life and salvation. The one who attracts minds to himself leads them to separate from the true Source of their strength.

It is not God's purpose that any human being should yield his mind and will to the control of another, becoming a passive instrument in his hands. No one is to merge his individuality in that of another. He is not to look to any human being as the source of healing. His dependence must be in God. In the dignity of his God-given manhood, he is to be controlled by God Himself, not by any human intelligence.

God desires to bring men into direct relation with Himself. In all His dealings with human beings He recognizes the principle of personal responsibility. He seeks to encourage a sense of personal dependence, and to impress the need of personal guidance. He desires to bring the human into association with the divine, that men may be transformed into the divine likeness. Satan works to thwart this purpose. He seeks to encourage dependence upon men. When minds are turned away from God, the tempter can bring them under his rule. He can control humanity.

The theory of mind controlling mind was originated by Satan to introduce himself as the chief worker, to put human philosophy where divine philosophy should be. Of all the errors that are finding acceptance among professedly Christian people, none is a more dangerous deception, none more certain to separate man from God, than is this. Innocent though it may appear, if exercised upon patients it will tend to their destruction, not to their restoration. It opens a door through which Satan will enter to take possession both of the mind that is given up to be controlled by another, and of the mind that controls.

Fearful is the power thus given to evil-minded men and women. What opportunities it affords to those who live by taking advantage of other's weaknesses or follies! How many, through control of minds feeble or diseased, will find a means of gratifying lustful passion or greed of gain!

There is something better for us to engage in than the control of humanity by humanity. The physician should educate the people to look from the human to the divine. Instead of teaching the sick to depend upon human beings for the cure of soul and body, he should direct them to the One who can save to the uttermost all who come unto Him. He who made man's mind knows what the mind needs. God alone is the one who can heal. Those whose minds and bodies are diseased are to behold in Christ the restorer. "Because I live," He says, "ye shall live also." This is the life we are to present to the sick, telling them that if they have faith in Christ as the restorer, if they co-operate with Him, obeying the laws of health and striving to perfect holiness in His fear, He will impart to them His life. When we present Christ to them in this way, we are imparting a power, a strength, that is of value; for it comes from above. This is the true science of healing for body and soul.

References for further study: *Testimonies for the Church,* vol. 3, pp. 168, 169; *The Ministry of Healing,* pages 246-260.

Christlike Compassion

I was shown that the physicians at our Institute should be men and women of faith and spirituality. They should make God their trust. There are many who come to the Institute who have, by their own sinful indulgence, brought upon themselves disease of almost every type. This class do not deserve the sympathy that they frequently require. And it is painful to the physicians to devote time and strength to this class, who are debased physically, mentally, and morally.

But there is a class who have, through ignorance, lived in violation of nature's laws. They have worked intemperately and have eaten intemperately, because it was the custom to do so. Some have suffered many things from many physicians, but have not been made better, but decidedly worse. At length they are torn from business, from society, and from their families; and as their last resort, they come to the Health Institute, with some faint hope that they may find relief. This class need sympathy. They should be treated with the greatest tenderness, and care should be taken to make clear to their understanding the laws of their being, that they may, by ceasing to violate them, and by governing themselves, avoid suffering and disease, the penalty of nature's violated law. . . .

Remember Christ, who came in direct contact with suffering humanity. Although, in many cases, the afflicted had brought disease upon themselves by their sinful course in violating natural law, Jesus pitied their weakness, and when they came to Him with disease the most loathsome,

Testimonies for the Church, vol. 3, pp. 178-184 (1872).

(347)

He did not stand aloof for fear of contamination; He touched them and bade disease give back.

Healing the Lepers

"And as He entered into a certain village, there met Him ten men that were lepers, which stood afar off: and they lifted up their voices, and said, Jesus, Master, have mercy on us. And when He saw them, He said unto them, Go show yourselves unto the priests. And it came to pass, that, as they went, they were cleansed. And one of them, when he saw that he was healed, turned back, and with a loud voice glorified God, and fell down on his face at His feet, giving Him thanks: and he was a Samaritan. And Jesus answering said, Were there not ten cleansed? but where are the nine? There are not found that returned to give glory to God, save this stranger. And He said unto him, Arise, go thy way: thy faith hath made thee whole." Luke 17:12-19.

Here is a lesson for us all. These lepers were so corrupted by disease that they had been restricted from society lest they should contaminate others. Their limits had been prescribed by the authorities. Jesus comes within their sight, and in their great suffering, they cry unto Him who alone has power to relieve them. Jesus bids them show themselves to the priests. They have faith to start on their way, believing in the power of Christ to heal them. As they go on their way, they realize that the horrible disease has left them. But only one has feelings of gratitude, only one feels his deep indebtedness to Christ for this great work wrought for him. This one returns praising God, and in the greatest humiliation falls at the feet of Christ, acknowledging with thankfulness the work wrought for him. And this man was a stranger; the other nine were Jews.

For the sake of this one man, who would make a right use of the blessing of health, Jesus healed the whole ten. The nine passed on without appreciating the work done and rendered no grateful thanks to Jesus for doing the work.

Thus will the physicians of the Health Institute have their efforts treated. But if, in their labor to help suffering humanity, one out of twenty makes a right use of the benefits received and appreciates their efforts in his behalf, the physicians should feel grateful and satisfied. If one life out of ten is saved, and one soul out of one hundred is saved in the kingdom of God, all connected with the Institute will be amply repaid for all their efforts. All their anxiety and care will not be wholly lost. If the King of glory, the Majesty of heaven, worked for suffering humanity, and so few appreciated His divine aid, the physicians and helpers at the Institute should blush to complain if their feeble efforts are not appreciated by all and seem to be thrown away on some. . . .

To deal with men and women whose minds as well as bodies are diseased is a nice work. Great wisdom is needed by the physicians at the Institute in order to cure the body through the mind. But few realize the power that the mind has over the body. A great deal of the sickness which afflicts humanity has its origin in the mind, and can only be cured by restoring the mind to health. There are very many more than we imagine who are sick mentally. Heart sickness makes many dyspeptics, for mental trouble has a paralyzing influence upon the digestive organs.

In order to reach this class of patients, the physician must have discernment, patience, kindness, and love. A sore, sick heart, a discouraged mind, needs mild treatment, and it is through tender sympathy that this class of minds can be healed. The physicians should first gain their confidence and then point them to the all-healing Physician. If their minds can be directed to the Burden Bearer and they can have faith that He will have an interest in them, the cure of their diseased bodies and minds will be sure.

Patience and Sympathy

There will ever be things arising to annoy, perplex, and try the patience of physicians and helpers. They must be prepared for this and not become excited or unbalanced. They must be calm and kind, whatever may occur. . . . They should ever consider that they are dealing with men and women of diseased minds, who frequently view things in a perverted light and yet are confident that they understand matters perfectly.

Physicians should understand that a soft answer turneth away wrath. Policy must be used in an institution where the sick are treated, in order to successfully control diseased minds and benefit the sick. If physicians can remain calm amid a tempest of inconsiderate, passionate words, if they can rule their own spirits when provoked and abused, they are indeed conquerors. "He that ruleth his spirit" is better "than he that taketh a city." Proverbs 16:32. To subdue self and bring the passions under the control of the will is the greatest conquest that men and women can achieve.—*Testimonies for the Church,* vol. 3, pp. 182, 183 (1872).

Reference for further study: *The Ministry of Healing,* pages 17-72, "The True Medical Missionary."

A Messenger of Mercy

The Christian physician is to be to the sick a messenger of mercy, bringing to them a remedy for the sin-sick soul as well as for the diseased body. As he uses the simple remedies that God has provided for the relief of physical suffering, he is to speak of Christ's power to heal the maladies of the soul.

How necessary that the physician live in close communion with the Saviour! The sick and suffering with whom he deals need the help that Christ alone can give. They need prayers indited by His Spirit. The afflicted one leaves himself to the wisdom and mercy of the physician, whose skill and faithfulness may be his only hope. Let the physician, then, be a faithful steward of the grace of God, a guardian of the soul as well as of the body.

The physician who has received wisdom from above, who knows that Christ is His personal Saviour, because he has himself been led to the Refuge, knows how to deal with the trembling, guilty, sin-sick souls who turn to him for help. He can respond with assurance to the inquiry, "What must I do to be saved?" He can tell the story of the Redeemer's love. He can speak from experience of the power of repentance and faith. As he stands by the bedside of the sufferer, striving to speak words that will bring to him help and comfort, the Lord works with him and through him. As the mind of the afflicted one is fastened on the Mighty Healer, the peace of Christ fills his heart, and the spiritual health that comes to him is used as the helping hand of God in restoring the health of the body.

Precious are the opportunities that the physician has of awakening in the hearts of those with whom he is

Testimonies for the Church, vol. 7, pp. 72-75 (1902).

brought in contact a sense of their great need of Christ. He is to bring from the treasure house of the heart things new and old, speaking the words of comfort and instruction that are longed for. Constantly he is to sow the seeds of truth, not presenting doctrinal subjects, but speaking of the love of the sin-pardoning Saviour. Not only should he give instruction from the word of God, line upon line, precept upon precept; he is to moisten this instruction with his tears and make it strong with his prayers, that souls may be saved from death.

In their earnest, feverish anxiety to avert the peril of the body, physicians are in danger of forgetting the peril of the soul. Physicians, be on your guard, for at the judgment seat of Christ you must meet those at whose deathbed you now stand.

The solemnity of the physician's work, his constant contact with the sick and the dying, require that, so far as possible, he be removed from the secular duties that others can perform. No unnecessary burdens should be laid on him, that he may have time to become acquainted with the spiritual needs of his patients. His mind should be ever under the influence of the Holy Spirit, that he may be able to speak in season the words that will awaken faith and hope.

At the bedside of the dying no word of creed or controversy is to be spoken. The sufferer is to be pointed to the One who is willing to save all who come to Him in faith. Earnestly, tenderly, strive to help the soul that is hovering between life and death.

Direct the Mind to Jesus

The physician should never lead his patients to fix their attention on him. He is to teach them to grasp with the hand of faith the outstretched hand of the Saviour.

Then the mind will be illuminated with the light radiating from the Sun of Righteousness. What physicians attempt to do, Christ did in deed and in truth. They try to save life; He is life itself.

The physician's effort to lead the minds of his patients to healthy action must be free from all human enchantment. It must not grovel to humanity, but soar aloft to the spiritual, grasping the things of eternity.

The physician should not be made the object of unkind criticism. This places on him an unnecessary burden. His cares are heavy, and he needs the sympathy of those connected with him in the work. He is to be sustained by prayer. The realization that he is appreciated will give him hope and courage.

Sin and Disease

The intelligent Christian physician has a constantly increasing realization of the connection between sin and disease. He strives to see more and more clearly the relation between cause and effect. He sees that those who are taking the nurses' course should be given a thorough education in the principles of health reform; that they should be taught to be strictly temperate in all things, because carelessness in regard to the laws of health is inexcusable in those set apart to teach others how to live.

When a physician sees that a patient is suffering from an ailment caused by improper eating and drinking, yet neglects to tell him of this, and to point out the need of reform, he is doing a fellow being an injury. Drunkards, maniacs, those who are given over to licentiousness—all appeal to the physician to declare clearly and distinctly that suffering is the result of sin. We have received great light on health reform. Why, then, are we not more decidedly in earnest in striving to counteract the causes that produce disease? Seeing the continual conflict with pain, laboring constantly to alleviate suffering, how can our physicians hold their peace? Can they refrain from lifting the voice in warning? Are they benevolent and merciful if they do not teach strict temperance as a remedy for disease?

Physicians, study the warning which Paul gave to the Romans: "I beseech you therefore, brethren, by the mercies of God, that ye present your bodies a living sacrifice, holy, acceptable unto God, which is your reasonable service. And be not conformed to this world: but be ye transformed by the renewing of your mind, that ye may prove what is that good, and acceptable, and perfect, will of God." Romans 12:1, 2.

Physicians to Conserve Their Strength

Physicians should not be overworked, and their nervous systems prostrated; for this condition of body will not be favorable to calm minds, steady nerves, and a cheerful, happy spirit. . . .

The privilege of getting away from the Health Institute should occasionally be accorded to all the physicians, especially to those who bear burdens and responsibilities. If there is such a scarcity of help that this cannot be done, more help should be secured. To have physicians overworked and thus disqualified to perform the duties of their profession is a thing to be dreaded. It should be prevented if possible, for its influence is against the interests of the Institute. The physicians should keep well. They must not get sick by overlabor, or by any imprudence on their part.—*Testimonies for the Church,* vol. 3, p. 182 (1872).

A Work That Will Endure

Saint Helena, California, June 25, 1903.

To Our Sanitarium Physicians—

My dear Brethren: Those who stand in responsible positions in the work of the Lord are represented as watchmen on the walls of Zion. God calls upon them to sound an alarm among the people. Let it be heard in all the plain. The day of woe, of wasting and destruction, is upon all who do unrighteousness. With special severity will the Lord's hand fall upon the watchmen who have failed to place before the people in clear lines their obligation to Him who by creation and by redemption is their owner.

My brethren, the Lord calls upon you to examine the heart closely. He calls upon you to adorn the truth in your daily practice, and in all your dealings with one another. He requires of you a faith that works by love and purifies the soul. It is dangerous for you to trifle with the sacred demands of conscience, dangerous for you to set an example that leads others in a wrong direction.

Christians should carry with them, wherever they go, the sweet fragrance of Christ's righteousness, showing that they are complying with the invitation, "Learn of Me; for I am meek and lowly in heart: and ye shall find rest unto your souls." Matthew 11:29, 30. Are you learning daily in the school of Christ—learning how to dismiss doubt and evil surmisings, learning how to be fair and noble in your dealings with your brethren, for your own sake and for Christ's sake?

Present Truth Leads Upward

Present truth leads onward and upward, gathering in the needy, the oppressed, the suffering, the destitute.

Testimonies for the Church, vol. 8, pp. 195-200 (1903).

All that will come are to be brought into the fold. In their lives there is to take place a reformation that will constitute them members of the royal family, children of the heavenly King. By hearing the message of truth, men and women are led to accept the Sabbath and to unite with the church by baptism. They are to bear God's sign by observing the Sabbath of creation. They are to know for themselves that obedience to God's commandments means eternal life.

Means and earnest labor may be safely invested in such a work as this, for it is a work that will endure. Thus those who have been dead in trespasses and sins are brought into fellowship with the saints and are made to sit in heavenly places with Christ. Their feet are placed on a sure foundation. They are enabled to reach a high standard, even the loftiest heights of faith, because Christians make straight paths for their feet, lest the lame be turned out of the way.

All to Act a Part

Every church should labor for the perishing within its own borders and for those outside its borders. The members are to shine as living stones in the temple of God, reflecting heavenly light. No random, haphazard, desultory work is to be done. To get fast hold of souls ready to perish means more than praying for a drunkard, and then, because he weeps and confesses the pollution of his soul, declaring him saved. Over and over again the battle must be fought.

Let the members of every church feel it their special duty to labor for those in their neighborhood. Let each one who claims to stand under the banner of Christ feel that he has entered into covenant relation with God, to do the work of the Saviour. Let not those who take up this work become weary in well-doing. When the re-deemed stand before God, precious souls will respond to their names who are there because of the faithful, patient efforts put forth in their behalf, the entreaties and earnest persuasions to flee to the Stronghold. Thus those who in this world have been laborers together with God will receive their reward.

The ministers of the popular churches will not allow the truth to be presented to the people from their pulpits. The enemy leads them to resist the truth with bitterness and malice. Falsehoods are manufactured. Christ's expe-rience with the Jewish rulers is repeated. Satan strives to eclipse every ray of light shining from God to His people. He works through the ministers as he worked through the priests and rulers in the days of Christ. Will those who know the truth join his party, to hinder, em-barrass, and turn aside those who are trying to work in God's appointed way to advance His work, to plant the standard of truth in the regions of darkness?

The Message for This Time

The third angel's message, embracing the messages of the first and second angels, is the message for this time. We are to raise aloft the banner on which is inscribed, "The commandments of God, and the faith of Jesus." The world is soon to meet the great Lawgiver over His broken law. This is not the time to put out of sight the great issues before us. God calls upon His people to mag-nify the law and make it honorable.

When the morning stars sang together and all the sons of God shouted for joy, the Sabbath was given to the world, that man might ever remember that in six days God created the world. He rested upon the seventh day, blessing it as the day of His rest, and gave it to the beings

He had created, that they might remember Him as the true and living God.

By His mighty power, notwithstanding the opposition of Pharaoh, God delivered His people from Egypt, that they might keep the law which had been given in Eden. He brought them to Sinai to hear the proclamation of this law.

By proclaiming the Ten Commandments to the children of Israel with His own voice, God demonstrated their importance. In awful grandeur He made known His majesty and authority as Ruler of the world. This He did to impress the people with the sacredness of His law and the importance of obeying it. The power and glory with which the law was given reveal its importance. It is the faith once delivered to the saints by Christ our Redeemer speaking from Sinai.

The Sign of Our Relationship to God

By the observance of the Sabbath, the children of Israel were to be distinguished from all other nations. "Verily My Sabbaths ye shall keep," Christ said, "for it is a sign between Me and you throughout your generations; that ye may know that I am the Lord that doth sanctify you." "It is a sign between Me and the children of Israel forever: for in six days the Lord made heaven and earth, and on the seventh day He rested, and was refreshed." "Wherefore the children of Israel shall keep the Sabbath, to observe the Sabbath throughout their generations, for a perpetual covenant." Exodus 31:13, 17, 16.

The Sabbath is a sign of the relationship existing between God and His people—a sign that they are His obedient subjects, that they keep holy His law. The observance of the Sabbath is the means ordained by God of preserving a knowledge of Himself and of distinguishing between His loyal subjects and the transgressors of His law.

This is the faith once delivered to the saints, who stand in moral power before the world, firmly maintaining this faith.

Opposition we shall have as we voice the message of the third angel. Satan will bring in every possible device to make of no effect the faith once delivered to the saints. "Many shall follow their pernicious ways; by reason of whom the way of truth shall be evil spoken of. And through covetousness shall they with feigned words make merchandise of you: whose judgment now of a long time lingereth not, and their damnation slumbereth not." 2 Peter 2:2, 3. But in spite of opposition, all are to hear the words of truth.

The law of God is the foundation of all enduring reformation. We are to present to the world in clear, distinct lines the need of obeying this law. Obedience to God's law is the greatest incentive to industry, economy, truthfulness, and just dealing between man and man.

The Foundation of Enduring Reformation

The law of God is to be the means of education in the family. Parents are under a most solemn obligation to obey this law, setting their children an example of the strictest integrity. Men in responsible positions, whose influence is far-reaching, are to guard well their ways and works, keeping the fear of the Lord ever before them. "The fear of the Lord is the beginning of wisdom." Psalm 111:10. Those who hearken diligently to the voice of the Lord and cheerfully keep His commandments will be among the number who see God. "The Lord commanded us to do all these statutes, to fear the Lord our God, for our good always, that He might preserve us alive, as it is at this day. And it shall be our righteousness, if we observe to do all these commandments before the Lord our God, as He hath commanded us." Deuteronomy 6:24, 25.

Our work as believers in the truth is to present before the world the immutability of the law of God. Ministers and teachers, physicians and nurses, are bound by covenant with God to present the importance of obeying His law. We are to be distinguished as a people who keep the commandments. The Lord has stated explicitly that He has a work to be done for the world. How shall it be done? Let us seek to find the best way and then perform the will of the Lord.

Each One in His Place

The physicians of the Health Institute should not feel compelled to do work that helpers can do. They should not serve in the bathroom or in the movement room, expending their vitality in doing what others might do. There should be no lack of helpers to nurse the sick and to watch with the feeble ones who need watchers. The physicians should reserve their strength for the successful performance of their professional duties. They should tell others what to do. If there is a want of those whom they can trust to do these things, suitable persons should be employed and properly instructed, and suitably remunerated for their services.—*Testimonies for the Church,* vol. 3, pp. 177, 178 (1872).

Reference for further study: *The Ministry of Healing,* pages 17-72, "The True Medical Missionary."

Dangers and Opportunities

Sanitarium, California, June 3, 1907.

The physician stands in a difficult place. Strong temptations will come to him, and unless kept by the power of God, that which he hears and sees in his work will discourage his heart and pollute his soul. His thoughts should be constantly uplifted to God. This is his only safety.

Countless are the opportunities that a physician has for winning souls to God, for cheering the discouraged and relieving the despair that comes to the soul when the body is tortured with pain.

But some who have chosen the medical profession are too easily led away from the duties resting upon the physician. Some by misuse enfeeble their powers, so that they cannot render to God perfect service. They place themselves where they cannot act with vigor, tact, and skill, and they do not realize that by disregard to physical laws they bring upon themselves inefficiency, and thus they rob and dishonor God.

Physicians should not allow their attention to be diverted from their work; neither should they confine themselves so closely to professional work that health will be injured. In the fear of God they should be wise in the use of strength that God has given them. Never should they disregard the means that God has provided for the preservation of health. It is their duty to bring under the control of reason every power that God has given them.

Value of Rest, Study, and Prayer

Of all men, the physician should, as far as possible, take regular hours for rest. This will give him power of endurance to bear the taxing burdens of his work. In his

Special Testimonies, Series B, No. 15, pp. 11-15 (1907).

busy life the physician will find that the searching of the Scriptures and earnest prayer will give vigor of mind and stability of character.

Seek to meet the expectations of Jesus Christ. He will help in every effort in the right direction. Remember that there is not an action of life, nor a motive of the heart, that is not open to the grace of the Saviour.

The way to the throne of God is always open. You cannot always be on your knees in prayer, but your silent petitions may constantly ascend to God for strength and guidance. When tempted, as you will be, you may flee to the secret place of the Most High. His everlasting arms will be underneath you. Let these words cheer you, "Thou hast a few names even in Sardis which have not defiled their garments; and they shall walk with Me in white: for they are worthy." Revelation 3:4.

When Christ is formed within, the hope of glory, you will be well balanced, and you will not be changeable, but will rise above the influences that discourage and discompose those who are not stayed upon Christ. You will be able to prove that it is possible to be a wise, successful physician, and at the same time an active Christian, serving the Lord in sincerity. Godliness is the foundation of true dignity and completeness of character.

Thoroughness and Promptness Essential

Unless the physicians in our sanitariums are men of thorough habits, unless they attend promptly to their duties, their work will become a reproach and the Lord's appointed agencies will lose their influence. By a course of negligence to duty the physician humiliates the Great Physician, of whom he should be a representative. Strict hours should be kept with all patients, high and low. No careless neglect should be allowed in any of the nurses. Ever be true to your word, prompt in meeting your appointments, for this means much to the sick.

Refinement and Delicacy

Among Christian physicians there should ever be a striving for the maintenance of the highest order of true refinement and delicacy, a preservation of those barriers of reserve that should exist between men and women.

We are living in a time when the world is represented as Noah's time, and as in the time of Sodom. I am constantly shown the great dangers to which youth, and men and women who have just reached manhood and womanhood, and also men and women of mature years, are exposed, and I dare not hold my peace. There is need of greater refinement, both in thought and association. There is need of Christians' being more elevated and delicate in words and deportment.

The work of the physician is of a character that if there is a coarseness in his nature, it will be revealed. Therefore, the physician should guard carefully his speech and avoid all commonness in his conversation. Every patient he treats is reading the traits of his character and the tone of his morals by his actions and conversation.

The light given me of the Lord regarding this matter is that as far as possible lady physicians should care for lady patients, and gentlemen physicians have the care of gentlemen patients. Every physician should respect the delicacy of the patients. Any unnecessary exposure of ladies before male physicians is wrong. Its influence is detrimental.

Delicate treatments should not be given by male physicians to women in our institutions. Never should a lady patient be alone with a gentleman physician, either for special examination or for treatment. Let the physicians be faithful in preserving delicacy and modesty under all circumstances.

In our medical institutions there ought always to be women of mature age and good experience who have been trained to give treatments to the lady patients. Women should be educated and qualified just as thoroughly as possible to become practitioners in the delicate diseases which afflict women, that their secret parts should not be exposed to the notice of men. There should be a much larger number of lady physicians, educated not only to act as trained nurses, but also as physicians. It is a most horrible practice, this revealing the secret parts of women to men, or men being treated by women.

Women physicians should utterly refuse to look upon the secret parts of men. Women should be thoroughly educated to work for women, and men to work for men. Let men know that they must go to their own sex and not apply to lady physicians. It is an insult to women, and God looks upon these things of commonness with abhorrence.

While physicians are called upon to teach social purity, let them practice that delicacy which is a constant lesson in practical purity. Women may do a noble work as practicing physicians; but when men ask a lady physician to give them examinations and treatments which demand the exposure of private parts, let her refuse decidedly to do this work.

In the medical work there are dangers which the physician should understand and constantly guard against. Truly converted men are the ones who should be employed as physicians in our sanitariums. Some physicians are self-sufficient and consider themselves able to guard their own ways; whereas if they but knew themselves, they would feel their great need of help from above, a higher intelligence.

Some medical men are unfit to act as physicians to women because of the attitude they assume toward them. They take liberties until it becomes a common thing with them to transgress the laws of chastity. Our physicians should have the highest regard for the direction given by God to His church when they were delivered from Egypt. This will keep them from becoming loose in manners and careless in regard to the laws of chastity. All who live by the laws given by God from Sinai may be safely trusted.

Skillful Midwives Needed

It is not in harmony with the instructions given at Sinai that gentlemen physicians should do the work of midwives. The Bible speaks of women at childbirth being attended by women, and thus it ought always to be. Women should be educated and trained to act skillfully as midwives and physicians to their sex. It is just as important that a line of study be given to educate women to deal with women's diseases, as it is that there should be gentlemen thoroughly trained to act as physicians and surgeons. And the wages of the woman should be proportionate to her services. She should be as much appreciated in her work as the gentleman physician is appreciated in his work.

Let us educate ladies to become intelligent in the work of treating the diseases of their sex. They will sometimes need the counsel and assistance of experienced gentlemen physicians. When brought into trying places let all be led by supreme wisdom. Let all bear in mind that they need and may have the wisdom of the Great Physician in their work.

We ought to have a school where women can be educated by women physicians, to do the best possible work in treating the diseases of women.

Among us as a people, the medical work should stand at its highest. Physicians should bear in mind that it is their work to fit souls as well as bodies for heavenly lives. Their service for God is to be uncorrupted by evil practices.

Every practitioner should study carefully the word of God. Read the story of the sons of Aaron in the tenth chapter of Leviticus, verses 1-11. Here was a case where the use of wine benumbed the senses. The Lord demands that the appetite and all the habits of life of the physician be kept under strict control. While dealing with the bodies of their patients, they are to constantly remember that the eye of God is upon their work.

The Causes of Disease to Be Understood

The most exalted part of the physician's work is to lead the men and women under his care to see that the cause of disease is the violation of the laws of health and to encourage them to higher and holier views of life. Instruction should be given that will provide an antidote for the diseases of the soul as well as for the sickness of the body. Only that sanitarium will be a healthful institution where right principles are established. The physician who, knowing the remedy for the diseases of the soul and body, neglects the educational part of his work, will have to give an account of his neglect in the day of judgment. Strict purity of language and every word and action is to be guarded

Dangers in Success

It is a dangerous age for any man who has talents which can be of value in the work of God; for Satan is constantly plying his temptations upon such a person, ever trying to fill him with pride and ambition; and when God would use him, in nine cases out of ten he becomes independent, self-sufficient, and feels capable of standing alone. This will be your danger, Dr. ——, unless you live a life of constant faith and prayer. You may have a deep and abiding sense of eternal things and that love for humanity which Christ has shown in His life. A close connection with Heaven will give the right tone to your fidelity and will be the ground of your success. Your feeling of dependence will drive you to prayer and your sense of duty summon you to effort. Prayer and effort, effort and prayer, will be the business of your life. You must pray as though the efficiency and praise were all due to God, and labor as though duty were all your own. If you want power you may have it, as it is awaiting your draft upon it. Only believe in God, take Him at His word, act by faith, and blessings will come.

In this matter, genius, logic, and eloquence will not avail. Those who have a humble, trusting, contrite heart, God accepts and hears their prayer; and when God helps, all obstacles will be overcome. How many men of great natural abilities and high scholarship have failed when placed in positions of responsibility, while those of feebler intellect, with less favorable surroundings, have been wonderfully successful. The secret was, the former trusted to themselves, while the latter united with Him who is won-

Special Testimonies to Physicians and Helpers, pages 15-17 (1879).

derful in counsel and mighty in working to accomplish what He will.

Your work being always urgent, it is difficult for you to secure time for meditation and prayer; but this you must not fail to do. The blessing of Heaven, obtained by daily supplication, will be as the bread of life to your soul and will cause you to increase in spiritual and moral strength, like a tree planted by the river of waters, whose leaf will be always green, and whose fruit will appear in due time.

Your neglect to attend the public worship of God is a serious error. The privileges of divine service will be as beneficial to you as to others and are fully as essential. You may be unable to avail yourself of these privileges as often as do many others. You will frequently be called, upon the Sabbath, to visit the sick, and may be obliged to make it a day of exhausting labor. Such labor to relieve the suffering was pronounced by our Saviour a work of mercy and no violation of the Sabbath. But when you regularly devote your Sabbaths to writing or labor, making no special change, you harm your own soul, give to others an example that is not worthy of imitation, and do not honor God.

You have failed to see the real importance, not only of attending religious meetings, but also of bearing testimony for Christ and the truth. If you do not obtain spiritual strength by the faithful performance of every Christian duty, thus coming into a closer and more sacred relation to your Redeemer, you will become weak in moral power.

The Bible Your Counselor

God would have all who profess to be gospel medical missionaries learn diligently the lessons of the Great Teacher. This they must do if they would find peace and rest. Learning of Christ, their hearts will be filled with the peace that He alone can give.

The one book that is essential for all to study is the Bible. Studied with reverence and godly fear, it is the greatest of all educators. In it there is no sophistry. Its pages are filled with truth. Would you gain a knowledge of God and Christ, whom He sent into the world to live and die for sinners? An earnest, diligent study of the Bible is necessary in order to gain this knowledge.

Many of the books piled up in the great libraries of earth confuse the mind more than they aid the understanding. Yet men spend large sums of money in the purchase of such books and years in their study, when they have within their reach a Book containing the words of Him who is the Alpha and Omega of wisdom. The time spent in a study of these books might better be spent in gaining a knowledge of Him whom to know aright is life eternal. Those only who gain this knowledge will at last hear the words, "Ye are complete in Him." Colossians 2:10.

Study the Bible more and the theories of the medical fraternity less, and you will have greater spiritual health. Your mind will be clearer and more vigorous. Much that is embraced in a medical course is positively unnecessary. Those who take a medical training spend a great deal of time in learning that which is worthless. Many of the theories that they learn may be compared in value to the traditions and maxims taught by the scribes and Pharisees.

Words of Counsel (1903).

Many of the intricacies with which they have to become familiar are an injury to their minds.

These things God has been opening before me for many years. In our medical schools and institutions we need men who have a deeper knowledge of the Scriptures, men who have learned the lessons taught in the word of God, and who can teach these lessons to others, clearly and simply, just as Christ taught His disciples the knowledge that He deemed most essential.

The Great Physician's Prescription for Rest

If our medical missionary workers would follow the Great Physician's prescription for obtaining rest, a healing current of peace would flow through their souls. Here is the prescription: "Come unto Me, all ye that labor and are heavy-laden, and I will give you rest. Take My yoke upon you, and learn of Me; for I am meek and lowly in heart: and ye shall find rest unto your souls. For My yoke is easy, and My burden is light." Matthew 11:28-30.

When our medical missionary workers follow this prescription, gaining from the Saviour power to reveal His characteristics, their scientific work will have greater soundness. Because the word of God has been neglected, strange things have been done in the medical missionary work of late. The Lord cannot accept the present showing.

Study the word, which God in His wisdom and love and goodness has made so plain and simple. The sixth chapter of John tells us what is meant by a study of the word. The principles revealed in the Scriptures are to be brought home to the soul. We are to eat the word of God; that is, we are not to depart from its precepts. We are to bring its truths into our daily lives, grasping the mysteries of godliness.

Pray to God. Commune with Him. Prove the very mind of God, as those who are striving for eternal life, and who must have a knowledge of His will. You can reveal the truth only as you know it in Christ. You are to receive and assimilate His words; they are to become part of yourselves. This is what is meant by eating the flesh and drinking the blood of the Son of God. You are to live by every word that proceedeth out of the mouth of God; that is, what God has revealed. Not all has been revealed; we could not bear such a revelation. But God has revealed all that is necessary for our salvation. We are not to leave His word for the suppositions of men.

Obtain an experimental knowledge of God by wearing the yoke of Christ. He gives wisdom to the meek and lowly, enabling them to judge of what is truth, bringing to light the why and wherefore, pointing out the result of certain actions. The Holy Spirit teaches the student of the Scriptures to judge all things by the standard of righteousness and truth and justice. The divine revelation supplies him with the knowledge that he needs.

And the needed knowledge will be given to all who come to Christ, receiving and practicing His teachings, making His words a part of their lives. Those who place themselves under the instruction of the great Medical Missionary, to be workers together with Him, will have a knowledge that the world, with all its traditional lore, cannot supply.

Make the Bible the man of your counsel. Your acquaintance with it will grow rapidly if you keep your mind free from the rubbish of the world. The more the Bible is studied, the deeper will be your knowledge of God. The truths of His word will be written in your soul, making an ineffaceable impression.

Not only will the student himself be benefited by a study of the word of God. His study is life and salvation to all with whom he associates. He will feel a sacred responsibility to impart the knowledge that he receives. His life will reveal the help and strength that he receives from communion with the word. The sanctification of the Spirit will be seen in thought, word, and deed. All that he says and does will proclaim that God is light and in Him is no darkness at all. Of such ones the Lord Jesus can indeed say, "Ye are laborers together with God."

Qualifications Needed

I was shown that physicians and helpers should be of the highest order, those who have an experimental knowledge of the truth, who will command respect, and whose word can be relied on. They should be persons who have not a diseased imagination, persons who have perfect self-control, who are not fitful or changeable, who are free from jealousy and evil surmising; persons who have a power of will that will not yield to slight indispositions, who are unprejudiced, who will think no evil, who think and move calmly, considerately, having the glory of God and the good of others ever before them. Never should one be exalted to a responsible position merely because he desires it. Those only should be chosen who are qualified for the position. Those who are to bear responsibilities should first be proved and given evidence that they are free from jealousy, that they will not take a dislike to this or that one, while they have a few favored friends and take no notice of others. God grant that all may move just right in that institution.—*Testimonies for the Church, vol. 1, p. 567 (1867).*

Praying for the Sick

In the matter of praying for the sick . . . I have been considering many things that have been presented to me in the past in reference to this subject.

Suppose that twenty men and women should present themselves as subjects for prayer at some of our camp meetings, this would not be unlikely, for those who are suffering will do anything in their power to obtain relief and to regain strength and health. Of these twenty, few have regarded the light on the subject of purity and health reform. They have neglected to practice right principles in eating and drinking and in taking care of their bodies, and some of those who are married have formed gross habits and indulged in unholy practice, while of those who are unmarried, some have been reckless of health and life, since in clear rays the light has shone upon them; but they have not had respect unto the light, nor have they walked circumspectly. Yet they solicit the prayers of God's people and call for the elders of the church.

Should they regain the blessing of health, many of them would pursue the same course of heedless transgression of nature's laws unless enlightened and thoroughly transformed. . . .

Sin has brought many of them where they are—to a state of feebleness of mind and debility of body. Shall prayer be offered to the God of heaven for His healing to come upon them then and there, without specifying any conditions? I say, No, decidedly no. What, then, shall be done? Present their cases before Him who knows every individual by name.

Present these thoughts to the persons who come asking for your prayers: We are human; we cannot read the

Our Camp Meetings, pages 44-48 (1892).

heart or know the secrets of your life. These are known only to yourself and God. If you now repent of your sin, if any of you can see that in any instance you have walked contrary to the light given you of God and have neglected to give honor to the body, the temple of God, but by wrong habits have degraded the body which is Christ's property, make confession of these things to God. Unless you are wrought upon by the Holy Spirit in special manner to confess your sins of private nature to man, do not breathe them to any soul.

Christ is your Redeemer; He will take no advantage of your humiliating confessions. If you have sin of a private character, confess it to Christ, who is the only Mediator between God and man. "If any man sin, we have an advocate with the Father, Jesus Christ the righteous." 1 John 2:1. If you have sinned by withholding from God His own in tithes and offerings, confess your guilt to God and to the church, and heed the injunction that He has given you: "Bring ye all the tithes into the storehouse." Malachi 3:10. . . .

A Most Solemn Experience

Praying for the sick is a most solemn thing, and we should not enter into this work in any careless, hasty way. Examination should be made as to whether those who would be blessed with health have indulged in evilspeaking, alienation, and dissension. Have they sowed discord among the brethren and sisters of the church? If these things have been committed they should be confessed before God and the church. When wrongs have been confessed the subjects for prayer may be presented before God in earnestness and faith, as the Spirit of God may move upon you.

But it is not always safe to ask for unconditional healing. Let your prayer include this thought: "Lord, Thou
knowest every secret of the soul. Thou art acquainted
with these persons; for Jesus, their advocate, gave His
life for them. He loves them better than we possibly can.
If, therefore, it is for Thy glory and the good of these
afflicted ones to raise them up to health, we ask Thee in
the name of Jesus, that health may be given them at this
time." In a petition of this kind, no lack of faith is manifested.

The Lord "doth not afflict willingly nor grieve the
children of men." Lamentations 3:33. "Like as a father
pitieth his children, so the Lord pitieth them that fear
Him. For He knoweth our frame; He remembereth that
we are dust." Psalm 103:13, 14. He knows our heart, for
He reads every secret of the soul. He knows whether or
not those for whom petitions are offered would be able
to endure the trial and test that would come upon them
if they lived. He knows the end from the beginning.
Many will be laid away to sleep before the fiery ordeal
of the time of trouble shall come upon our world. This
is another reason why we should say after our earnest
petition: "Nevertheless not my will, but Thine, be done."
Luke 22:42. Such a petition will never be registered in
heaven as a faithless prayer.

The apostle was bidden to write, "Blessed are the dead
which die in the Lord from henceforth: Yea, saith the
Spirit, that they may rest from their labors; and their
works do follow them." Revelation 14:13. From this we
can see that all are not to be raised up; and if they are
not raised to health they should not be judged as unworthy of eternal life. If Jesus, the world's Redeemer,
prayed, "O My Father, if it be possible, let this cup pass

from Me," and added, "nevertheless not as I will, but as
Thou wilt" (Matthew 26:39), how very appropriate it is
for finite mortals to make the same surrender to the wisdom and will of God.

According to His Will

In praying for the sick, we are to pray that, if it is
God's will, they may be raised to health; but if not, that
He will give them His grace to comfort, His presence to
sustain them in their suffering.

Many who should set their house in order neglect to
do it when they have hope that they will be raised to
health in answer to prayer. Buoyed up by a false hope,
they do not feel the need of giving words of exhortation
and counsel to their children, parents, or friends, and it is
a great misfortune. Accepting the assurance that they
would be healed when prayed for, they dare not make a
reference as to how their property shall be disposed of,
how their family is to be cared for, or express any wish
concerning matters of which they would speak if they
thought they would be removed by death. In this way
disasters are brought upon the family and friends, for
many things that should be understood are left unmentioned because they fear expression on these points would
be denial of their faith. Believing they will be raised to
health by prayer, they fail to use hygienic measures which
are within their power to use, fearing it would be a denial
of their faith.

I thank the Lord that it is our privilege to co-operate
with Him in the work of restoration, availing ourselves
of all the possible advantages in the recovery of health.
It is no denial of our faith to place ourselves in the condition most favorable for recovery.

Reference for further study: *The Ministry of Healing,* pages 225-
233, "Prayer for the Sick."

Submission and Faith

In such cases of affliction, where Satan has control of the mind, before engaging in prayer there should be the closest self-examination to discover if there are not sins which need to be repented of, confessed, and forsaken. Deep humility of soul before God is necessary, and firm, humble reliance upon the merits of the blood of Christ alone. Fasting and prayer will accomplish nothing while the heart is estranged from God by a wrong course of action. Read Isaiah 58:6, 7, 9-11.

It is heart work that the Lord requires, good works springing from a heart filled with love. All should carefully and prayerfully . . . investigate their motives and actions. The promise of God to us is on condition of obedience, compliance with all His requirements. Read Isaiah 58:1-3. . . .

Faith and Calmness

I was shown that in case of sickness, where the way is clear for the offering up of prayer for the sick, the case should be committed to the Lord in calm faith, not with a storm of excitement. He alone is acquainted with the past life of the individual and knows what his future will be. He who is acquainted with the hearts of all men knows whether the person, if raised up, would glorify His name or dishonor Him by backsliding and apostasy. All that we are required to do is to ask God to raise the sick up if in accordance with His will, believing that He hears the reasons which we present and the fervent prayers offered. If the Lord sees it will best honor Him, He will answer our prayers. But to urge recovery without submission to His will is not right.

Testimonies for the Church, vol. 2, pp. 146-149 (1868).

What God promises He is able at any time to perform, and the work which He gives His people to do He is able to accomplish by them. If they will live according to every word He has spoken, every good word and promise will be fulfilled unto them. But if they come short of perfect obedience, the great and precious promises are afar off and they cannot reach the fulfillment.

All that can be done in praying for the sick is to earnestly importune God in their behalf, and in perfect confidence rest the matter in His hands. If we regard iniquity in our hearts the Lord will not hear us. He can do what He will with His own. He will glorify Himself by working in and through them who wholly follow Him so that it shall be known that it is the Lord, and that their works are wrought in God.

Faith and Obedience

Said Christ, "If any man serve Me, him will My Father honor." When we come to Him we should pray that we might enter into and accomplish His purpose, and that our desires and interests might be lost in His. We should acknowledge our acceptance of His will, not praying Him to concede to ours. It is better for us that God does not always answer our prayers just when we desire and in just the manner we wish. He will do more and better for us than to accomplish all our wishes; for our wisdom is folly.

We have united in earnest prayer around the sickbed of men, women, and children, and have felt that they were given back to us from the dead in answer to our earnest prayers. In these prayers we thought we must be positive, and if we exercised faith, that we must ask for nothing less than life. We dared not say, "If it will glorify God," fearing it would admit a semblance of doubt. We have anxiously watched those who have been given back, as it were, from the dead. We have seen some of these, especially youth, raised to health, and they have forgotten God, become dissolute in life, causing sorrow and anguish to parents and friends, and have become a shame to those who feared to pray. They lived not to honor and glorify God, but to curse Him with their lives of vice.

We no longer mark out a way, nor seek to bring the Lord to our wishes. If the life of the sick can glorify Him, we pray that they may live, nevertheless, not as we will but as He will. Our faith can be just as firm, and more reliable, by committing the desire to the all-wise God and, without feverish anxiety, in perfect confidence trusting all to Him. We have the promise. We know that He hears us if we ask according to His will.

Our petitions must not take the form of a command, but of intercession for Him to do the things we desire of Him. When the church are united, they will have strength and power; but when part of them are united to the world and many are given to covetousness, which God abhors, He can do but little for them. Unbelief and sin shut them away from God. We are so weak that we cannot bear much spiritual prosperity, lest we take the glory and accredit goodness and righteousness to ourselves as the reason of the signal blessing of God, when it was all because of the great mercy and loving-kindness of our compassionate heavenly Father and not because any good was found in us.

Reference for further study: *The Ministry of Healing,* pages 59-72, "The Touch of Faith."

13—C.O.H.

Faith and Works

In praying for the sick, it is essential to have faith; for it is in accordance with the word of God. "The effectual fervent prayer of a righteous man availeth much." James 5:16. So we cannot discard praying for the sick, and we should feel very sad if we could not have the privilege of approaching God, to lay before Him all our weaknesses and our infirmities, to tell the compassionate Saviour all about these things, believing that He hears our petitions. Sometimes answers to our prayers come immediately; sometimes we have to wait patiently and continue earnestly to plead for the things that we need, our cases being illustrated by the case of the importunate solicitor for bread. "Which of you shall have a friend, and shall go unto him at midnight," etc. This lesson means more than we can imagine. We are to keep on asking, even if we do not realize the immediate response to our prayers. "I say unto you, Ask, and it shall be given you; seek, and ye shall find; knock, and it shall be opened unto you. For everyone that asketh receiveth; and he that seeketh findeth; and to him that knocketh it shall be opened." Luke 11:9, 10.

We need grace, we need divine enlightenment, that through the Spirit we may know how to ask for such things as we need. If our petitions are indited by the Lord they will be answered.

There are precious promises in the Scriptures to those who wait upon the Lord. We all desire an immediate answer to our prayers and are tempted to become discouraged if our prayer is not immediately answered. Now, my experience has taught me that this is a great mistake. The delay is for our special benefit. We have a chance to

Health, Philanthropic, and Medical Missionary Work, pages 51-54 (1892).

see whether our faith is true and sincere or changeable like the waves of the sea. We must bind ourselves upon the altar with the strong cords of faith and love, and let patience have her perfect work. Faith strengthens through continual exercise. This waiting does not mean that because we ask the Lord to heal there is nothing for us to do. On the contrary, we are to make the very best use of the means which the Lord in His goodness has provided for us in our necessities.

I have seen so much of carrying matters to extremes, in praying for the sick, that I have felt that this part of our experience requires much solid, sanctified thinking, lest we shall make movements that we may call faith, but which are really nothing less than presumption. Persons worn down with affliction need to be counseled wisely, that they may move discreetly; and while they place themselves before God to be prayed for that they may be healed, they are not to take the position that methods of restoration to health in accordance with nature's laws are to be neglected.

If they take the position that in praying for healing they must not use the simple remedies provided by God to alleviate pain and to aid nature in her work, lest it be a denial of faith, they are taking an unwise position. This is not a denial of faith; it is in strict harmony with the plans of God. When Hezekiah was sick, the prophet of God brought him the message that he should die. He cried unto the Lord, and the Lord heard His servant and worked a miracle in his behalf, sending him a message that fifteen years should be added to his life. Now, one word from God, one touch of the divine finger, would have cured Hezekiah instantly, but special directions were given to take a fig and lay it upon the affected part, and Hezekiah was raised to life. In everything we need to move along the line of God's providence.

The human agent should have faith and should cooperate with the divine power, using every facility, taking advantage of everything that, according to his intelligence, is beneficial, working in harmony with natural laws; and in doing this he neither denies nor hinders faith.

Gratitude for Health

How often those who are in health forget the wonderful mercies that are continued to them day by day, year after year. They render no tribute of praise to God for all His benefits. But when sickness comes, God is remembered. The strong desire for recovery leads to earnest prayer, and this is right. God is our refuge in sickness as in health. But many do not leave their cases with Him; they encourage weakness and disease by worrying about themselves. If they would cease repining and rise above depression and gloom, their recovery would be more sure. They should remember with gratitude how long they enjoyed the blessing of health; and should this precious boon be restored to them, they should not forget that they are under renewed obligations to their Creator. When the ten lepers were healed, only one returned to find Jesus and give Him glory. Let us not be like the unthinking nine whose hearts were untouched by the mercy of God. —*Testimonies for the Church,* vol. 5, p. 315 (1885).

The Physician's Influence

I have been shown that the physicians should come into a closer connection with God and stand and work earnestly in His strength. They have a responsible part to act. Not only the lives of the patients, but their souls also, are at stake. Many who are benefited physically, may, at the same time, be greatly helped spiritually. Both the health of the body and the salvation of the soul are in a great degree dependent upon the course of the physicians. It is of the utmost consequence that they are right, that they have not only scientific knowledge, but the knowledge of God's will and ways. Great responsibilities rest upon them.

My brethren, you should see and feel your responsibility, and, in view of it, humble your souls before God and plead with Him for wisdom. You have not realized how much the salvation of the souls of those whose bodies you are seeking to relieve from suffering, depends upon your words, your actions and deportment. You are doing work which must bear the test of the judgment. You must guard your own souls from the sins of selfishness, self-sufficiency, and self-confidence.

Draw Water From the Hidden Spring

You should preserve a true Christian dignity, but avoid all affectation. Be strictly honest in heart and life. Let faith, like the palm tree, strike its penetrating roots beneath the things which do appear, and obtain spiritual refreshment from the living springs of God's grace and mercy. There is a well of water which springeth up into everlasting life. You must draw your life from this hid-

Testimonies for the Church, vol. 4, pp. 566-569 (1881).

den spring. If you divest yourselves of selfishness and strengthen your souls by constant communion with God, you may promote the happiness of all with whom you come in contact. You will notice the neglected, inform the ignorant, encourage the oppressed and desponding, and, as far as possible, relieve the suffering. And you will not only point the way to heaven, but will walk in that way yourselves.

Be not satisfied with superficial knowledge. Be not elated by flattery nor depressed by faultfinding. Satan will tempt you to pursue such a course that you may be admired and flattered; but you should turn away from his devices. You are servants of the living God.

Your intercourse with the sick is an exhausting process and would gradually dry up the very springs of life if there were no change, no opportunity for recreation, and if angels of God did not guard and protect you. If you could see the many perils through which you are conducted safely every day by these messengers of Heaven, gratitude would spring up in your hearts and find expression from your lips. If you make God your strength, you may, under the most discouraging circumstances, attain a height and breadth of Christian perfection which you hardly think it possible to reach. Your thoughts may be elevated, you may have noble aspirations, clear perceptions of truth, and purposes of action which shall raise you above all sordid motives.

Both thought and action will be necessary if you would attain to perfection of character. While brought in contact with the world you should be on your guard that you do not seek too ardently for the applause of men and live for their opinion. Walk carefully, if you would walk safely; cultivate the grace of humility and hang your helpless souls upon Christ. You may be, in every sense, men of God. In the midst of confusion and temptation in the worldly crowd you may, with perfect sweetness, keep the independence of the soul.

Daily Communion With God

If you are in daily communion with God, you will learn to place His estimate upon men, and the obligations resting upon you to bless suffering humanity will meet with a willing response. You are not your own; your Lord has sacred claims upon your supreme affections and the very highest services of your life. He has a right to use you in your body and in your spirit, to the fullest extent of your capabilities, for His own honor and glory. Whatever crosses you may be required to bear, whatever labors or sufferings are imposed upon you by His hand, you are to accept without a murmur.

Those for whom you labor are your brethren in distress, suffering from physical disorders and the spiritual leprosy of sin. If you are any better than they, it is to be credited to the cross of Christ. Many are without God and without hope in the world. They are guilty, corrupt, and degraded, enslaved by Satan's devices. Yet these are the ones whom Christ came from heaven to redeem. They are subjects for tenderest pity, sympathy, and tireless effort, for they are on the verge of ruin. They suffer from ungratified desires, disordered passions, and the condemnation of their own consciences; they are miserable in every sense of the word, for they are losing their hold on this life and have no prospect for the life to come.

Be Active and Vigilant

You have an important field of labor, and you should be active and vigilant, rendering cheerful and unqualified obedience to the Master's calls. Ever bear in mind that your efforts to reform others should be made in the spirit of unwavering kindness. Nothing is ever gained by holding yourselves aloof from those whom you would help. You should keep before the minds of patients the fact that in suggesting reforms of their habits and customs you are presenting before them that which is not to ruin but to save them; that, while yielding up what they have hitherto esteemed and loved, they are to build on a more secure foundation. While reform must be advocated with firmness and resolution, all appearance of bigotry or an overbearing spirit should be carefully shunned. Christ has given us precious lessons of patience, forbearance, and love. Rudeness is not energy; nor is domineering, heroism. The Son of God was persuasive. He was manifested to draw all men unto Him. His followers must study His life more closely and walk in the light of His example, at whatever sacrifice to self. Reform, continual reform, must be kept before the people, and your example should enforce your teachings.

Obedience and Happiness

Let it ever be kept before the mind that the great object of hygienic reform is to secure the highest possible development of mind and soul and body. All the laws of nature—which are the laws of God—are designed for our good. Obedience to them will promote our happiness in this life and will aid us in a preparation for the life to come.—*Christian Temperance,* page 120 (1890).

NURSES AND HELPERS

Christ's Methods to Be Followed

From Christ's methods of labor we may learn many valuable lessons. He did not follow merely one method; in various ways He sought to gain the attention of the multitude and, having succeeded in this, He proclaimed to them the truths of the gospel. His chief work lay in ministering to the poor, the needy, and the ignorant. In simplicity He opened before them the blessings they might receive, and thus He aroused their soul's hunger for the truth, the bread of life.

Christ's life is an example to all His followers, showing the duty of those who have learned the way of life to teach others what it means to believe in the word of God. There are many now in the shadow of death who need to be instructed in the truths of the gospel. Nearly the whole world is lying in wickedness. To every believer in Christ, words of hope have been given for those who sit in darkness: "The land of Zabulon, and the land of Nephthalim, by the way of the sea, beyond Jordan, Galilee of the Gentiles; the people which sat in darkness saw great light; and to them which sat in the region and shadow of death light is sprung up." Matthew 4:15, 16.

Earnest, devoted young people are needed to enter the work as nurses. As these young men and women use conscientiously the knowledge they gain, they will increase in capability, becoming better and better qualified to be the Lord's helping hand.

Review and Herald, Dec. 24, 1914.

The Lord wants wise men and women, who can act in the capacity of nurses, to comfort and help the sick and suffering. O that all who are afflicted might be ministered to by Christian physicians and nurses who could help them to place their weary, pain-racked bodies in the care of the Great Healer, in faith looking to Him for restoration! If through judicious ministration the patient is led to give his soul to Christ and to bring his thoughts into obedience to the will of God, a great victory is gained. . . .

There are many lines of work to be carried forward by the missionary nurse. There are opportunities for well-trained nurses to go into homes and there endeavor to awaken an interest in the truth. In almost every community there are large numbers who will not listen to the teaching of God's word or attend any religious service. If these are reached by the gospel, it must be carried to their homes. Often the relief of their physical needs is the only avenue by which they can be approached.

Missionary nurses who care for the sick and relieve the distress of the poor will find many opportunities to pray with them, to read to them from God's word, and to speak of the Saviour. They can pray with and for the helpless ones who have not strength of will to control the appetites that passion has degraded. They can bring a ray of hope into the lives of the defeated and disheartened. The revelation of unselfish love, manifested in acts of disinterested kindness, will make it easier for these suffering ones to believe in the love of Christ.

Many have no faith in God and have lost confidence in man. But they appreciate acts of sympathy and helpfulness. As they see one with no inducement of earthly praise or compensation coming to their homes to minister to the sick, to feed the hungry, to clothe the naked, and to comfort the sad, and ever tenderly pointing all to Him of whose love and pity the human worker is but the messenger—as they see this, their hearts are touched. Gratitude springs up; faith is kindled. They see that God cares for them and they are prepared to listen to the teaching of His word.

Gospel Workers to Minister to the Sick

Whether in foreign missions or in the home field, all missionaries, both men and women, will gain much more ready access to the people, and will find their usefulness greatly increased, if they are able to minister to the sick. Women who go as missionaries to heathen lands may thus find opportunity for giving the gospel to the women of those lands, when every other door of access is closed. All gospel workers should know how to give the simple treatments that do so much to relieve pain and remove disease.

Gospel workers should be able also to give instruction in the principles of healthful living. There is sickness everywhere, and much of it might be prevented by attention to the laws of health. The people need to see the bearing of health principles upon their well-being, both for this life and for the life to come. They need to be awakened to their responsibility for the human habitation fitted up by their Creator as His dwelling place, and over which He desires them to be faithful stewards.

Thousands need and would gladly receive instruction concerning the simple methods of treating the sick, methods that are taking the place of the use of poisonous drugs. There is great need of instruction in regard to dietetic reform. Wrong habits of eating and the use of unhealthful food are in no small degree responsible for the intemperance and crime and wretchedness that curse the world.

In teaching health principles, keep before the mind the great object of reform—that its purpose is to secure the highest development of body and mind and soul. Show that the laws of nature, being the laws of God, are designed for our good; that obedience to them promotes happiness in this life, and aids in the preparation for the life to come.

Encourage the people to study that marvelous organism, the human system, and the laws by which it is governed. Those who perceive the evidences of God's love, who understand something of the wisdom and beneficence of His laws and the results of obedience, will come to regard their duties and obligations from an altogether different point of view. Instead of looking upon an observance of the laws of health as a matter of sacrifice or self-denial, they will regard it as it really is, an inestimable blessing.

Teach the Health Reform Principles

Every gospel worker should feel that to teach the principles of healthful living is a part of his appointed work. Of this work there is great need, and the world is open for it.

Christ commits to His followers an individual work —a work that cannot be done by proxy. Ministry to the sick and the poor, the giving of the gospel to the lost, is not to be left to committees or organized charities. Individual responsibility, individual effort, personal sacrifice, are the requirement of the gospel.

"Go out into the highways and hedges, and compel them to come in," is Christ's demand, "that My house may be filled." Luke 14:23. He brings men into touch with those whom they may benefit. "Bring the poor that are cast out to thy house," He says. "When thou seest the naked, ... cover him." Isaiah 58:7. "They shall lay hands on the sick, and they shall recover." Mark 10:18. Through direct contact, through personal ministry, the blessings of the gospel are to be communicated.

Those who take up their appointed work will not only bless others, but will themselves be blessed. The consciousness of duty well done will have a reflex influence upon their own souls. The despondent will forget their despondency, the weak will become strong, the ignorant intelligent, and all will find an unfailing helper in Him who has called them.

House-to-House Work

Those who engage in house-to-house labor will find opportunities for ministry in many lines. They should pray for the sick and should do all in their power to relieve them from suffering. They should work among the lowly, the poor, and the oppressed. We should pray for and with the helpless ones who have not strength of will to control the appetites that passion has degraded. Earnest, persevering effort must be made for the salvation of those in whose hearts an interest is awakened. Many can be reached only through acts of disinterested kindness. Their physical wants must first be relieved. As they see evidence of our unselfish love, it will be easier for them to believe in the love of Christ.

Missionary nurses are best qualified for this work, but others should be connected with them. These, although not specially educated and trained in nursing, can learn from their fellow workers the best manner of labor.—*Testimonies for the Church,* vol. 6, pp. 83, 84 (1900).

A Plea for Medical Missionaries

We are living in the last days. The end of all things is at hand. The signs foretold by Christ are fast fulfilling. There are stormy times before us, but let us not utter one word of unbelief or discouragement. He who understands the necessities of the situation arranges that advantages should be brought to the workers in various places, to enable them more effectively to arouse the attention of the people. He knows the needs and the necessities of the feeblest of His flock, and He sends His own message into the highways and the byways. He loves us with an everlasting love. Let us remember that we bear a message of healing to a world filled with sin-sick souls. May the Lord increase our faith and help us to see that He desires us all to become acquainted with His ministry of healing and with the mercy seat. He desires the light of His grace to shine forth from many places.

Sanitariums As Missionary Agencies

There are souls in many places who have not yet heard the message. Henceforth medical missionary work is to be carried forward with an earnestness with which it has never yet been carried. This work is the door through which the truth is to find entrance to the large cities, and sanitariums are to be established in many places.

Sanitarium work is one of the most successful means of reaching all classes of people. Our sanitariums are the right hand of the gospel, opening ways whereby suffering humanity may be reached with the glad tidings of healing through Christ. In these institutions the sick may be taught to commit their cases to the Great Physician,

Testimonies for the Church, vol. 9, pp. 167-172 (1909).

who will co-operate with their earnest efforts to regain health, bringing to them healing of soul as well as healing of body.

Christ is no longer in this world in person, to go through our cities and towns and villages, healing the sick; but He has commissioned us to carry forward the medical missionary work that He began. In this work we are to do our very best. Institutions for the care of the sick are to be established where men and women suffering from disease may be placed under the care of God-fearing physicians and nurses and be treated without drugs.

I have been instructed that we are not to delay to do the work that needs to be done in health reform lines. Through this work we are to reach souls in the highways and byways. I have been given special light that in our sanitariums many souls will receive and obey present truth. In these institutions men and women are to be taught how to care for their own bodies, and at the same time how to become sound in the faith. They are to be taught what is meant by eating the flesh and drinking the blood of the Son of God. Said Christ, "The words that I speak unto you, they are spirit, and they are life." John 6:63.

Our sanitariums are to be schools in which instruction shall be given in medical missionary lines. They are to bring to sin-sick souls the leaves of the tree of life, which will restore to them peace and hope and faith in Christ Jesus.

The Work in Large Cities

Let the Lord's work go forward. Let the medical missionary and the educational work go forward. I am sure that this is our great lack—earnest, devoted, intelligent, capable workers. In every large city there should be a representation of true medical missionary work. Let many now ask, "Lord, what wilt Thou have me to do?" Acts 9:6. It is the Lord's purpose that His method of healing without drugs shall be brought into prominence in every large city through our medical institutions. God invests with holy dignity those who go forth farther and still farther, in every place to which it is possible to obtain entrance. Satan will make the work as difficult as possible, but divine power will attend all truehearted workers. Guided by our heavenly Father's hand, let us go forward, improving every opportunity to extend the work of God.

The Lord speaks to all medical missionaries, saying, Go, work today in My vineyard to save souls. God hears the prayers of all who seek Him in truth. He has the power that we all need. He fills the heart with love and joy and peace and holiness. Character is constantly being developed. We cannot afford to spend the time working at cross-purposes with God.

There are physicians who, because of a past connection with our sanitariums, find it profitable to locate close to these institutions; and they close their eyes to the great field, neglected and unworked, in which unselfish labor would be a blessing to many. Missionary physicians can exert an uplifting, refining, sanctifying influence. Physicians who do not do this abuse their power and do a work that the Lord repudiates.

Training for a Quick Work

If ever the Lord has spoken by me, He speaks when I say that the workers engaged in educational lines, in ministerial lines, and in medical missionary lines, must stand as a unit, all laboring under the supervision of God, one helping the other, each blessing each.

Those connected with our schools and sanitariums are to labor with earnest alacrity. The work that is done under the ministration of the Holy Spirit, out of love for God and for humanity, will bear the divine signature and will make its impression on human minds.

The Lord calls upon our young people to enter our schools and quickly fit themselves for service. In various places, outside of cities, schools are to be established where our youth can receive an education that will prepare them to go forth to do evangelical work and medical missionary work.

The Lord must be given an opportunity to show men their duty and to work upon their minds. No one is to bind himself to serve for a term of years under the direction of one group of men or in one specified branch of the Master's work, for the Lord Himself will call men, as of old He called the humble fishermen, and will Himself give them instruction regarding their field of labor and the methods they should follow. He will call men from the plow and from other occupations, to give the last note of warning to perishing souls. There are many ways in which to work for the Master, and the Great Teacher will open the understanding of these workers, enabling them to see wondrous things in His word.

Nurses As Evangelists

Christ, the great Medical Missionary, is our example. Of Him it is written that He "went about all Galilee, teaching in their synagogues, and preaching the gospel of the kingdom, and healing all manner of sickness and all manner of disease among the people." Matthew 4:23.

He healed the sick and preached the gospel. In His service, healing and teaching were linked closely together. Today they are not to be separated.

The nurses who are trained in our institutions are to be fitted up to go out as medical missionary evangelists, uniting the ministry of the word with that of physical healing.

We must let our light shine amid the moral darkness. Many who are now in darkness, as they see a reflection of the Light of the world, will realize that they have a hope of salvation. Your light may be small, but remember that it is what God has given you, and that He holds you responsible to let it shine forth. Someone may light his taper from yours, and his light may be the means of leading others out from the darkness.

All around us are doors open for service. We should become acquainted with our neighbors and seek to draw them to Christ. As we do this, He will approve and cooperate with us.

Often the inhabitants of a city where Christ labored wished Him to stay with them and continue to work among them. But He would tell them that He must go to cities that had not heard the truths that He had to present. After He had given the truth to those in one place, He left them to build upon what He had given them, while He went to another place. His methods of labor are to be followed today by those to whom He has left His work. We are to go from place to place, carrying the message. As soon as the truth has been proclaimed in one place, we are to go to warn others.

Organization of Companies

There should be companies organized and educated most thoroughly to work as nurses, as evangelists, as ministers, as canvassers, as gospel students, to perfect a character after the divine similitude. To prepare to receive the higher education in the school above is now to be our purpose.

From the instruction that the Lord has given me from time to time, I know that there should be workers who make medical evangelistic tours among the towns and villages. Those who do this work will gather a rich harvest of souls, from both the higher and lower classes. The way for this work is best prepared by the efforts of the faithful canvasser.

Many will be called into the field to labor from house to house, giving Bible readings, and praying with those who are interested.

Let our ministers, who have gained an experience in preaching the word, learn how to give simple treatments and then labor intelligently as medical missionary evangelists.

An Urgent Work

Workers—gospel medical missionaries—are needed now. You cannot afford to spend years in preparation. Soon doors now open to the truth will be forever closed. Carry the message now. Do not wait, allowing the enemy to take possession of the fields now open before you. Let little companies go forth to do the work to which Christ appointed His disciples. Let them labor as evangelists, scattering our publications and talking of the truth to those they meet. Let them pray for the sick, ministering to their necessities, not with drugs, but with nature's remedies, and teaching them how to regain health and avoid disease.

Duties and Privileges of Sanitarium Workers

The management of so large and important an institution as the sanitarium necessarily involves great responsibility, both in temporal and spiritual matters. It is of the highest importance that this asylum for those who are diseased in body and mind shall be such that Jesus, the Mighty Healer, can preside among them, and all that is done may be under the control of His Spirit. All connected with this institution should qualify themselves for the faithful discharge of their God-given responsibilities. They should attend to every little duty with as much fidelity as to matters of greater importance. All should study prayerfully how they can themselves become most useful and make this retreat for the sick a grand success.

We do not realize with what anxiety patients with their various diseases come to the sanitarium, all desiring help, but some doubtful and distrusting, while others are more confident that they shall be relieved. Those who have not visited the institution are watching with interest every indication of the principles which are cherished by its managers.

All who profess to be children of God should unceasingly bear in mind that they are missionaries, in their labors brought in connection with all classes of minds. There will be the refined and the coarse, the humble and the proud, the religious and the skeptical, the confiding and the suspicious, the liberal and the avaricious, the pure and the corrupt, the educated and the ignorant, the rich and the poor; in fact, almost every grade of character and condition will be found among the patients at the sanitarium. Those who come to this asylum come because

Testimonies for the Church, vol. 4, pp. 554-562 (1881).

they need help; and thus, whatever their station or condition, they acknowledge that they are not able to help themselves. These varied minds cannot be treated alike; yet all, whether they are rich or poor, high or low, dependent or independent, need kindness, sympathy, and love. By mutual contact, our minds should receive polish and refinement. We are dependent upon one another, closely bound together by the ties of human brotherhood.

> Heaven, forming each on other to depend,
> A master, or a servant, or a friend,
> Bids each on other for assistance call,
> Till one man's weakness grows the strength of all.

Value of Social Relations

It is through the social relations that Christianity comes in contact with the world. Every man or woman who has tasted of the love of Christ and has received into the heart the divine illumination, is required of God to shed light on the dark pathway of those who are unacquainted with the better way. Every worker in that sanitarium should become a witness for Jesus. Social power, sanctified by the Spirit of Christ, must be improved to win souls to the Saviour.

He who has to deal with persons differing so widely in character, disposition, and temperament will have trials, perplexities, and collisions, even when he does his best. He may be disgusted with the ignorance, pride, and independence which he will meet; but this should not discourage him. He should stand where he will sway rather than be swayed. Firm as a rock to principle, with an intelligent faith, he should stand uncorrupted by surrounding influences. The people of God should not be transformed by the various influences to which they must necessarily be exposed; but they must stand up for Jesus, and by the aid of His Spirit exert a transforming power upon minds deformed by false habits and defiled by sin.

The Beauty of Holiness

Christ is not to be hid away in the heart and locked in as a coveted treasure, sacred and sweet, to be enjoyed solely by the possessor. We are to have Christ in our hearts as a well of water, springing up into everlasting life, refreshing all who come in contact with us. We must confess Christ openly and bravely, exhibiting in our characters his meekness, humility, and love, till men shall be charmed by the beauty of holiness. It is not the best way to preserve our religion as we bottle perfumes, lest the fragrance should escape.

The very conflicts and rebuffs we meet are to make us stronger and give stability to our faith. We are not to be swayed, like a reed in the wind, by every passing influence. Our souls, warmed and invigorated by the truths of the gospel and refreshed by divine grace, are to open and expand and shed their fragrance upon others. Clad in the whole armor of righteousness, we can meet any influence and our purity remain untarnished.

All should consider that God's claims upon them are paramount to all others. God has given to every person capabilities to improve, that he may reflect glory to the Giver. Every day some progress should be made. If the workers leave the sanitarium as they entered it, without making decided improvement, gaining in knowledge and spiritual strength, they have met with loss. God designs that Christians shall grow continually—grow up into the full stature of men and women in Christ. All who do not grow stronger and become more firmly rooted and grounded in the truth are continually retrograding.

A Light to the World

A special effort should be made to secure the services of conscientious, Christian workers. It is the purpose of God that a health institution should be organized and controlled exclusively by Seventh-day Adventists; and when unbelievers are brought in to occupy responsible positions, an influence is presiding there that will tell with great weight against the sanitarium. God did not intend that this institution should be carried on after the order of any other health institute in the land, but that it should be one of the most effectual instrumentalities in His hands of giving light to the world. It should stand forth with scientific ability, with moral and spiritual power, and as a faithful sentinel of reform in all its bearings; and all who act a part in it should be reformers, having respect to its rules, and heeding the light of health reform now shining upon us as a people.

All can be a blessing to others, if they will place themselves where they will correctly represent the religion of Jesus Christ. But there has been greater anxiety to make the outward appearance in every way presentable, that it may meet the minds of worldly patients, than to maintain a living connection with Heaven, to watch and pray, that this instrumentality of God may be wholly successful in doing good to the bodies and also to the souls of men.

A Molding Power

What can be said, and what can be done, to awaken conviction in the hearts of all connected with this important institution? How can they be led to see and feel the danger of making wrong moves unless they daily have a living experience in the things of God? The physicians are in a position where, should they exert an influence in accordance with their faith, they would have a molding power upon all connected with the institution. This is one of the best missionary fields in the world, and all in responsible positions should become acquainted with God and ever be receiving light from Heaven. . . .

There are some who are not what the Lord would have them to be. They are abrupt and harsh and need the softening, subduing influence of the Spirit of God. It is never convenient to take up the cross and follow in the path of self-denial, and yet this must be done. God wants all to have His grace and His Spirit to make fragrant their life. Some are too independent, too self-sufficient, and do not counsel with others as they should. . . .

There must be, with all who have any influence in the sanitarium, a conforming to God's will, a humiliation of self, an opening of the heart to the precious influence of the Spirit of Christ. The gold tried in the fire represents love and faith. Many are nearly destitute of love. Self-sufficiency blinds their eyes to their great need. There is a positive necessity for a daily conversion to God, a new, deep, and daily experience in the religious life.

There should be awakened in the hearts of the physicians, especially, a most earnest desire to have that wisdom which God alone can impart; for as soon as they become self-confident they are left to themselves, to follow the impulses of the unsanctified heart. When I see what these physicians may become, in connection with Christ, and what they will fail to become if they do not daily connect with Him, I am filled with apprehension that they will be content with reaching a worldly standard and have no ardent longings, no hungering and thirsting for the beauty of holiness, the ornament of a meek and quiet spirit, which is in the sight of God of great price.

The peace of Christ, the peace of Christ—money cannot buy it, brilliant talent cannot command it, intellect cannot secure it; it is the gift of God. The religion of Christ—how shall I make all understand their great loss if they fail to carry its holy principles into the daily life? The meekness and lowliness of Christ is the Christian's power. It is indeed more precious than all things which genius can create or wealth can buy. Of all things that are sought, cherished, and cultivated, there is nothing so valuable in the sight of God as a pure heart, a disposition imbued with thankfulness and peace.

If the divine harmony of truth and love exists in the heart, it will shine forth in words and actions. The most careful cultivation of the outward proprieties and courtesies of life has not sufficient power to shut out all fretfulness, harsh judgment, and unbecoming speech. The spirit of genuine benevolence must dwell in the heart. Love imparts to its possessor grace, propriety, and comeliness of deportment. Love illuminates the countenance and subdues the voice; it refines and elevates the entire man. It brings him into harmony with God, for it is a heavenly attribute.

Many are in danger of thinking that in the cares of labor, in writing and practicing as physicians, or performing the duties of the various departments, they are excusable if they lay down prayer, neglect the Sabbath, and neglect religious service. Sacred things are thus brought down to meet their convenience, while duties, denials, and crosses are left untouched. Neither physicians nor helpers should attempt to perform their work without taking time to pray. God would be the helper of all who profess to love Him, if they would come to Him in faith and, with a sense of their own weakness, crave His power. When they separate from God their wisdom will be found to be foolishness. When they are small in their own eyes and lean heavily upon their God, then He will be the arm of their power, and success will attend their efforts; but when they allow the mind to be diverted from God, then Satan comes in and controls the thoughts and perverts the judgment. . . .

Brethren, I entreat you to move with an eye single to the glory of God. Let His power be your dependence, His grace your strength. By study of the Scriptures and earnest prayer seek to obtain clear conceptions of your duty, and then faithfully perform it. It is essential that you cultivate faithfulness in little things, and in so doing you will acquire habits of integrity in greater responsibilities. The little incidents of everyday life often pass without our notice, but it is these things that shape the character. Every event of life is great for good or for evil. The mind needs to be trained by daily tests, that it may acquire power to stand in any difficult position. In the days of trial and of peril you will need to be fortified to stand firmly for the right, independent of every opposing influence.

Advance in Knowledge

God is willing to do much for you, if you will only feel your need of Him. Jesus loves you. Ever seek to walk in the light of God's wisdom; and through all the changing scenes of life, do not rest unless you know that your will is in harmony with the will of your Creator. Through faith in Him you may obtain strength to resist every temptation of Satan and thus increase in moral power with every test from God.

You may become men of responsibility and influence if, by the power of your will, united with divine strength, you earnestly engage in the work. Exercise the mental powers and in no case neglect the physical. Let not intellectual slothfulness close up your path to greater knowledge. Learn to reflect as well as to study, that your minds may expand, strengthen, and develop. Never think that you have learned enough and that you may now relax your efforts. The cultivated mind is the measure of the man. Your education should continue during your lifetime; every day you should be learning and putting to practical use the knowledge gained.

You are rising in true dignity and moral worth as you practice virtue and cherish uprightness in heart and life. Let not your character be affected by a taint of the leprosy of selfishness. A noble soul, united with a cultivated intellect, will make you men whom God will use in positions of sacred trust.

It should be the first work of all connected with this institution to be right before God themselves, and then to stand in the strength of Christ, unaffected by the wrong influences to which they will be exposed. If they make the broad principles of the word of God the foundation of the character, they may stand wherever the Lord in His providence may call them, surrounded by any deleterious influence, and yet not be swayed from the path of right.

Cheerfulness

In sanitariums and hospitals, where nurses are constantly associated with large numbers of sick people, it requires a decided effort to be always pleasant and cheerful and to show thoughtful consideration in every word and act. In these institutions it is of the utmost importance that the nurses strive to do their work wisely and well. They need ever to remember that in the discharge of their daily duties they are serving the Lord Christ.

A Ready Mind

The sick need to have wise words spoken to them. Nurses should study the Bible daily, that they may be able to speak words that will enlighten and help the suffering. Angels of God are in the rooms where these suffering ones are being ministered to, and the atmosphere surrounding the soul of the one giving treatment should be pure and fragrant. Physicians and nurses are to cherish the principles of Christ. In their lives His virtues are to be seen. Then, by what they do and say, they will draw the sick to the Saviour.

The Christian nurse, while administering treatment for the restoration of health, will pleasantly and successfully draw the mind of the patient to Christ, the healer of the soul as well as of the body. The thoughts presented, here a little and there a little, will have their influence. The older nurses should lose no favorable opportunity of calling the attention of the sick to Christ. They should be ever ready to blend spiritual healing with physical healing.

In the kindest and tenderest manner nurses are to teach that he who would be healed must cease to transgress the

The Ministry of Healing, pages 222-224 (1905).

(406)

law of God. He must cease to choose a life of sin. God cannot bless the one who continues to bring upon himself disease and suffering by a willful violation of the laws of heaven. But Christ, through the Holy Spirit, comes as a healing power to those who cease to do evil and learn to do well.

Efficiency Depends Upon Vigor

The efficiency of the nurse depends, to a great degree, upon physical vigor. The better the health, the better will she be able to endure the strain of attendance upon the sick and the more successfully can she perform her duties. Those who care for the sick should give special attention to diet, cleanliness, fresh air, and exercise. Like carefulness on the part of the family will enable them also to endure the extra burdens brought upon them and will help to prevent them from contracting disease. . . .

Nurses, and all who have to do with the sickroom, should be cheerful, calm, and self-possessed. All hurry, excitement, or confusion should be avoided. Doors should be opened and shut with care and the whole household be kept quiet. In cases of fever, special care is needed when the crisis comes and the fever is passing away. Then constant watching is often necessary. Ignorance, forgetfulness, and recklessness have caused the death of many who might have lived had they received proper care from judicious, thoughtful nurses.—*The Ministry of Healing,* pages 219-222 (1905).

Integrity Among Workers

The helpers at the sanitarium should not feel at liberty to appropriate to their own use articles of food provided for the patients. The temptation is especially strong to indulge in things allowed to newcomers, who must be induced gradually to correct pernicious habits. Some of the workers, like the children of Israel, allow perverted appetite and old habits of indulgence to clamor for victory. They long, as did ancient Israel, for the leeks and onions of Egypt. All connected with this institution should strictly adhere to the laws of life and health, and thus give no countenance, by their example, to the wrong habits of others, which have made it necessary for them to come to the sanitarium for relief.

Employees have no right to help themselves to crackers, nuts, raisins, dates, sugar, oranges or fruit of any kind; for, in the first place, in eating these things between meals, as is generally done, they are injuring the digestive organs. No food should pass the lips between the regular meals. Again, those who partake of these things are taking that which is not theirs. Temptation is continually before them to taste the food which they are handling; and here is an excellent opportunity for them to gain control of the appetite. But food seems to be very abundant, and they forget that it all represents so much money value. One and another thoughtlessly indulge the habit of tasting and helping themselves, until they fancy that there is no real sin in the practice.

All should beware of cherishing this view of the matter, for conscience is thus losing its sensitiveness. One may reason, "The little I have taken does not amount

Special Testimonies to Physicians and Helpers, pages 59-65 (1879).

to much;" but the question comes home, Did the smallness of the amount lessen the sin of the act? Again, the little which one person takes may not amount to much, but when five act on the same plan, five littles are taken. Then ten, twenty, or even more, may presume in the same way, until every day the workers may, to their own injury, appropriate many littles that they have no right to touch. Many littles make much in the end. But the greatest loss is sustained by the ones who digress, for they are violating the principles of right and learning to look upon transgression in small matters as no transgression at all. They forget the words of Christ. "He that is faithful in that which is least is faithful also in much: and he that is unjust in the least is unjust also in much." Luke 16:10.

When an effort is made to correct these practices, it is generally received as an evidence of stinginess on the part of the managers; and some will make no change, but go on hardening the conscience, until it becomes seared as with a hot iron. They rise up against any restriction and act and talk defiantly, as though their rights had been invaded. But God looks upon all these things as theft, and so the record is carried up to heaven.

All fraud and deceit is forbidden in the word of God. Direct theft and outright falsehood are not sins into which persons of respectability are in danger of falling. It is transgression in the little things that first leads the soul away from God. By their one sin in partaking of the forbidden fruit, Adam and Eve opened the floodgates of woe upon the world. Some may regard that transgression as a very little thing; but we see that its consequences were anything but small. The angels in heaven have a wider and more elevated sphere of action than we; but right with them and right with us are one and the same thing.

The managers of the sanitarium are not actuated by a mean, penurious spirit in reproving the wrongs that have been mentioned, and requiring what is due to such an institution. It is no stepping down from proper dignity to guard the interests of the sanitarium in these matters. Officers who are faithful themselves, naturally look for faithfulness in others. Strict integrity should govern the dealings of the managers and should be enforced upon all who labor under their direction.

Men of principle need not the restriction of locks and keys; they do not need to be watched and guarded. They will deal truly and honorably at all times—alone, with no eye upon them, as well as in public. They will not bring a stain upon their souls for any amount of gain or selfish advantage. They scorn a mean act. Although no one else might know it, they would know it themselves, and this would destroy their self-respect. Those who are not conscientious and faithful in little things would not be reformed, were there laws and restrictions and penalties upon the point. . . .

Those who do not overcome in little things will have no moral power to withstand greater temptations. All who seek to make honesty the ruling principle in the daily business of life will need to be on their guard that they "covet no man's silver, or gold, or apparel." While they are content with convenient food and clothing, it will be found an easy matter to keep the heart and hands from the defilement of covetousness and dishonesty. . . .

Those who are employed at our sanitarium have in many respects the best advantages for the formation of correct habits. None will be placed beyond the reach of temptation; for in every character there are weak points that are in danger when assailed. . . . All should feel the necessity of keeping the moral nature braced by constant watchfulness. Like faithful sentinels, they should guard the citadel of the soul, never feeling that they may relax their vigilance for a moment. In earnest prayer and living faith is their only safety.

Those who begin to be careless of their steps will find that before they are aware of it, their feet are entangled in a web from which it is impossible for them to extricate themselves. It should be a fixed principle with all to be truthful and honest. Whether they are rich or poor, whether they have friends or are left alone, come what will, they should resolve in the strength of God that no influence shall lead them to commit the least wrong act. One and all should realize that upon them, individually, depends in a measure the prosperity of the sanitarium.

Steadfastness

The mind must be trained through daily tests to habits of fidelity, to a sense of the claims of right and duty above inclination and pleasure. Minds thus trained do not waver between right and wrong, as the reed trembles in the wind; but as soon as matters come before them, they discern at once that principle is involved, and they instinctively choose the right without long debating the matter. They are loyal because they have trained themselves to habits of faithfulness and truth.—*Testimonies for the Church,* vol. 3, p. 22 (1872).

A Sad Picture

As the condition of the sanitarium was presented before me in vision, an angel of God seemed to conduct me from room to room in the different departments. The conversation I was made to hear in the rooms of the helpers was not of a character to elevate and strengthen mind or morals. The frivolous talk, the foolish jesting, the meaningless laugh, fell painfully upon the ear. . . .

I was astonished as I saw the jealousy indulged and listened to the words of envy, the reckless talk, which made angels of God ashamed. Words and actions and motives were recorded. And how little did these light, superficial heads and hard hearts realize that an angel of God stood at the door, writing down the manner in which these precious moments were employed. God will bring to light every word and every action. He is in every place. These messengers, although unseen, are visitors in the bedchamber. The hidden works of darkness will be brought to light. The thoughts, the intents and purposes of the heart, will stand revealed. All things are naked and open to the eyes of Him with whom we have to do.

I was conducted to a few rooms from which came the voice of prayer. How welcome was the sound! A bright light shone upon the face of my guide as his hand traced every word of the petition. "The eyes of the Lord are over the righteous, and His ears are open unto their prayers." 1 Peter 3:12.

Disagreeable Criticism

From still other rooms came the most disagreeable sallies of low wit and vain talk. Some were making sport

---

Special Testimonies to Physicians and Helpers, pages 87-89 (1879).

of individuals and even imitating the words uttered in meeting; sacred things were made the subject of jest. Young men and young women were severely criticized; courtship and marriage were dwelt upon in a low, disgusting manner. There was scarcely a serious word spoken; the conversation was of a character to debase the mind and taint the morals, and all retired without committing themselves to God.

Waves of Influence

You may never know the result of your influence from day to day, but be sure that it is exerted for good or evil. Many who have a kind heart and good impulses permit their attention to be absorbed in worldly business or pleasure, while the souls that look to them for guidance drift on to hopeless wreck. Such persons may have a high profession and may stand well in the opinion of men, even as Christians, but in the day of God, when our works shall be compared with the divine law, then it will be found that they have not come up to the standard. Others who saw their course fell a little below them, and still others fell below the latter class, and thus the work of degeneracy went on.

Throw a pebble into the lake and a wave is formed, and another and another; and as they increase, the circle widens until they reach the very shore. Thus our influence, though apparently insignificant, may continue to extend far beyond our knowledge or control.—*Review and Herald,* Jan. 24, 1882.

The Power of Association

In our institutions, where many are laboring together, the influence of association is very great. It is natural to seek companionship. Everyone will find companions or make them. And just in proportion to the strength of the friendship, will be the amount of influence which friends will exert over one another for good or for evil. All will have associates, and will influence and be influenced in their turn.

The link is a mysterious one which binds human hearts together, so that the feelings, tastes, and principles of two individuals are closely blended. One catches the spirit, and copies the ways and acts, of the other. As wax retains the figure of the seal, so the mind retains the impression produced by intercourse and association. The influence may be unconscious, yet it is no less powerful.

If the youth could be persuaded to associate with the pure, the thoughtful, and the amiable, the effect would be most salutary. If choice is made of companions who fear the Lord, the influence will lead to truth, to duty, and to holiness. A truly Christian life is a power for good. But, on the other hand, those who associate with men and women of questionable morals, of bad principles and practices, will soon be walking in the same path. The tendencies of the natural heart are downward. He who associates with the skeptic will soon become skeptical; he who chooses the companionship of the vile will most assuredly become vile. To walk in the counsel of the ungodly is the first step toward standing in the way of sinners and sitting in the seat of the scornful.

Testimonies for the Church, vol. 4, pp. 587-591 (1881).

(414)

Choose Noble Associates

Let all who would form a right character choose associates who are of a serious, thoughtful turn of mind, and who are religiously inclined. Those who have counted the cost and wish to build for eternity must put good material into their building. If they accept of rotten timbers, if they are content with deficiencies of character, the building is doomed to ruin. Let all take heed how they build. The storm of temptation will sweep over the building, and unless it is firmly and faithfully constructed it will not stand the test.

A good name is more precious than gold. There is an inclination with the youth to associate with those who are inferior in mind and morals. What real happiness can a young person expect from a voluntary connection with persons who have a low standard of thoughts, feelings, and deportment? Some are debased in taste and depraved in habits, and all who choose such companions will follow their example. We are living in times of peril that should cause the hearts of all to fear. We see the minds of many wandering through the mazes of skepticism. The causes of this are ignorance, pride, and a defective character. Humility is a hard lesson for fallen man to learn. There is something in the human heart which rises in opposition to revealed truth on subjects connected with God and sinners, the transgression of the divine law and pardon through Christ.

Study the Scriptures

My brethren and sisters, old and young, when you have an hour of leisure open the Bible and store the mind with its precious truths. When engaged in labor, guard the mind, keep it stayed upon God, talk less and meditate more. Remember, "Every idle word that men shall speak, they shall give account thereof in the day of judgment." Matthew 12:36. Let your words be select; this will close a door against the adversary of souls. Let your day be entered upon with prayer; work as in God's sight. His angels are ever by your side, making a record of your words, your deportment, and the manner in which your work is done.

If you turn from good counsel and choose to associate with those who you have reason to suspect are not religiously inclined, although they profess to be Christians, you will soon become like them. You place yourself in the way of temptation, on Satan's battleground, and will, unless constantly guarded, be overcome by his devices. There are persons who have for some time made a profession of religion, who are, to all intents and purposes, without God and without a sensitive conscience. They are vain and trifling; their conversation is of a low order. Courtship and marriage occupy the mind to the exclusion of higher and nobler thoughts.

The associations chosen by the workers are determining their destiny for this world and for the next. Some who were once conscientious and faithful have sadly changed; they have disconnected from God, and Satan has allured them to his side. They are now irreligious and irreverent, and they have an influence upon others who are easily molded. Evil associations are deteriorating character; principle is being undermined. "He that walketh with wise men shall be wise: but a companion of fools shall be destroyed." Proverbs 13:20.

Avoid Flirtation

The young are in danger, but they are blind to discern the tendencies and result of the course they are pursuing.

Many of them are engaged in flirtation. They seem to be infatuated. There is nothing noble, dignified, or sacred in these attachments; as they are prompted by Satan, the influence is such as to please him. Warnings to these persons fall unheeded. They are headstrong, self-willed, defiant. They think the warning, counsel, or reproof does not apply to them. Their course gives them no concern. They are continually separating themselves from the light and love of God. They lose all discernment of sacred and eternal things; and while they may keep up a dry form of Christian duties, they have no heart in these religious exercises. All too late, these deceived souls will learn that "strait is the gate, and narrow is the way, which leadeth unto life, and few there be that find it." Matthew 7:14.

Words and actions and motives are recorded; but how little do these light, superficial heads and hard hearts realize that an angel of God stands writing down the manner in which their precious moments are employed. God will bring to light every word and every action. He is in every place. His messengers, although unseen, are visitors in the workroom and in the sleeping apartment. The hidden works of darkness will be brought to light. The thoughts, the intents and purposes of the heart, will stand revealed. All things are naked and open to the eyes of Him with whom we have to do.

The workers should take Jesus with them in every department of their labor. Whatever is done should be done with an exactness and thoroughness that will bear inspection. The heart should be in the work. Faithfulness is as essential in life's common duties as in those involving greater responsibility. Some may receive the idea that their work is not ennobling; but this is just as they choose to make it. They alone are capable of degrad-

ing or elevating their employment. We wish that every
drone might be compelled to toil for his daily bread, for
work is a blessing, not a curse. Diligent labor will keep
us from many of the snares of Satan, who "finds some
mischief still for idle hands to do."

Be Not Ashamed of Work

None of us should be ashamed of work, however small
and servile it may appear. Labor is ennobling. All who
toil with head or hands are working men or working
women. And all are doing their duty and honoring their
religion as much while working at the washtub or washing the dishes, as they are in going to meeting. While the
hands are engaged in the most common labor, the mind
may be elevated and ennobled by pure and holy thoughts.
When any of the workers manifest a lack of respect for
religious things, they should be separated from the work.
Let none feel that the institution is dependent upon them.

Those who have been employed in our institutions
should now be responsible workers, reliable in every place,
as faithful to duty as the compass to the pole. Had they
rightly improved their opportunities, they might now
have symmetrical characters and a deep, living experience in religious things. But some of these workers have
separated from God. Religion is laid aside. It is not an
inwrought principle, carefully cherished wherever they
go, into whatever society they are thrown, proving as an
anchor to the soul. I wish all the workers carefully to
consider that success in this life, and success in gaining
the future life, depend largely upon faithfulness in little
things. Those who long for higher responsibilities should
manifest faithfulness in performing the duties just where
God has placed them.

The perfection of God's work is as clearly seen in the tiniest insect as in the king of birds. The soul of the little child that believes in Christ is as precious in His sight as are the angels about His throne. "Be ye therefore perfect, even as your Father which is in heaven is perfect." Matthew 5:48. As God is perfect in His sphere, so man may be perfect in his sphere. Whatever the hand finds to do should be done with thoroughness and dispatch. Faithfulness and integrity in little things, the performance of little duties and little deeds of kindness, will cheer and gladden the pathway of life; and when our work on earth is ended, every one of the little duties performed with fidelity will be treasured as a precious gem before God.

In Our Schools

In our schools missionary nurses should receive lessons from well-qualified physicians, and as a part of their education should learn how to battle with disease and to show the value of nature's remedies. This work is greatly needed. Cities and towns are steeped in sin and moral corruption, yet there are Lots in every Sodom. The poison of sin is at work at the heart of society, and God calls for reformers to stand in defense of the law which He has established to govern the physical system. They should at the same time maintain an elevated standard in the training of the mind and the culture of the heart, that the Great Physician may co-operate with the human helping hand in doing a work of mercy and necessity in the relief of suffering.—*Testimonies for the Church,* vol. 6, p. 136 (1900).

A Lack of Economy

As my guide conducted me through the different departments, the lack of economy everywhere stirred my soul with grief, for I had a full sense of the debt hanging over the institution. The petty dishonesty, the selfish neglect of duty, were marked by the recording angel. The waste permitted here and there, in the course of a year amounts to a considerable sum. Much of this might be saved by the helpers; but each will say, "It does not belong to me to look after these things." Would they pass these things by so indifferently if the loss was to be sustained by themselves? No, they would know exactly what to do and how to do it; but it makes all the difference, now that it belongs to the institution. This is the fruit of selfishness and is registered against them under the heading of unfaithfulness.

In the dining room and kitchen I saw marks of negligence and untidiness. The floors were not cleanly, and there was a great lack of thoroughness, of nicety and order. These things speak to all who have access to these rooms, of the character of the workers. The impression would not be made that the sanitarium had a class of neat, faithful, orderly helpers. Some have labored faithfully, while others have done their work mechanically, as though they had no interest in it except to get through as quickly as possible. Order and thoroughness were neglected, because no one was near to watch them and criticize their work. Unfaithfulness was written against their names.

The matron looked upon the same that I saw, but she good-naturedly passed it by and seemed to have no sense of the true state of things. I saw a few trying to change

Special Testimonies to Physicians and Helpers, pages 90, 91 (1879).

things for the better and pleading for a faithful discharge of duty; but an indignant protest was raised, and most unmerciful thrusts were given those who ventured to take this responsibility. Unpleasant remarks were unsparingly made, and feelings of jealousy and envy indulged, and those who would have been true and faithful found numbers so large against them that they were compelled to allow things to drift on as before. These are some of the existing evils at the sanitarium.

Our Influence

Every act of our lives affects others for good or evil. Our influence is tending upward or downward; it is felt, acted upon, and to a greater or less degree reproduced by others. If by our example we aid others in the development of good principles, we give them power to do good. In their turn they exert the same beneficial influence upon others, and thus hundreds and thousands are affected by our unconscious influence. If we by acts strengthen or force into activity the evil powers possessed by those around us, we share their sin and will have to render an account for the good we might have done them and did not do, because we made not God our strength, our guide, our counselor.—*Testimonies for the Church,* vol. 2, p. 133 (1868).

Need of Opportunity for Christian Culture

No soul can prosper without time to pray, to search the Scriptures; and all should, as far as possible, have the privilege of attending public worship. All need to keep the oil of grace in their vessels with their lamps. Above all others, the workers who are thrown into the society of worldlings need to have Jesus held up before them, that they may behold the Lamb of God that taketh away the sin of the world. The godless element to which they are exposed makes it essential that personal labor should be bestowed upon them. Who could be closely related to these patients, and hear them talk, and breathe in the atmosphere that surrounds their souls, without running some risk? Counteracting influences should always be exerted, lest, through the tempting allurements of Satan, the worldly element shall steal away hearts from God. Never let the worldly class be honored and great deference be paid to them above those who love God and are seeking to do His will.

Those who, from whatever cause, are obliged to work on the Sabbath, are always in peril; they feel the loss, and from doing works of necessity they fall into the habit of doing things on the Sabbath that are not necessary. The sense of its sacredness is lost, and the holy commandment is of no effect. A special effort should be made to bring about a reform in regard to Sabbath observance. The workers in the sanitarium do not always do for themselves what is their privilege and duty. Often they feel so weary that they become demoralized. This should not be. The soul can be rich in grace only as it shall abide in the presence of God. God is the great proprietor of

Health, Philanthropic, and Medical Missionary Work, pages 13-16 (1890).

the sanitarium, of the Review and Herald office, of the Pacific Press, of our colleges. In all these institutions the managers must receive their directions from above. And wherever the temptations that come through association with the ungodly are strongest, there the greatest care must be exercised to place the workers in close connection with Christ and the influences proceeding from Him. His word must be our guide in all things; and if poverty comes because we abide by a plain "Thus saith the Lord," we must abide by it, even at the loss of all things else. Better have poverty in temporal things, and abide in Christ and be nourished by His word, which is spirit and life. "Man shall not live by bread alone, but by every word that proceedeth out of the mouth of God." Matthew 4:4. The world may smile as we repeat this to them, but it is the word of the Son of God. He says, "Whoso eateth My flesh [the word that Christ speaks to us] . . . hath eternal life; and I will raise him up at the last day." John 6:54.

We cannot always be on our knees in prayer, but the way to the mercy seat is always open. While engaged in active labor, we may ask for help; and we are promised by One who will not deceive us, "Ye shall receive." The Christian can and will find time to pray. Daniel was a statesman; heavy responsibilities rested upon him; yet three times a day he sought God, and the Lord gave him the Holy Spirit. So today men may resort to the sacred pavilion of the Most High and feel the assurance of His promise, "My people shall dwell in a peaceable habitation, and in sure dwellings, and in quiet resting places." Isaiah 32:18. All who really desire it can find a place for communion with God, where no ear can hear but the one open to the cries of the helpless, distressed, and needy—

the One who notices even the fall of the little sparrow. He says, "Ye are of more value than many sparrows." Matthew 10:31.

If the rush of work is allowed to drive us from our purpose of seeking the Lord daily, we shall make the greatest mistakes; we shall incur losses, for the Lord is not with us; we have closed the door so that He cannot find access to our souls. But if we pray even when our hands are employed, the Saviour's ear is open to hear our petitions. If we are determined not to be separated from the Source of our strength, Jesus will be just as determined to be at our right hand to help us, that we may not be put to shame before our enemies. The grace of Christ can accomplish for us that which all our efforts will fail to do. Those who love and fear God may be surrounded with a multitude of cares, and yet not falter or make crooked paths for their feet. God takes care of you in the place where it is your duty to be. But be sure, as often as possible, to go where prayer is wont to be made. The Saviour says, "Thou hast a few names even in Sardis which have not defiled their garments; and they shall walk with Me in white: for they are worthy." Revelation 3:4. These souls overcame by the blood of the Lamb and the word of their testimony. Amid the moral pollution that prevailed on every hand, they held fast their integrity. And why? They were partakers of the divine nature, and thus they escaped the corruption that is in the world through lust. They became rich in faith, heirs to an inheritance of more value than the gold of Ophir. Only a life of constant dependence upon the Saviour is a life of holiness.

TEACHING HEALTH PRINCIPLES

The Church Should Awake

We have come to a time when every member of the church should take hold of medical missionary work. The world is a lazar house filled with victims of both physical and spiritual disease. Everywhere people are perishing for lack of a knowledge of the truths that have been committed to us. The members of the church are in need of an awakening, that they may realize their responsibility to impart these truths. Those who have been enlightened by the truth are to be light bearers to the world. To hide our light at this time is to make a terrible mistake. The message to God's people today is, "Arise, shine; for thy light is come, and the glory of the Lord is risen upon thee." Isaiah 60:1.

On every hand we see those who have had much light and knowledge deliberately choosing evil in the place of good. Making no attempt to reform, they are growing worse and worse. But the people of God are not to walk in darkness. They are to walk in the light, for they are reformers.

Before the true reformer, the medical missionary work will open many doors. No one need wait until called to some distant field before beginning to help others. Wherever you are, you can begin at once. Opportunities are within the reach of everyone. Take up the work for which you are held responsible—the work that should be done in your home and in your neighborhood. Wait

Testimonies for the Church, vol. 7, pp. 62-67 (1902).

not for others to urge you to action. In the fear of God go forward without delay, bearing in mind your individual responsibility to Him who gave His life for you. Act as if you heard Christ calling upon you personally to do your utmost in His service. Look not to see who else is ready. If you are truly consecrated, God will, through your instrumentality, bring into the truth others whom He can use as channels to convey light to many that are groping in darkness.

All Can Act a Part

All can do something. In an effort to excuse themselves, some say, "My home duties, my children, claim my time and my means." Parents, your children should be your helping hand, increasing your power and ability to work for the Master. Children are the younger members of the Lord's family. They should be led to consecrate themselves to God, whose they are by creation and by redemption. They should be taught that all their powers of body, mind, and soul are His. They should be trained to help in various lines of unselfish service. Do not allow your children to be hindrances. With you the children should share spiritual as well as physical burdens. By helping others they increase their own happiness and usefulness.

Let our people show that they have a living interest in medical missionary work. Let them prepare themselves for usefulness by studying the books that have been written for our instruction in these lines. These books deserve much more attention and appreciation than they have received. Much that is for the benefit of all to understand has been written for the special purpose of instruction in the principles of health. Those who study and practice these principles will be greatly blessed, both physically and spiritually. An understanding of the philosophy of health will be a safeguard against many of the evils that are continually increasing.

Home Study

Many who desire to obtain knowledge in medical missionary lines have home duties that will sometimes prevent them from meeting with others for study. These may learn much in their own homes in regard to the expressed will of God concerning these lines of missionary work, thus increasing their ability to help others. Fathers and mothers, obtain all the help you can from the study of our books and publications. . . . Take time to read to your children from the health books, as well as from the books treating more particularly on religious subjects. Teach them the importance of caring for the body—the house they live in. Form a home reading circle, in which every member of the family shall lay aside the busy cares of the day and unite in study. Fathers, mothers, brothers, sisters, take up this work heartily, and see if the home church will not be greatly improved.

Especially will the youth who have been accustomed to reading novels and cheap storybooks receive benefit by joining in the evening family study. Young men and young women, read the literature that will give you true knowledge, and that will be a help to the entire family. Say firmly: "I will not spend precious moments in reading that which will be of no profit to me, and which only unfits me to be of service to others. I will devote my time and my thoughts to acquiring a fitness for God's service. I will close my eyes to frivolous and sinful things. My ears are the Lord's, and I will not listen to the subtle reasoning of the enemy. My voice shall not in any way be subject to a will that is not under the influence of the

Spirit of God. My body is the temple of the Holy Spirit, and every power of my being shall be consecrated to worthy pursuits."

The Youth, God's Helping Hand

The Lord has appointed the youth to be His helping hand. If in every church they would consecrate themselves to Him, if they would practice self-denial in the home, relieving their careworn mother, the mother could find time to make neighborly visits, and, when opportunity offered, they could themselves give assistance by doing little errands of mercy and love. Books and papers treating on the subject of health and temperance could be placed in many homes. The circulation of this literature is an important matter; for thus precious knowledge can be imparted in regard to the treatment of disease —knowledge that would be a great blessing to those who cannot afford to pay for a physician's visits.

The Study of Physiology

Parents should seek to interest their children in the study of physiology. There are but few among the youth who have any definite knowledge of the mysteries of life. The study of the wonderful human organism, the relation and dependence of its complicated parts, is one in which many parents take little interest. Although God says to them, "Beloved, I wish above all things that thou mayest prosper and be in health, even as thy soul prospereth" (3 John 2), yet they do not understand the influence of the body upon the mind or of the mind upon the body. Needless trifles occupy their attention, and then they plead a lack of time as an excuse for not obtaining the information necessary to enable them properly to instruct their children.

If all would obtain a knowledge of this subject and would feel the importance of putting it to practical use, we should see a better condition of things. Parents, teach your children to reason from cause to effect. Show them that, if they violate the laws of health, they must pay the penalty by suffering. Show them that recklessness in regard to bodily health tends to recklessness in morals. Your children require patient, faithful care. It is not enough for you to feed and clothe them; you should seek also to develop their mental powers, and to imbue their hearts with right principles. But how often are beauty of character and loveliness of temper lost sight of in the eager desire for outward appearance! O parents, be not governed by the world's opinion; labor not to reach its standard. Decide for yourselves what is the great aim of life, and then bend every effort to reach that aim. You cannot with impunity neglect the proper training of your children. Their defective characters will publish your unfaithfulness. The evils that you permit to pass uncorrected, the coarse, rough manners, the disrespect and disobedience, the habits of indolence and inattention, will bring dishonor to your names and bitterness into your lives. The destiny of your children rests to a great extent in your hands. If you fail in duty, you may place them in the ranks of the enemy and make them his agents in ruining others; on the other hand, if you faithfully instruct them, if in your own lives you set before them a godly example, you may lead them to Christ, and they in turn will influence others, and thus many may be saved through your instrumentality.

Instruct the Children

Fathers and mothers, do you realize the importance of the responsibility resting upon you? Do you realize the necessity of guarding your children from careless, demoralizing habits? Allow your children to form only such associations as will have a right influence upon their characters. Do not allow them to be out in the evening unless you know where they are and what they are doing. Instruct them in the principles of moral purity. If you have neglected to teach them line upon line, precept upon precept, here a little and there a little, begin at once to do your duty. Take up your responsibilities and work for time and for eternity. Let not another day pass without confessing your neglect to your children. Tell them that you mean now to do your God-appointed work. Ask them to take hold with you in the reform. Make diligent efforts to redeem the past. No longer remain in the condition of the Laodicean church. In the name of the Lord I call upon every family to show its true colors. Reform the church in your own home.

As you faithfully do your duty in the home, the father as a priest of the household, the mother as a home missionary, you are multiplying agencies for doing good outside of the home. As you improve your own powers, you are becoming better fitted to labor in the church and in the neighborhood. By binding your children to yourselves and to God, fathers and mothers and children become laborers together with God.

As a means of overcoming prejudice and gaining access to minds, medical missionary work must be done, not in one or two places only, but in many places where the truth has not yet been proclaimed. We are to work as gospel medical missionaries, to heal the sin-sick souls by giving them the message of salvation.—*Testimonies for the Church,* vol. 9, p. 211 (1909).

Gospel Workers to Teach Health Reform

Our ministers should become intelligent on health reform. They need to become acquainted with physiology and hygiene; they should understand the laws that govern physical life and their bearing upon the health of mind and soul.

Thousands upon thousands know little of the wonderful body God has given them or of the care it should receive, and they consider it of more importance to study subjects of far less consequence. The ministers have a work to do here. When they take a right position on this subject, much will be gained. In their own lives and homes they should obey the laws of life, practicing right principles and living healthfully. Then they will be able to speak correctly on this subject, leading the people higher and still higher in the work of reform. Living in the light themselves, they can bear a message of great value to those who are in need of just such a testimony.

There are precious blessings and a rich experience to be gained if ministers will combine the presentation of the health question with all their labors in the churches. The people must have the light on health reform. . . .

The presidents of our conferences need to realize that it is high time they were placing themselves on the right side of this question. Ministers and teachers are to give to others the light they have received. Their work in every line is needed. God will help them; He will strengthen His servants who stand firmly, and will not be swayed from truth and righteousness in order to accommodate self-indulgence.—*Testimonies for the Church,* vol. 6, pp. 376, 377 (1900).

The Temperance Reform

There needs to be a great reformation on the subject of temperance. The world is filled with self-indulgence of every kind. Because of the benumbing influence of stimulants and narcotics the minds of many are unable to discern between the sacred and the common. Their mental powers are weakened, and they cannot discern the deep spiritual things of the word of God.

The Christian will be temperate in all things—in eating, in drinking, in dress, and in every phase of life. "Every man that striveth for the mastery is temperate in all things. Now they do it to obtain a corruptible crown; but we an incorruptible." 1 Corinthians 9:25. We have no right to indulge in anything that will result in a condition of mind that hinders the Spirit of God from impressing us with the sense of our duty. It is a masterpiece of satanic skill to place men where they can with difficulty be reached with the gospel.

Shall there not be among us as a people a revival of the temperance work? Why are we not putting forth much more decided efforts to oppose the liquor traffic, which is ruining the souls of men and is causing violence and crime of every description? With the great light that God has entrusted to us, we should be in the forefront of every true reform. The use of drugged liquors is making men mad and leading them to commit the most horrible crimes. Because of the wickedness that follows largely as the result of the use of liquor, the judgments of God are falling upon our earth today. Have we not a solemn responsibility to put forth earnest efforts in opposition to this great evil?—*Review and Herald,* Aug. 29, 1907.

At the Camp Meetings

Every true reform has its place in the work of the third angel's message. Especially does the temperance reform demand our attention and support. At our camp meetings we should call attention to this work and make it a living issue. We should present to the people the principles of true temperance and call for signers to the temperance pledge. Careful attention should be given to those who are enslaved by evil habits. We must lead them to the cross of Christ.

Our camp meetings should have the labors of medical men. These should be men of wisdom and sound judgment, men who respect the ministry of the word and who are not victims of unbelief. These men are the guardians of the health of the people, and they are to be recognized and respected. They should give instruction to the people in regard to the dangers of intemperance. This evil must be more boldly met in the future than it has been in the past. Ministers and doctors should set forth the evils of intemperance. Both should work in the gospel with power to condemn sin and exalt righteousness. Those ministers or doctors who do not make personal appeals to the people are remiss in their duty. They fail of doing the work which God has appointed them.

In other churches there are Christians who are standing in defense of the principles of temperance. We should seek to come near to these workers and make a way for them to stand shoulder to shoulder with us. We should call upon great and good men to second our efforts to save that which is lost.

If the work of temperance were carried forward by us as it was begun thirty years ago, if at our camp meetings we presented before the people the evils of intemper-

Testimonies for the Church, vol. 6, pp. 110, 111 (1900).

ance in eating and drinking, and especially the evil of liquor drinking, if these things were presented in connection with the evidences of Christ's soon coming, there would be a shaking among the people. If we showed a zeal in proportion to the importance of the truths we are handling, we might be instrumental in rescuing hundreds, yea thousands, from ruin.

A Good Work Made Difficult

Present truth lies in the work of health reform as verily as in other features of gospel work. No one branch when separated from others can be a perfect whole.

The gospel of health has able advocates, but their work has been made very hard because so many ministers, presidents of conferences, and others in positions of influence have failed to give the question of health reform its proper attention. They have not recognized it in its relation to the work of the message as the right arm of the body. While very little respect has been shown to this department by many of the people and by some of the ministers, the Lord has shown His regard for it by giving it abundant prosperity. When properly conducted, the health work is an entering wedge, making a way for other truths to reach the heart. When the third angel's message is received in its fullness, health reform will be given its place in the councils of the conference, in the work of the church, in the home, at the table, and in all the household arrangements. Then the right arm will serve and protect the body.—*Testimonies for the Church,* vol. 6, p. 327 (1900).

References for further study: *Testimonies for the Church,* vol. 5, pp. 354-361, "Manufacture of Wine and Cider;" *The Ministry of Healing,* pages 171-182, "Working for the Intemperate."

Disseminating Temperance Principles

God bids His people blend harmoniously in their service for Him, that they may work in Christ's lines. This last message of warning must be brought to the world, and there are continual calls for those who will go forth and carry the message to the missionary fields that are calling for help. There are some who cannot themselves go to these fields, but they can help with their means in support of the work.

Many can engage in the work of selling our periodicals. Thus they can earn means for the work in foreign fields while sowing seeds of truth in the byways and hedges in the home field. Such labor will be blessed of God, and it will not be done in vain.

Wherever you are, let your light shine forth. Hand out papers and pamphlets to those with whom you associate, when you are riding on the cars, visiting, conversing with your neighbors; and improve every opportunity to speak a word in season. The Holy Spirit will make the seed productive in some hearts.

As a people we should cultivate kindliness and courtesy in our association with those whom we meet. Let us avoid any abruptness of manner, and strive always to present the truth in an easy way. This truth means life, eternal life to the receiver. Study therefore to pass easily and courteously from subjects of a temporal nature to the spiritual and eternal. A most courteous manner characterized the work of the Saviour. Seek in the most gentle way to introduce your mission. While walking by the way, or seated by the wayside, you may drop into some heart the seed of truth.

I have words of encouragement to speak in regard to

Review and Herald, June 18, 1908.

the special number of the Watchman, which the Southern Publishing House is soon to bring out. I shall rejoice to see our conferences help in this work by taking a large number of this issue for circulation. Let there be no forbiddings placed upon the effort, but let all take hold to give this temperance number a wide circulation.

There could be no better time than now for a movement of this kind, when the temperance question is creating such widespread interest. Let our people everywhere take hold decidedly to let it be seen where we stand on the temperance question. Let everything possible be done to circulate strong, stirring appeals for the closing of the saloon. Let this paper be made a power for good. Our work for temperance is to be more spirited, more decided.

Precious light will be given in the publications you scatter through the towns and cities. Your humble prayers, your unselfish activity, will be blessed of God, and the truth as it is in Jesus will come to those who need it. The words that Christ spoke to men while He was in the world He will speak again through His humble, faithful followers. Through them He will give to men the bread of life and the waters of salvation. Brethren, take up this work in humility of heart. The simplicity of true godliness will cause you to be respected and will lead men and women to seek the source of your power. Believe, and you will receive the things you ask for.

Co-operating With Christian Temperance Workers

The Woman's Christian Temperance Union is an organization with whose efforts for the spread of temperance principles we can heartily unite. The light has been given me that we are not to stand aloof from them, but while there is to be no sacrifice of principle on our part, as far as possible we are to unite with them in laboring for temperance reforms. My husband and I, in our labors, united with these temperance workers, and we had the joy of seeing several unite with us in the observance of the true Sabbath. Among them there is a strong prejudice against us, but we shall not remove this prejudice by standing aloof. God is testing us. We are to work with them when we can, and we can assuredly do this on the question of utterly closing the saloon.

As the human agent submits his will to the will of God, the Holy Spirit will make the impression upon the hearts of those to whom he ministers. I have been shown that we are not to shun the W.C.T.U. workers. By uniting with them in behalf of total abstinence, we do not change our position regarding the observance of the seventh day, and we can show our appreciation of their position regarding the subject of temperance. By opening the door and inviting them to unite with us on the temperance question, we secure their help along temperance lines; and they, by uniting with us, will hear new truths which the Holy Spirit is waiting to impress upon hearts.

My brethren, be workers together with Christ. Make every possible effort in season and out of season to spread the light of present truth. The Lord has taught us how safe is the cable that anchors us to the living Rock. Here is an opportunity to labor for those who have truth on some points, but who on other points are not safely anchored. Keep in touch with the people wherever you can. "Let your light so shine before men, that they may see your good works, and glorify your Father which is in heaven." Matthew 5:16.

Reference for further study: *The Ministry of Healing,* pages 337-346, "The Liquor Traffic and Prohibition."

Teach With Wisdom

We must go no faster than we can take those with us whose consciences and intellects are convinced of the truths we advocate. We must meet the people where they are. Some of us have been many years in arriving at our present position in health reform. It is slow work to obtain a reform in diet. We have powerful appetites to meet, for the world is given to gluttony. If we should allow the people as much time as we have required to come up to the present advanced state in reform, we would be very patient with them and allow them to advance step by step, as we have done, until their feet are firmly established upon the health-reform platform. But we should be very cautious not to advance too fast, lest we be obliged to retrace our steps. In reforms, we would better come one step short of the mark than to go one step beyond it. And if there is error at all, let it be on the side next to the people.

Above all things, we should not with our pens advocate positions that we do not put to a practical test in our own families, upon our own tables. . . .

If we come to persons who have not been enlightened in regard to health reform, and present our strongest positions at first, there is danger of their becoming discouraged as they see how much they have to give up, so that they will make no effort to reform. We must lead the people along patiently and gradually, remembering the hole of the pit whence we were digged.—*Testimonies for the Church,* vol. 3, pp. 20, 21 (1872).

The Right Exercise of the Will

The victims of evil habit must be aroused to the necessity of making an effort for themselves. Others may put forth the most earnest endeavor to uplift them, the grace of God may be freely offered, Christ may entreat, His angels may minister; but all will be in vain unless they themselves are roused to fight the battle in their own behalf.

The last words of David to Solomon, then a young man, and soon to receive the crown of Israel, were, "Be thou strong, . . . and show thyself a man." 1 Kings 2:2. To every child of humanity, the candidate for an immortal crown, are these words of inspiration spoken, "Be thou strong, and show thyself a man."

The self-indulgent must be led to see and feel that great moral renovation is necessary if they would be men. God calls upon them to arouse, and in the strength of Christ win back the God-given manhood that has been sacrificed through sinful indulgence.

Feeling the terrible power of temptation, the drawing of desire that leads to indulgence, many a man cries in despair, "I cannot resist evil." Tell him that he can, that he must resist. He may have been overcome again and again, but it need not be always thus. He is weak in moral power, controlled by the habits of a life of sin. His promises and resolutions are like ropes of sand. The knowledge of his broken promises and forfeited pledges weakens his confidence in his own sincerity and causes him to feel that God cannot accept him or work with his efforts. But he need not despair.

The Ministry of Healing, pages 174-179 (1905).

Those who put their trust in Christ are not to be enslaved by any hereditary or cultivated habit or tendency. Instead of being held in bondage to the lower nature, they are to rule every appetite and passion. God has not left us to battle with evil in our own finite strength. Whatever may be our inherited or cultivated tendencies to wrong, we can overcome through the power that He is ready to impart. . . .

Through the right exercise of the will an entire change may be made in the life. By yielding up the will to Christ, we ally ourselves with divine power. We receive strength from above to hold us steadfast. A pure and noble life, a life of victory over appetite and lust, is possible to everyone who will unite his weak, wavering human will to the omnipotent, unwavering will of God.

Those who are struggling against the power of appetite should be instructed in the principles of healthful living. They should be shown that violation of the laws of health, by creating diseased conditions and unnatural cravings, lays the foundation of the liquor habit. Only by living in obedience to the principles of health can they hope to be freed from the craving for unnatural stimulants. While they depend upon divine strength to break the bonds of appetite, they are to co-operate with God by obedience to His laws, both moral and physical. . . .

For every soul struggling to rise from a life of sin to a life of purity, the great element of power abides in the only "name under heaven, given among men, whereby we must be saved." "If any man thirst," for restful hope, for deliverance from sinful propensities, Christ says, "let him come unto Me, and drink." The only remedy for vice is the grace and power of Christ.

Sign the Pledge

As Christians, we should stand firmly in defense of temperance. There is no class of persons capable of accomplishing more in the cause of temperance, than our God-fearing youth. If the young men who live in our cities would unite in a firm, decided army, and set their faces as a flint against every form of selfish, health-destroying indulgence, what a power they might be for good! How many they might save from becoming demoralized by visiting the halls and gardens that are fitted up with music and every attraction to allure the youth! Intemperance, Licentiousness, and Profanity are sisters.

Let every God-fearing youth gird on the armor and press to the front. Let no excuse be offered when you are asked to put your name to the temperance pledge, but sign every pledge presented and induce others to sign with you. Work for the good of your own souls and the good of others. Never let an opportunity pass to cast your influence on the side of strict temperance.

We thank the Lord that a victory has been gained, but we hope to carry our brethren and sisters up to a still higher standard, where they will sign the pledge to abstain from coffee and the herb that comes from China.

Coffee is a hurtful indulgence. It temporarily excites the mind to unwonted action, but the aftereffect is sad —prostration and exhaustion of the physical, mental, and moral forces. The mind becomes enervated, and unless through determined effort the habit is overcome, the activity of the brain is greatly lessened.

A leaflet; written April 19, 1887.

In some cases it is as difficult to break up this tea-and-coffee habit as it is for the inebriate to discontinue the use of liquor. The money used for tea and coffee as a common drink is worse than wasted. It does the user, be it man or woman, harm, and that continually.

All these nerve irritants are wearing away the life forces, and the restlessness, the impatience, the mental feebleness caused by shattered nerves become a warring element, ever working against spiritual progress. Shall Christians bring their appetite under the control of reason, or will they continue its indulgence because they feel so "let down" without it, like the drunkard without his stimulant? Shall not those who advocate temperance reform awake in regard to these injurious things also? And shall not the pledge embrace coffee and tea as hurtful stimulants?

Premature Tests

The Lord desires our ministers, physicians, and church members to be careful not to urge those who are ignorant of our faith to make sudden changes in diet, thus bringing men to a premature test. Hold up the principles of health reform and let the Lord lead the honest in heart. They will hear and believe. Nor does the Lord require His messengers to present the beautiful truths of healthful living in a way that will prejudice minds. Let no one put stumbling blocks before the feet that are walking in the dark paths of ignorance. Even in praising a good thing, it is well not to be too enthusiastic, lest you turn out of the way those who come to hear. Present the principles of temperance in their most attractive form.— *Gospel Workers,* page 233 (1915).

Keep Health Reform to the Front

As a people we have been given the work of making known the principles of health reform. There are some who think that the question of diet is not of sufficient importance to be included in their evangelistic work. But such make a great mistake. God's word declares, "Whether therefore ye eat, or drink, or whatsoever ye do, do all to the glory of God." 1 Corinthians 10:31. The subject of temperance, in all its bearings, has an important place in the work of salvation.

Instruction Connected With City Missions

In connection with our city missions there should be suitable rooms where those in whom an interest has been awakened can be gathered for instruction. This necessary work is not to be carried on in such a meager way that an unfavorable impression will be made on the minds of the people. All that is done should bear favorable witness to the Author of truth, and should properly represent the sacredness and importance of the truths of the third angel's message.

Cooking schools are to be held. The people are to be taught how to prepare wholesome food. They are to be shown the need of discarding unhealthful foods. But we should never advocate a starvation diet. It is possible to have a wholesome, nutritious diet without the use of tea, coffee, and flesh food. The work of teaching the people how to prepare a dietary that is at once wholesome and appetizing is of the utmost importance.

The work of health reform is the Lord's means for lessening suffering in our world and for purifying His

Testimonies for the Church, vol. 9, pp. 112, 113 (1909).

15—C.O.H.

church. Teach the people that they can act as God's help-ing hand, by co-operating with the Master Worker in restoring physical and spiritual health. This work bears the signature of Heaven and will open doors for the en-trance of other precious truths. There is room for all to labor who will take hold of this work intelligently.

Keep the work of health reform to the front is the message I am instructed to bear. Show so plainly its value that a widespread need for it will be felt. Abstinence from all hurtful food and drink is the fruit of true religion. He who is thoroughly converted will abandon every in-jurious habit and appetite. By total abstinence he will overcome his desire for health-destroying indulgences.

Go Forward

I am instructed to say to health-reform educators, Go forward. The world needs every jot of the influence you can exert to press back the tide of moral woe. Let those who teach the third angel's message stand true to their colors. "I beseech you therefore, brethren, by the mercies of God, that ye present your bodies a living sacrifice, holy, acceptable unto God, which is your reasonable service. And be not conformed to this world: but be ye trans-formed by the renewing of your mind, that ye may prove what is that good, and acceptable, and perfect, will of God." Romans 12:1, 2. May the Lord arm those who labor in word and doctrine, with the clearest messages of truth. If His workers will give these messages with simplicity, assurance, and all authority, the Lord will work with them.

Continual Reform Must Be Advocated

The circulation of our health publications is a most important work. It is a work in which all who believe the special truths for this time should have a living interest. God desires that now, as never before, the minds of the people shall be deeply stirred to investigate the great temperance question and principles underlying true health reform. The physical life is to be carefully educated, cultivated, and developed, that through men and women the divine nature may be revealed in its fullness. Both the physical and the mental powers, with the affections, are to be so trained that they can reach the highest efficiency.

Reform, continual reform, must be kept before the people, and by our example we must enforce our teachings. True religion and the laws of health go hand in hand. It is impossible to work for the salvation of men and women without presenting to them the need of breaking away from sinful gratifications, which destroy the health, debase the soul, and prevent divine truth from impressing the mind. Men and women must be taught to take a careful review of every habit and practice, and at once put away those things that cause an unhealthy condition of the body, and thus cast a dark shadow over the mind.

God's People to Be Light Bearers

God desires His people to be light bearers to a world lying in midnight darkness. But if they refuse to go forward in the light which He causes to shine on their pathway, the light will finally become to them darkness; and instead of being light bearers to the world, they

The Circulation of Our Health Journals, pages 1-4 (1901).

themselves will be lost in the blackness that surrounds them. God desires His light bearers ever to keep a high standard before them. By precept and example they must hold this perfect standard high above Satan's false standard, which, if followed, will lead to misery, degradation, disease, and death for both body and soul.

Those who act as teachers are to be intelligent in regard to disease and its causes, understanding that every action of the human agent should be in perfect harmony with the laws of life. The light God has given on health reform is for our salvation and the salvation of the world. Men and women should be informed in regard to the human habitation fitted up by our Creator as His dwelling place, and over which He desires us to be faithful stewards. These grand truths must be given to the world. We must reach the people where they are and by example and precept lead them to see the beauties of the better way.

The world is in sad need of instruction along these lines. The time has come when each soul must be staunch and true to every ray of light God has given, and begin in earnest to give this gospel of health to the people. We shall have strength and power to do this, if we practice these truths in our own lives. If we all followed the light we have received, the blessing of God would rest on us and we should be anxious to place these truths before those who know them not. . . .

In all our work caution should be used that no one branch be made a specialty, while other interests are left to suffer. There has not been that interest taken in the circulation of our health journals that there should be. The circulation of these journals must not be neglected, or the people will suffer great loss.

Let none think that the circulation of the health journals is a minor matter. All should take hold of this work with more interest and make greater efforts in this direction. God will greatly bless those who take hold of it in earnest, for it is a work that should receive attention at this time.

Ministers can and should do much to urge the circulation of the health journals. Every member of the church should work as earnestly for these journals as for our other periodicals. There should be no friction between the two. Both are essential, and both should occupy the field at the same time. Each is the complement of the other, and can in no wise take its place. The circulation of the health journals will be a powerful agency in preparing the people to accept those special truths that are to fit them for the soon coming of the Son of man.

Sanitariums Needed in Washington and Other Places

Sanitarium, California, July 5, 1903.

My dear Brethren:

Our people far and near need to ask themselves how the Lord regards their neglect of important centers in America. There are many places in this country in which the truth has never been proclaimed. Many years ago there should have been a sanitarium in Washington, D.C. But men have chosen their way in many things, and the places to which the truth should have found entrance, by the establishment of medical missionary work, have been neglected. . . .

Why have not those who have taken a leading part in medical missionary work been burdened to carry to Washington the message of temperance in eating, drinking, and dressing? There would have been less difficulty in giving the message in this place than in some other places.

There are many places that need gospel medical missionary work. Plants should be made in these places. God designs that our sanitariums shall be a means of reaching high and low, rich and poor. They are to be so conducted that by their work attention will be called to the message that God has sent to the world. Many will not heed the call of mercy; nevertheless it is to be given to all, that whosoever will may come to the water of life and drink.—*Review and Herald,* Aug. 11, 1903.

(448)

Educate, Educate, Educate

We should educate ourselves, not only to live in harmony with the laws of health, but to teach others the better way. Many, even of those who profess to believe the special truths for this time, are lamentably ignorant with regard to health and temperance. They need to be educated, line upon line, precept upon precept. The subject must be kept fresh before them. This matter must not be passed over as nonessential, for nearly every family needs to be stirred up on the question. The conscience must be aroused to the duty of practicing the principles of true reform. God requires that His people shall be temperate in all things. Unless they practice true temperance, they will not, they cannot, be susceptible to the sanctifying influence of the truth.

Our ministers should become intelligent upon this question. They should not ignore it, nor be turned aside by those who call them extremists. Let them find out what constitutes true health reform and teach its principles, both by precept and by a quiet, consistent example. At our large gatherings instruction should be given upon health and temperance. Seek to arouse the intellect and the conscience. Bring into service all the talent at command, and follow up the work with publications upon the subject. "Educate, educate, educate," is the message that has been impressed upon me.

In all our missions, women of intelligence should have charge of the domestic arrangements—women who know how to prepare food nicely and healthfully. The table should be abundantly supplied with food of the best quality. If any have a perverted taste that craves tea, coffee, condiments, and unhealthful dishes, enlighten them. Seek

Christian Temperance, pages 117-122 (1890).

to arouse the conscience. Set before them the principles of the Bible upon hygiene. Where plenty of good milk and fruit can be obtained, there is rarely any excuse for eating animal food; it is not necessary to take the life of any of God's creatures to supply our ordinary needs. In certain cases of illness or exhaustion it may be thought best to use some meat, but great care should be taken to secure the flesh of healthy animals. It has come to be a very serious question whether it is safe to use flesh food at all in this age of the world. It would be better never to eat meat than to use the flesh of animals that are not healthy. . . .

Again and again I have been shown that God is trying to lead us back, step by step, to His original design—that man should subsist upon the natural products of the earth. Among those who are waiting for the coming of the Lord, meat eating will eventually be done away; flesh will cease to form a part of their diet. We should ever keep this end in view, and endeavor to work steadily toward it. . . .

A Knowledge of Healthful Cooking

One reason why many have become discouraged in practicing health reform is that they have not learned how to cook so that proper food, simply prepared, would supply the place of the diet to which they have been accustomed. They become disgusted with the poorly prepared dishes, and next we hear them say that they have tried the health reform and cannot live in that way. Many attempt to follow out meager instructions in health reform and make such sad work that it results in injury to digestion and in discouragement to all concerned in the attempt. You profess to be health reformers, and for this very reason you should become good cooks. Those who can avail themselves of the advantages of properly conducted hygienic cooking schools will find it a great benefit both in their own practice and in teaching others.

Teach Wisely and by Example

Do not catch hold of isolated ideas and make them a test, criticizing others whose practice may not agree with your opinion; but study the subject broadly and deeply, and seek to bring your own ideas and practices into perfect harmony with the principles of true Christian temperance.

There are many who try to correct the lives of others by attacking what they regard as wrong habits. They go to those whom they think in error and point out their defects, but do not seek to direct the mind to true principles. Such a course often comes far short of securing the desired results. When we make it evident that we are trying to correct others, we too often arouse their combativeness and do more harm than good. And there is danger to the reprover also. He who takes it upon himself to correct others is likely to cultivate a habit of fault-finding, and soon his whole interest will be in picking flaws and finding defects. Do not watch others, to pick at their faults or expose their errors. Educate them to better habits by the power of your own example. . . .

The Physician a Teacher

A great amount of good can be done by enlightening all to whom we have access, as to the best means, not only of curing the sick, but of preventing disease and suffering. The physician who endeavors to enlighten his patients as to the nature and causes of their maladies, and to teach them how to avoid disease, may have uphill work; but if he is a conscientious reformer, he will talk plainly of the ruinous effects of self-indulgence in eating, drinking, and dressing, of the overtaxation of the vital forces that has brought his patients where they are. He will not increase the evil by administering drugs till exhausted nature gives up the struggle, but will teach the patients how to form correct habits and to aid nature in her work of restoration by a wise use of her own simple remedies.

In all our health institutions it should be made a special feature of the work to give instruction in regard to the laws of health. The principles of health reform should be carefully and thoroughly set before all, both patients and helpers. This work requires moral courage, for while many will profit by such efforts, others will be offended. But the true disciple of Christ, he whose mind is in harmony with the mind of God, while constantly learning, will be teaching as well, leading the minds of others upward, away from the prevailing errors of the world.

The Work of the Church

Much of the prejudice that prevents the truth of the third angel's message from reaching the hearts of the people might be removed if more attention were given to health reform. When people become interested in this subject, the way is often prepared for the entrance of other truths. If they see that we are intelligent with regard to health, they will be more ready to believe that we are sound in Bible doctrines.

This branch of the Lord's work has not received due attention, and through this neglect much has been lost. If the church would manifest a greater interest in the reforms through which God Himself is seeking to fit them for His coming, their influence would be far greater than it now is. God has spoken to His people and He designs that they shall hear and obey His voice. Although the health reform is not the third angel's message, it is closely connected with it. Those who proclaim the message should teach health reform also. It is a subject that we must understand in order to be prepared for the events that are close upon us, and it should have a prominent place.

Indifference and Unbelief

I was shown that the work of health reform has scarcely been entered upon yet. While some feel deeply, and act out their faith in the work, others remain indifferent and have scarcely taken the first step in reform. There seems to be in them a heart of unbelief, and as this reform restricts the lustful appetite, many shrink back. They have other gods before the Lord. Their taste, their appetite, is their god, and when the ax is laid at the root of the tree, and those who have indulged their depraved appetites at the expense of health are touched, their sin pointed out, their idols shown them, they do not wish to be convinced; and although God's voice should speak directly to them to put away those health-destroying indulgences, some would still cling to the hurtful things which they love. They seem joined to their idols, and God will soon say to His angels, Let them alone.... I saw that we as a people must make an advance move in this great work. Ministers and people must act in concert. God's people are not prepared for the loud cry of the third angel. They have a work to do for themselves which they should not leave for God to do for them. He has left this work for them to do. It is an individual work; one cannot do it for another.—*Testimonies for the Church,* vol. 1, p. 486 (1865).

A Warning Against Spiritualist Physicians

From time to time I have received letters from both ministers and lay members of the church, inquiring if I think it wrong to consult spiritualist and clairvoyant physicians. So numerous are these agents of Satan becoming, and so general is the practice of seeking counsel from them, that it seems needful to utter words of warning.

God has placed it in our power to obtain a knowledge of the laws of health. He has made it a duty to preserve our physical powers in the best possible condition, that we may render to Him acceptable service. Those who refuse to improve the light and knowledge that have been mercifully placed within their reach are rejecting one of the means which God has granted them to promote spiritual as well as physical life. They are placing themselves where they will be exposed to the delusions of Satan.

Not a few in this Christian age and Christian nation resort to evil spirits, rather than trust to the power of the living God. The mother watching by the sickbed of her child, exclaims, "I can do no more. Is there no physician who has power to restore my child?" She is told of the wonderful cures performed by some clairvoyant or magnetic healer, and she trusts her dear one to his charge, placing it as verily in the hands of Satan as if he were standing by her side. In many instances the future life of the child is controlled by a satanic power which it seems impossible to break.

I have heard a mother pleading with an infidel physician to save the life of her child; but when I entreated her to seek help from the Great Physician, who is able

Christian Temperance, pages 111-116 (1890).

to save to the uttermost all who come to Him in faith, she turned away with impatience.

The Experience of Ahaziah

When Ahaziah, king of Israel, was sick, "he sent messengers, and said unto them, Go, inquire of Baalzebub the god of Ekron whether I shall recover of this disease." On the way they met Elijah, and instead of a message from the idol, the king heard the awful denunciation from the God of Israel, "Thou shalt not come down from that bed on which thou art gone up, but shalt surely die." 2 Kings 1:2, 6.

It was Christ that bade Elijah speak these words to the apostate king. Jehovah Immanuel had cause to be greatly displeased at Ahaziah's impiety. What had Christ not done to win the hearts of Israel and to inspire them with unwavering confidence in Himself? For ages He had visited His people with manifestations of the most condescending kindness and unexampled love. From the time of the patriarchs, He had shown how His "delights were with the sons of men." Proverbs 8:31. He had been a very present help to all who sought Him in sincerity. "In all their affliction He was afflicted, and the Angel of His presence saved them: in His love and in His pity He redeemed them." Isaiah 63:9. Yet Israel had revolted from God and turned for help to the Lord's worst enemy.

The Hebrews were the only nation favored with a knowledge of the true God. When the king of Israel sent to inquire of a pagan oracle, he proclaimed to the heathen that he had more confidence in their idols than in the God of his people, the Creator of the heavens and the earth. In the same manner do those who profess to have a knowledge of God's word dishonor Him when they turn from the Source of strength and wisdom, to ask help or counsel from the powers of darkness. If God's wrath was kindled by such a course on the part of a wicked, idolatrous king, how must He regard a similar course pursued by those who profess to be His servants?

Unwise Confidence

Many are unwilling to put forth the needed effort to obtain a knowledge of the laws of life and the simple means to be employed for the restoration of health. They do not place themselves in right relation to life. When sickness is the result of their transgression of natural law, they do not seek to correct their errors and then ask the blessing of God, but they resort to the physicians. If they recover health, they give to drugs and doctors all the honor. They are ever ready to idolize human power and wisdom, seeming to know no other god than the creature —dust and ashes.

It is not safe to trust to physicians who have not the fear of God before them. Without the influence of divine grace, the hearts of men are "deceitful above all things, and desperately wicked." Jeremiah 17:9. Self-aggrandizement is their aim. Under cover of the medical profession, what iniquities have been practiced, what delusions supported! The physician may claim to possess great wisdom and marvelous skill, while at the same time his character is abandoned, and his practice contrary to the laws of health. The Lord our God assures us that He is waiting to be gracious; He invites us to call upon Him in the day of trouble.

Furthermore, the teaching of these physicians is continually leading away from the principles God has given us in regard to health, especially on the diet question. They say we are not living as we ought and prescribe changes that are contrary to the light God has sent. Brethren, how can the Lord let His blessing rest upon us when we are going right upon the enemy's ground?

God the Helper of His People

Why is it that men are so unwilling to trust Him who created man and who can, by a touch, a word, a look, heal all manner of disease? Who is more worthy of our confidence than the One who has made so great a sacrifice for our redemption? Our Lord has given us definite instruction, through the apostle James, as to our duty in case of sickness. When human help fails, God will be the helper of His people. "Is any sick among you? let him call for the elders of the church; and let them pray over him, anointing him with oil in the name of the Lord: and the prayer of faith shall save the sick, and the Lord shall raise him up." James 5:14, 15. If the professed followers of Christ would, with purity of heart, exercise as much faith in the promises of God as they repose in satanic agencies, they would realize, in soul and body, the life-giving power of the Holy Spirit.

God has granted to this people great light, yet we are not placed beyond the reach of temptation. Who among us are seeking help from the gods of Ekron? Look on this picture—a picture not drawn from imagination. In how many, even among Seventh-day Adventists, may its leading characteristics be seen! An invalid, apparently very conscientious, yet bigoted and self-sufficient, freely avows his contempt for the laws of life and health, which divine mercy has led us as a people to accept. His food must be prepared in a manner to satisfy his morbid cravings. Rather than sit at a table where wholesome food is provided, he will patronize restaurants, because he can there indulge appetite without restraint. A fluent advocate of temperance, he disregards its foundation principles. He wants relief, but refuses to obtain it at the price of self-denial.

That man is worshipping at the shrine of perverted appetite. He is an idolater. The powers which, sanctified and ennobled, might be employed to honor God, are weakened and rendered of little service. An irritable temper, a confused brain, and unstrung nerves are among the results of his disregard of nature's laws. He is inefficient and unreliable. Whoever has the courage and honesty to warn him of danger thereby incurs his displeasure. The slightest remonstrance or opposition is sufficient to rouse his combative spirit. But now an opportunity is presented to seek help from one whose power comes through the medium of witchcraft. To this source he applies with eagerness, freely expending time and money in the hope of securing the proffered boon. He is deceived, infatuated. The sorcerer's power is made the theme of praise, and others are influenced to seek his aid. Thus the God of Israel is dishonored, while Satan's power is revered and exalted.

In the name of Christ I would address His professed followers: Abide in the faith which you have received from the beginning. "Shun profane and vain babblings." 2 Timothy 2:16. Instead of putting your trust in witchcraft, have faith in the living God. Cursed is the path that leads to Endor or to Ekron. The feet will stumble and fall that venture upon this forbidden ground. There is a God in Israel, with whom is deliverance for all who are oppressed. Righteousness is the foundation of His throne.

There is danger in departing in the least from the Lord's instruction. When we deviate from the plain path of duty, a train of circumstances will arise that seems irresistibly to draw us farther and farther from the right. Needless intimacies with those who have no respect for God will seduce us ere we are aware. The fear of offending worldly friends will deter us from expressing our gratitude to God or acknowledging our dependence upon Him.

We must keep close to the word of God. We need its warnings and encouragement, its threatenings and promises. We need the perfect example given only in the life and character of our Saviour. Angels of God will preserve His people while they walk in the path of duty, but there is no assurance of such protection for those who deliberately venture upon Satan's ground. An agent of the great deceiver will say and do anything to gain his object. It matters little whether he calls himself a spiritualist, an "electric physician," or a "magnetic healer." By specious pretenses he wins the confidence of the unwary. He pretends to read the life history and to understand all the difficulties and afflictions of those who resort to him. Disguising himself as an angel of light, while the blackness of the pit is in his heart, he manifests great interest in women who seek his counsel. He tells them that all their troubles are due to an unhappy marriage. This may be too true, but such counsel does not better their condition. He tells them that they need love and sympathy. Pretending great interest in their welfare, he casts a spell over his unsuspecting victims, charming them as the serpent charms the trembling bird. Soon they are completely in his power, and sin, disgrace, and ruin are the terrible sequel.

Our only safety is in preserving the ancient landmarks. "To the law and to the testimony: if they speak not according to this word, it is because there is no light in them." Isaiah 8:20.

The Ruin Wrought by Satan

Through spiritualism, Satan appears as a benefactor of the race, healing the diseases of the people and professing to present a new and more exalted system of religious faith; but at the same time he works as a destroyer. His temptations are leading multitudes to ruin. Intemperance dethrones reason; sensual indulgence, strife, and bloodshed follow. Satan delights in war, for it excites the worst passions of the soul and then sweeps into eternity its victims steeped in vice and blood. It is his object to incite the nations to war against one another; for he can thus divert the minds of the people from the work of preparation to stand in the day of God.

Satan works through the elements also to garner his harvest of unprepared souls. He has studied the secrets of the laboratories of nature, and he uses all his power to control the elements as far as God allows. When he was suffered to afflict Job, how quickly flocks and herds, servants, houses, children, were swept away, one trouble succeeding another as in a moment. It is God that shields His creatures and hedges them in from the power of the destroyer. But the Christian world have shown contempt for the law of Jehovah, and the Lord will do just what He has declared that He would—He will withdraw His blessings from the earth and remove His protecting care from those who are rebelling against His law and teaching and forcing others to do the same. Satan has control of all whom God does not especially guard. He will favor and prosper some, in order to further his own designs; and he will bring trouble upon others and lead men to believe that it is God who is afflicting them.

The Great Controversy, pages 589, 590 (1888).
(460)

While appearing to the children of men as a great physician who can heal all their maladies, he will bring disease and disaster, until populous cities are reduced to ruin and desolation. Even now he is at work. In accidents and calamities by sea and by land, in great conflagrations, in fierce tornadoes and terrific hailstorms, in tempests, floods, cyclones, tidal waves, and earthquakes, in every place and in a thousand forms, Satan is exercising his power. He sweeps away the ripening harvest, and famine and distress follow. He imparts to the air a deadly taint, and thousands perish by the pestilence. These visitations are to become more and more frequent and disastrous. Destruction will be upon both man and beast. "The earth mourneth and fadeth away," "The haughty people . . . do languish. The earth also is defiled under the inhabitants thereof; because they have transgressed the laws, changed the ordinance, broken the everlasting covenant." Isaiah 24:4, 5.

Some will be tempted to receive these wonders as from God. The sick will be healed before us. Miracles will be performed in our sight. Are we prepared for the trial which awaits us when the lying wonders of Satan shall be more fully exhibited? Will not many be ensnared and taken? By departing from the plain precepts and commandments of God and giving heed to fables, the minds of many are preparing to receive these lying wonders. We must all now seek to arm ourselves for the contest in which we must soon engage. Faith in God's word, prayerfully studied and practically applied, will be our shield from Satan's power and will bring us off conquerors through the blood of Christ.—*Testimonies for the Church,* vol. 1, p. 302 (1862).

The Canvasser a Teacher

The temperance question is to receive decided support from God's people. Intemperance is striving for the mastery; self-indulgence is increasing, and the publications treating on health reform are greatly needed. Literature bearing on this point is the helping hand of the gospel, leading souls to search the Bible for a better understanding of the truth. The note of warning against the great evil of intemperance should be sounded; and that this may be done, every Sabbathkeeper should study and practice the instruction contained in our health periodicals and our health books. And they should do more than this: they should make earnest efforts to circulate these publications among their neighbors.

The sale of our health literature will in no way hinder the sale of publications dealing with other phases of the third angel's message. All are to prepare the way for the coming of the Lord.

Value of Our Publications

Canvassers should call the attention of those they visit to our health publications, telling them of the valuable instruction these periodicals contain regarding the care of the sick and treatment of diseases. Tell them this instruction, studied and practiced, will bring health to the family. Explain how important it is for every family to understand the science of life. Direct their minds to Him who formed and who keeps in motion the wonderful machinery of the body. Tell them that it is our part to co-operate with God, caring wisely for all our faculties and organs. The proper care of the body is a great respon-

Review and Herald, June 23, 1903.

sibility and requires an intelligent knowledge of its parts. Tell them that God is dishonored when, for the gratification of appetite and passion, man misuses the machinery of the body, so that it does its work feebly and with difficulty. Tell them that the books you have for sale give much valuable instruction regarding health and that by practicing this instruction much suffering, and also much of the money spent in paying doctors' bills, will be saved. Tell them that in these books there is advice which they cannot possibly obtain from their physician during the short visits he makes.

Teaching by Example

In his association with those whom he meets, the canvasser can do much to show the value of healthful living. Instead of staying at a hotel, he should, if possible, obtain lodging with a private family. As he sits at the table with the family, let him practice the instruction given in the health works he is selling, holding up the banner of strict temperance. As opportunity is offered, let him speak of the value of a healthful diet. He should never be ashamed to say, "No, thank you; I do not eat meat." If tea is offered, let him refuse it, explaining that it is harmful, that though for a time stimulating, the stimulating effect passes off, and a corresponding depression is left. Let him explain the injurious effect of intoxicating drinks, and of tobacco, tea, and coffee, on the digestive organs and the brain.

Ministering to the Sick

As the canvasser goes from place to place, he will find many who are sick. He should have a practical knowledge of the causes of disease and should understand how to give simple treatments, that he may relieve the suffering ones. More than this, he should pray in faith and simplicity for the sick, pointing them to the Great Physician. As he thus walks and works with God, ministering angels are beside him, giving him access to hearts. What a wide field for missionary effort lies before the faithful, consecrated canvasser; what a blessing will be his in the diligent performance of his work.

A Sacred and Important Work

Young men, young women, you are called by the Master to take up His work. His requirements are too sacred to be tampered with. In the name of the Lord I ask you to conquer every unlawful appetite and passion and to purify your souls by a belief in the truth. Overcome by the blood of the Lamb and the word of your testimony. Discharge faithfully your obligations, looking to God for strength.

Church members, awake to the importance of the circulation of our literature and devote more time to this work. Place in the homes of the people papers, tracts, and books that will preach the gospel in its several lines. There is no time to be lost. Let many give themselves willingly and unselfishly to the canvassing work, and thus help to sound a warning that is greatly needed. When the church takes up her appointed work, she will go forth "fair as the moon, clear as the sun, and terrible as an army with banners." Song of Solomon 6:10.

Hand Out the Literature

Several speakers had addressed large and attentive congregations at the camp meeting at Rome, N.Y., on First day, September 12, 1875. The following night I dreamed that a young man of noble appearance came into the room where I was, immediately after I had been speaking. This same person has appeared before me in important dreams to instruct me from time to time during the past twenty-six years. Said he: You have called the attention of the people to important subjects, which, to a large number, are strange and new. To some they are intensely interesting. The laborers in word and doctrine have done what they could in presenting the truth, which has raised inquiry in minds and awakened an interest. But unless there is a more thorough effort made to fasten these impressions upon minds, your efforts now made will prove nearly fruitless. Satan has many attractions ready to divert the mind, and the cares of this life and the deceitfulness of riches all combine to choke the seed of truth sown in the heart, and in most cases it bears no fruit.

In every effort such as you are now making, much more good would result from your labors if you had appropriate reading matter ready for circulation. Tracts upon the important points of truth for the present time should be handed out freely to all who will accept them, without money and without price, which might eventually result in a hundredfold return to the treasury. You are to sow beside all waters.

The press is a powerful means to move the minds and hearts of the people. And the men of this world seize

Signs of the Times, Nov. 11, 1875.

the press and make the most of every opportunity to get poisonous literature before the people. If men under the influence of the spirit of the world and of Satan are earnest to circulate books, tracts, and papers of a corrupting nature, you should be more earnest to get reading matter of an elevating and saving character before the people.

Tracts on Health Reform

There should be more earnest efforts made to enlighten the people upon the great subject of health reform. Tracts of four, eight, twelve, sixteen, and more pages, containing pointed, well-written articles on this great question, should be scattered like the leaves of autumn.

Tracts in Many Languages

Small tracts on the different points of Bible truth applicable to the present time should be printed in different languages and scattered where there is any probability that they would be read. God has placed at the command of His people advantages in the press, which, combined with other agencies, will be successful in extending the knowledge of the truth. Tracts, papers, and books, as the case demands, should be circulated in all the cities and villages in the land. Here is missionary work for all to engage in.

The Invitation

"The Spirit and the bride say, Come. And let him that heareth say, Come. And let him that is athirst come. And whosoever will, let him take the water of life freely."

Object Lessons in Health Reform

The large gatherings of our people afford an excellent opportunity of illustrating the principles of health reform. Some years ago at these gatherings much was said in regard to health reform and the benefits of a vegetarian diet; but at the same time flesh meats were furnished at the tables in the dining tent, and various unhealthful articles of food were sold at the provision stand. Faith without work is dead; and the instruction upon health reform, denied by practice, did not make the deepest impression. At later camp meetings those in charge have educated by practice as well as by precept. No meat has been furnished at the dining tent, but fruits, grains, and vegetables have been supplied in abundance. As visitors ask questions in regard to the absence of meat, the reason is plainly stated, that flesh is not the most healthful food.

As we near the close of time, we must rise higher and still higher upon the question of health reform and Christian temperance, presenting it in a more positive and decided manner. We must strive continually to educate the people, not only by our words but by our practice. Precept and practice combined have a telling influence.

At the camp meeting, instruction on health topics should be given to the people. At our meetings in Australia, lectures on health subjects were given daily, and a deep interest was aroused. A tent for the use of physicians and nurses was on the ground, medical advice was given freely and was sought by many. Thousands of people attended the lectures, and at the close of the camp meeting the people were not satisfied to let the matter drop with what they had already learned. In several cities

Testimonies for the Church, vol. 6, pp. 112, 113 (1900).

where camp meetings were held, some of the leading citizens urged that a branch sanitarium be established, promising their co-operation. In several cities the work has been started, with good success. A health institution, rightly conducted, gives character to our work in new fields. And not only is it a benefit to the people, but the workers connected with it can be a help to the laborers in evangelistic lines.

In every city where we have a church, there is need of a place where treatment can be given. Among the homes of our church members there are few that afford room and facilities for the proper care of the sick. A place should be provided where treatment may be given for common ailments. The building might be inelegant and even rude, but it should be furnished with facilities for giving simple treatments. These, skillfully employed, would prove a blessing, not only to our own people, but to their neighbors, and might be the means of calling the attention of many to health principles.

It is the Lord's purpose that in every part of our world health institutions shall be established as a branch of the gospel work. These institutions are to be His agencies for reaching a class whom nothing else will reach. They need not be large buildings, but should be so arranged that effective work may be done.

Beginnings might be made in every prominent place where camp meetings are held. Make small beginnings and enlarge as circumstances may demand. Count the cost of every undertaking, that you may be sure of being able to finish. Draw as little as possible from the treasury. Men of faith and financial ability are needed to plan economically. Our sanitariums must be erected with a limited outlay of means. Buildings in which to begin the work can often be secured at low cost.

Why Conduct Sanitariums?

In letters received from our brethren, the questions are asked, "Why do we expend so much effort in establishing sanitariums? Why do we not pray for the healing of the sick, instead of having sanitariums?"

There is more to these questions than is at first apparent. In the early history of our work, many were healed by prayer. And some, after they were healed, pursued the same course in the indulgence of appetite that they had followed in the past. They did not live and work in such a way as to avoid sickness. They did not show that they appreciated the Lord's goodness to them. Again and again they were brought to suffering through their own careless, thoughtless course of action. How could the Lord be glorified in bestowing on them the gift of health?

When the light came that we should begin sanitarium work, the reasons were plainly given. There were many who needed to be educated in regard to healthful living. As the work developed, we were instructed that suitable places were to be provided, to which we could bring the sick and suffering who knew nothing of our people and scarcely anything of the Bible, and there teach them how to regain health by rational methods of treatment without having recourse to poisonous drugs, and at the same time surround them with uplifting spiritual influences. As a part of the treatment, lectures were to be given on right habits of eating and drinking and dressing. Instruction was to be given regarding the choice and the preparation of food, showing that food may be prepared so as to be wholesome and nourishing and at the same time appetizing and palatable.

Special Testimonies, Series B, No. 13, pp. 9, 10 (1905).

In all our medical institutions, patients should be systematically and carefully instructed how to prevent disease by a wise course of action. Through lectures and the consistent practice of the principles of healthful living on the part of consecrated physicians and nurses, the blinded understanding of many will be opened, and truths never before thought of will be fastened on the mind. Many of the patients will be led to keep the body in the most healthy condition possible, because it is the Lord's purchased possession. . . .

When we have shown the people that we have right principles regarding health reform, we should then take up the temperance question in all its bearings, and drive it home to the hilt.

It is to save the souls, as well as to cure the bodies, of men and women, that at much expense our sanitariums are established. God designs that by means of these agencies of His own planting, the rich and the poor, the high and the low, shall find the bread of heaven and the water of life. He designs that they shall be educated in right habits of living, spiritual and physical. The salvation of many souls is at stake. In the providence of God, many of the sick are to be given the opportunity of separating for a time from harmful associations and surroundings and of placing themselves in institutions where they may receive health-restoring treatments and wise instruction from Christian nurses and physicians. The establishment of sanitariums is a providential arrangement, whereby people from all churches are to be reached and made acquainted with the truth for this time.

HEALTH FOOD WORK

The Preparation of Healthful Foods

Cooranbong, N.S.W., March 10, 1900.

During the past night many things have been opened before me. The manufacture and sale of health foods will require careful and prayerful consideration.

There are many minds in many places to whom the Lord will surely give knowledge of how to prepare foods that are healthful and palatable, if He sees that they will use this knowledge righteously. Animals are becoming more and more diseased, and it will not be long until animal food will be discarded by many besides Seventh-day Adventists. Foods that are healthful and life-sustaining are to be prepared, so that men and women will not need to eat meat.

The Lord will teach many in all parts of the world to combine fruits, grains, and vegetables into foods that will sustain life and will not bring disease. Those who have never seen the recipes for making the health foods now on the market will work intelligently, experimenting with the food productions of the earth, and will be given light regarding the use of these productions. The Lord will show them what to do.

He who gives skill and understanding to His people in one part of the world will give skill and understanding to His people in other parts of the world. It is His design that the food treasures of each country shall be so prepared that they can be used in the countries for which they are suited. As God gave manna from heaven to sustain the children of Israel, so He will now give His people in different places skill and wisdom to use the productions of these countries in preparing foods to take the place of meat. These foods should be made in the different countries; for to transport them from one country to another makes them so expensive that the poor cannot afford them. It will never pay to depend upon America for the supply of health foods for other countries. Great difficulty will be found in handling the imported goods without financial loss.

All who handle the health foods are to work unselfishly for the benefit of their fellow men. Unless men allow the Lord to guide their minds, untold difficulties will arise as different ones engage in this work. When the Lord gives one skill and understanding, let that one remember that this wisdom was not given for his benefit only, but that with it he might help others.

Knowledge to Be Imparted to Others

No man is to think that he is the possessor of all knowledge regarding the preparation of health foods, or that he has the sole right to use the Lord's treasures of earth and tree in this work. No man is to feel free to use according to his own pleasure the knowledge God has given him on this subject. "Freely ye have received, freely give." Matthew 10:8.

It is our wisdom to prepare simple, inexpensive, healthful foods. Many of our people are poor, and healthful foods are to be provided that can be supplied at prices that the poor can afford to pay. It is the Lord's design that the poorest people in every place shall be supplied with inexpensive, healthful foods. In many places industries for the manufacture of these foods are to be established. That which is a blessing to the work in one place will be a blessing in another place where money is very much harder to obtain.

God is working in behalf of His people. He does not desire them to be without resources. He is bringing them back to the diet originally given to man. Their diet is to consist of the foods made from the materials He has provided. The materials principally used in these foods will be fruits and grains and nuts, but various roots will also be used.

The profits on these foods are to come principally from the world, rather than from the Lord's people. God's people have to sustain His work; they have to enter new fields and establish churches. On them rest the burdens of many missionary enterprises. No unnecessary burdens are to be placed upon them. To His people God is a present help in every time of need.

Great care should be exercised by those who prepare recipes for our health journals. Some of the specially prepared foods now being made can be improved, and our plans regarding their use will have to be modified. Some have used the nut preparations too freely. Many have written to me, "I cannot use the nut foods; what shall I use in the place of meat?" One night I seemed to be standing before a company of people, telling them that nuts are used too freely in their preparation of foods, that the system cannot take care of them when used as in some of the recipes given, and that, if used more sparingly, the results would be more satisfactory.

The Value of Fresh Fruits

The Lord desires those living in countries where fresh fruit can be obtained during a large part of the year, to awake to the blessing they have in this fruit. The more we depend upon the fresh fruit just as it is plucked from the tree, the greater will be the blessing. Some, after adopting a vegetarian diet, return to the use of flesh meat.

This is foolish indeed, and reveals a lack of knowledge of how to provide proper food in the place of meat.

Cooking schools, conducted by wise instructors, are to be held in America and in other lands. Everything that we can do should be done to show the people the value of the reform diet.

There is danger that our restaurants will be conducted in such a way that our helpers will work very hard day after day and week after week, and yet not be able to point to any good accomplished. This matter needs careful consideration. We have no right to bind our young people up in a work that yields no fruit to the glory of God.

There is danger that the restaurant work, though regarded as a wonderfully successful way of doing good, will be so conducted that it will promote merely the physical well-being of those whom it serves. A work may apparently bear the features of supreme excellence, but it is not good in God's sight unless it is performed with an earnest desire to do His will and fulfill His purpose. If God is not recognized as the author and end of our actions, they are weighed in the balances of the sanctuary, and found wanting.—*Testimonies for the Church,* vol. 7, p. 120 (1902).

Practical Piety

The world will be convinced, not by what the pulpit teaches, but by what the church lives. The minister in the desk announces the theory of the gospel; the practical piety of the church demonstrates its power.—*Testimonies for the Church,* vol. 7, p. 16 (1902).

Educate the People

Saint Helena, California, August 20, 1902.

Wherever the truth is proclaimed, instruction should be given in the preparation of healthful foods. God desires that in every place the people shall be taught to use wisely the products that can be easily obtained. Skillful teachers should show the people how to utilize to the very best advantage the products that they can raise or secure in their section of the country. Thus the poor, as well as those in better circumstances, can learn to live healthfully.

From the beginning of the health-reform work, we have found it necessary to educate, educate, educate. God desires us to continue this work of educating the people. We are not to neglect it because of the effect we may fear it will have on the sales of the health foods prepared in our factories. That is not the most important matter. Our work is to show the people how they can obtain and prepare the most wholesome food, how they can co-operate with God in restoring His moral image in themselves.

Our workers should exercise their ingenuity in the preparation of healthful foods. None are to pry into Dr. Kellogg's secrets, but all should understand that the Lord is teaching many minds in many places to make healthful foods. There are many products which, if properly prepared and combined, can be made into foods that will be a blessing to those who cannot afford to purchase the more expensive, specially prepared health foods. He who in the building of the tabernacle gave skill and understanding in all manner of cunning work, will give skill and understanding to His people in the combining of natural food products, thus showing them how to secure a healthful diet.

Testimonies for the Church, vol. 7, pp. 132-137 (1902).

Knowledge in regard to the preparation of healthful foods is God's property, and has been communicated to man, in order that he may communicate it to his fellow men. In saying this, I do not refer to the special preparations that it has taken Dr. Kellogg and others long study and much expense to perfect. I refer especially to the simple preparations that all can make for themselves, instruction in regard to which should be given freely to those who desire to live healthfully, and especially to the poor.

It is the Lord's design that in every place men and women shall be encouraged to develop their talents by preparing healthful foods from the natural products of their own section of the country. If they look to God, exercising their skill and ingenuity under the guidance of His Spirit, they will learn how to prepare natural products into healthful foods. Thus they will be able to teach the poor how to provide themselves with foods that will take the place of flesh meat. Those thus helped can in turn instruct others. Such a work will yet be done with consecrated zeal and energy. If it had been done before, there would today be many more people in the truth, and many more who could give instruction. Let us learn what our duty is, and then do it. We are not to be dependent and helpless, waiting for others to do the work that God has committed to us.

The Selection of Foods

In the use of foods we should exercise good, sound common sense. When we find that a certain food does not agree with us, we need not write letters of inquiry to learn the cause of the disturbance. Change the diet; use less of some foods; try other preparations. Soon we shall know the effect that certain combinations have on us.

As intelligent human beings, let us individually study the principles and use our experience and judgment in deciding what foods are best for us.

The foods used should be suited to the occupation in which we are engaged and the climate in which we live. Some foods that are suitable in one country will not do in another.

There are some who would be benefited more by abstinence from food for a day or two every week than by any amount of treatment or medical advice. To fast one day a week would be of incalculable benefit to them.

The Use of Nut Foods

I have been instructed that the nut foods are often used unwisely, that too large a proportion of nuts is used, that some nuts are not as wholesome as others. Almonds are preferable to peanuts; but peanuts, in limited quantities, may be used in connection with grains to make nourishing and digestible food.

Olives may be so prepared as to be eaten with good results at every meal. The advantages sought by the use of butter may be obtained by the eating of properly prepared olives. The oil in the olives relieves constipation, and for consumptives, and for those who have inflamed, irritated stomachs, it is better than any drug. As food it is better than any oil coming secondhand from animals.

It would be well for us to do less cooking and to eat more fruit in its natural state. Let us teach the people to eat freely of the fresh grapes, apples, peaches, pears, berries, and all other kinds of fruit that can be obtained. Let these be prepared for winter use by canning, using glass, as far as possible, instead of tin.

Concerning flesh meat, we should educate the people to let it alone. Its use is contrary to the best development of the physical, mental, and moral powers. And we should bear a clear testimony against the use of tea and coffee. It is also well to discard rich desserts. Milk, eggs, and butter should not be classed with flesh meat. In some cases the use of eggs is beneficial. The time has not come to say that the use of milk and eggs should be wholly discarded. There are poor families whose diet consists largely of bread and milk. They have little fruit and cannot afford to purchase the nut foods. In teaching health reform, as in all other gospel work, we are to meet the people where they are. Until we can teach them how to prepare health-reform foods that are palatable, nourishing, and yet inexpensive, we are not at liberty to present the most advanced propositions regarding health-reform diet.

Let Reform Be Progressive

Let the diet reform be progressive. Let the people be taught how to prepare food without the use of milk or butter. Tell them that the time will soon come when there will be no safety in using eggs, milk, cream, or butter, because disease in animals is increasing in proportion to the increase of wickedness among men. The time is near when, because of the iniquity of the fallen race, the whole animal creation will groan under the diseases that curse our earth.

God will give His people ability and tact to prepare wholesome food without these things. Let our people discard all unwholesome recipes. Let them learn how to live healthfully, teaching to others what they have learned. Let them impart this knowledge as they would Bible instruction. Let them teach the people to preserve the health and increase the strength by avoiding the large amount of cooking that has filled the world with chronic invalids. By precept and example make it plain that the food which God gave Adam in his sinless state is the best for man's use as he seeks to regain that sinless state.

Teach With Wisdom

Those who teach the principles of health reform should be intelligent in regard to disease and its causes, understanding that every action of the human agent should be in perfect harmony with the laws of life. The light God has given on health reform is for our salvation and the salvation of the world. Men and women should be informed in regard to the human habitation, fitted up by our Creator as His dwelling place and over which He desires us to be faithful stewards. "For ye are the temple of the living God; as God hath said, I will dwell in them, and walk in them; and I will be their God, and they shall be My people." 2 Corinthians 6:16.

Hold up the principles of health reform, and let the Lord lead the honest in heart. Present the principles of temperance in their most attractive form. Circulate the books that give instruction in regard to healthful living.

The people are in sad need of the light shining from the pages of our health books and journals. God desires to use these books and journals as mediums through which flashes of light shall arrest the attention of the people and cause them to heed the warning of the message of the third angel. Our health journals are instrumentalities in the field to do a special work in disseminating the light that the inhabitants of the world must have in this day of God's preparation. They wield an untold influence in the interests of health and temperance and social-purity reform, and will accomplish great good in presenting these subjects in a proper manner and in their true light to the people.

The Lord has been sending us line upon line, and if we reject these principles, we are not rejecting the messenger who teaches them, but the One who has given us the principles.

Be Light Bearers

Reform, continual reform, must be kept before the people, and by our example we must enforce our teaching. True religion and the laws of health go hand in hand. It is impossible to work for the salvation of men and women without presenting to them the need of breaking away from sinful gratifications, which destroy the health, debase the soul, and prevent divine truth from impressing the mind. Men and women must be taught to take a careful view of every habit and every practice and at once put away those things that cause an unhealthy condition of the body, and thus cast a dark shadow over the mind. God desires His light bearers ever to keep a high standard before them. By precept and example they must hold their perfect standard high above Satan's false standard, which, if followed, will lead to misery, degradation, disease, and death for both body and soul. Let those who have obtained a knowledge of how to eat and drink and dress so as to preserve health, impart this knowledge to others. Let the poor have the gospel of health preached unto them from a practical point of view, that they may know how to care properly for the body, which is the temple of the Holy Spirit.

The Restaurant Work

We must do more than we have done to reach the people of our cities. We are not to erect large buildings in the cities, but over and over again the light has been given me that we should establish in all our cities small plants which shall be centers of influence.

The Lord has a message for our cities, and this message we are to proclaim in our camp meetings and by other public efforts, and also through our publications. In addition to this, hygienic restaurants are to be established in the cities, and by them the message of temperance is to be proclaimed. Arrangements should be made to hold meetings in connection with our restaurants. Whenever possible, let a room be provided where the patrons can be invited to lectures on the science of health and Christian temperance, where they can receive instruction on the preparation of wholesome food and on other important subjects. In these meetings there should be prayer and singing and talks, not only on health and temperance topics, but also on other appropriate Bible subjects. As the people are taught how to preserve physical health, many opportunities will be found to sow the seeds of the gospel of the kingdom.

The subjects should be presented in such a way as to impress the people favorably. There should be in the meetings nothing of a theatrical nature. The singing should not be done by a few only. All present should be encouraged to join in the song service. There are those who have a special gift of song, and there are times when a special message is borne by one singing alone or by several uniting in song. But the singing is seldom to be

Testimonies for the Church, vol. 7, pp. 115-120 (1902).

done by a few. The ability to sing is a talent of influence, which God desires all to cultivate and use to His name's glory.

Use of Reading Matter

Those who come to our restaurants should be supplied with reading matter. Their attention should be called to our literature on temperance and dietetic reform, and leaflets treating on the lessons of Christ should also be given them. The burden of supplying this reading matter should be shared by all our people. All who come should be given something to read. It may be that many will leave the tract unread, but some among those in whose hands you place it may be searching for light. They will read and study what you give them, and then pass it on to others.

The workers in our restaurants should live in such close connection with God that they will recognize the promptings of His Spirit to talk personally about spiritual things to such and such a one who comes to the restaurant. When self is crucified and Christ is formed within, the hope of glory, we shall reveal in thought, word, and deed the reality of our belief in the truth. The Lord will be with us, and through us the Holy Spirit will work to reach those who are out of Christ.

The Lord has instructed me that this is the work to be done by those conducting our restaurants. The pressure and rush of business must not lead to a neglect of the work of soul saving. It is well to minister to the physical wants of our fellow men, but if ways are not found to let the light of the gospel shine forth to those who come day by day for their meals, how is God glorified by our work?

When the restaurant work was started, it was expected that it would be the means of reaching many with the message of present truth. Has it done this? To the workers in our restaurants the question was asked by One in authority: "To how many have you spoken regarding their salvation? How many have heard from your lips earnest appeals to accept Christ as a personal Saviour? How many have been led by your words to turn from sin to the service of the living God?"

As in our restaurants people are supplied with temporal food, let not the workers forget that they themselves and those whom they serve need to be constantly supplied with the bread of heaven. Let them watch constantly for opportunities to speak of the truth to those who know it not.

Care of the Helpers

The managers of our restaurants are to work for the salvation of the employees. They must not overwork, because by doing so they will place themselves where they have neither strength nor inclination to help the workers spiritually. They are to devote their best powers to instructing their employees in spiritual lines, explaining the Scriptures to them and praying with them and for them. They are to guard the religious interests of the helpers as carefully as parents are to guard the religious interests of their children. Patiently and tenderly they are to watch over them, doing all in their power to help them in the perfection of Christian characters. Their words are to be like apples of gold in pictures of silver; their actions are to be free from every trace of selfishness and harshness. They are to stand as minutemen, watching for souls as they that must give an account. They are to strive to keep their helpers standing on vantage ground, where their courage will constantly grow stronger and their faith in God constantly increase.

Unless our restaurants are conducted in this way, it will be necessary to warn our people against sending their children to them as workers. Many of those who patronize our restaurants do not bring with them the angels of God; they do not desire the companionship of these holy beings. They bring with them a worldly influence, and to withstand this influence the workers need to be closely connected with God. The managers of our restaurants must do more to save the young people in their employ. They must put forth greater efforts to keep them alive spiritually, so that their young minds will not be swayed by the worldly spirit with which they are constantly brought in contact. The girls and the young women in our restaurants need a shepherd. Every one of them needs to be sheltered by home influences.

There is danger that the youth, entering our institutions as believers, and desiring to help in the cause of God, will become weary and disheartened, losing their zeal and courage, and growing cold and indifferent. We cannot crowd these youth into small, dark rooms, and deprive them of the privileges of home life, and then expect them to have a wholesome religious experience.

It is important that wise plans be laid for the care of the helpers in all our institutions, and especially for those employed in our restaurants. Good helpers should be secured, and every advantage should be provided that will aid them to grow in grace and in the knowledge of Christ. They are not to be left to the mercy of haphazard circumstances, with no regular time for prayer, and no time at all for Bible study. When left thus, they become heedless and careless, indifferent to eternal realities.

With every restaurant there should be connected a man and his wife who can act as guardians of the helpers, a man and woman who love the Saviour and the souls for whom He died, and who keep the way of the Lord.

The young women should be under the care of a wise, judicious matron, a woman who is thoroughly converted, who will carefully guard the workers, especially the younger ones.

The workers are to feel that they have a home. They are God's helping hand, and they are to be treated as carefully and tenderly as Christ declared that the little child whom He set in the midst of His disciples was to be treated. "Whoso shall offend one of these little ones which believe in Me," He said, "it were better for him that a millstone were hanged about his neck, and that he were drowned in the depth of the sea." "Take heed that ye despise not one of these little ones; for I say unto you, That in heaven their angels do always behold the face of My Father which is in heaven." Matthew 18:6, 10. The care that should be given to these employees is one of the reasons in favor of having in a large city several small restaurants instead of one large one. But this is not the only reason why it will be best to establish several small restaurants in different parts of our large cities.

Advantages in Small Restaurants

The smaller restaurants will recommend the principles of health reform just as well as the larger establishment, and will be much more easily managed. We are not commissioned to feed the world, but we are instructed to educate the people. In the smaller restaurants there will not be so much work to do, and the helpers will have more time to devote to the study of the word, more time to learn how to do their work well, and more time to answer the inquiries of the patrons who are desirous of learning about the principles of health reform.

If we fulfill the purpose of God in this work, the righteousness of Christ will go before us, and the glory of the Lord will be our rearward. But if there is no ingathering of souls, if the helpers themselves are not spiritually benefited, if they are not glorifying God in word and deed, why should we open and maintain such establishments? If we cannot conduct our restaurants to God's glory, if we cannot exert through them a strong religious influence, it would be better for us to close them up and use the talents of our youth in other lines of work. But our restaurants can be so conducted that they will be the means of saving souls. Let us seek the Lord earnestly for humility of heart, that He may teach us how to walk in the light of His counsel, how to understand His word, how to accept it, and how to put it into practice.

Teach Children to Cook

Do not neglect to teach your children how to cook. In so doing you impart to them principles which they must have in their religious education. In giving your children lessons in physiology, and teaching them how to cook with simplicity and yet with skill, you are laying the foundation for the most useful branches of education. Skill is required to make good light bread. There is religion in good cooking, and I question the religion of that class who are too ignorant and too careless to learn to cook.—*Testimonies for the Church*, vol. 2, p. 537 (1870).

Restaurants in Large Cities

While in New York in the winter of 1901, I received light in regard to the work in that great city. Night after night the course that our brethren should pursue passed before me. In Greater New York the message is to go forth as a lamp that burneth. God will raise up laborers for this work, and His angels will go before them. Though our large cities are fast reaching a condition similar to the condition of the world before the Flood, though they are as Sodom for wickedness, yet there are in them many honest souls who, as they listen to the startling truths of the advent message, will feel the conviction of the Spirit. New York is ready to be worked. In that great city the message of truth will be given with the power of God. The Lord calls for workmen. He calls upon those who have gained an experience in the cause to take up and carry forward in His fear the work to be done in New York and in other large cities of America. He calls also for means to be used in this work.

It was presented to me that we should not rest satisfied because we have a vegetarian restaurant in Brooklyn, but that others should be established in other sections of the city. The people living in one part of Greater New York do not know what is going on in other parts of that great city. Men and women who eat at the restaurants established in different places will become conscious of an improvement in health. Their confidence once gained, they will be more ready to accept God's special message of truth.

Wherever medical missionary work is carried on in our large cities, cooking schools should be held; and wherever a strong educational missionary work is in progress, a hygienic restaurant of some sort should be

Testimonies for the Church, vol. 7, pp. 54-56 (1902)

established, which shall give a practical illustration of the proper selection and the healthful preparation of foods.

When in Los Angeles, I was instructed that not only in various sections of that city, but in San Diego and in other tourist resorts of Southern California, health restaurants and treatment rooms should be established. Our efforts in these lines should include the great seaside resorts. As the voice of John the Baptist was heard in the wilderness, "Prepare ye the way of the Lord," so must the voice of the Lord's messengers be heard in the great tourist and seaside resorts.

Restaurants and Treatment Rooms

I have been given light that in many cities it is advisable for a restaurant to be connected with treatment rooms. The two can co-operate in upholding right principles. In connection with these, it is sometimes advisable to have rooms that will serve as lodgings for the sick. These establishments will serve as feeders to the sanitariums located in the country and would better be conducted in rented buildings. We are not to erect in the cities large buildings in which to care for the sick, because God has plainly indicated that the sick can be better cared for outside of the cities. In many places it will be necessary to begin sanitarium work in the cities, but, as much as possible, this work should be transferred to the country as soon as suitable locations can be secured.—*Testimonies for the Church,* vol. 7, p. 60.

Closing on the Sabbath

The question has been asked, "Should our restaurants be opened on the Sabbath?" My answer is, No, no! The observance of the Sabbath is our witness to God—the mark, or sign, between Him and us that we are His people. Never is this mark to be obliterated.

Were the workers in our restaurants to provide meals on the Sabbath the same as they do through the week, for the mass of people who would come, where would be their day of rest? What opportunity would they have to recruit their physical and spiritual strength?

Not long since, special light was given me on this subject. I was shown that efforts would be made to break down our standard of Sabbath observance, that men would plead for the opening of our restaurants on the Sabbath; but that this must never be done.

A scene passed before me. I was in our restaurant in San Francisco. It was Friday. Several of the workers were busily engaged in putting up packages of such foods as could be easily carried by the people to their homes, and a number were waiting to receive these packages. I asked the meaning of this, and the workers told me that some among their patrons were troubled because, on account of the closing of the restaurant, they could not on the Sabbath obtain food of the same kind as that which they used during the week. Realizing the value of the wholesome foods obtained at the restaurant, they protested against being denied them on the seventh day and pleaded with those in charge of the restaurant to keep it open every day in the week, pointing out what they

---

Testimonies for the Church, vol. 7, pp. 121-123 (1902).

would suffer if this were not done. "What you see today," said the workers, "is our answer to this demand for the health foods upon the Sabbath. These people take on Friday food that lasts over the Sabbath, and in this way we avoid condemnation for refusing to open the restaurant on the Sabbath."

The line of demarcation between our people and the world must ever be kept unmistakably plain. Our platform is the law of God, in which we are enjoined to observe the Sabbath day, for, as is distinctly stated in the thirty-first chapter of Exodus, the observance of the Sabbath is a sign between God and His people. "Verily My Sabbaths ye shall keep," He declares; "for it is a sign between Me and you *throughout your generations;* that ye may know that I am the Lord that doth sanctify you. Ye shall keep the Sabbath therefore; for it is holy unto you. . . . It is a sign between Me and the children of Israel *forever:* for in six days the Lord made heaven and earth, and on the seventh day He rested, and was refreshed."

We are to heed a "thus saith the Lord," even though by our obedience we cause great inconvenience to those who have no respect for the Sabbath. On one hand we have man's supposed necessities; on the other, God's commands. Which have the greatest weight with us?

In our sanitariums, the family of patients, with the physicians, nurses, and helpers, must be fed upon the Sabbath, as any other family, with as little labor as possible. But our restaurants should not be opened on the Sabbath. Let the workers be assured that they will have this day for the worship of God. The closed doors on the Sabbath stamp the restaurant as a memorial for God, a memorial which declares that the seventh day is the Sabbath and that on it no unnecessary work is to be done.

I have been instructed that one of the **principal** reasons why hygienic restaurants and treatment rooms should be established in the centers of large cities is that by this means the attention of leading men will be called to the third angel's message. Noticing that these restaurants are conducted in a way altogether different from the way in which ordinary restaurants are conducted, men of intelligence will begin to inquire into the reasons for the difference in business methods and will investigate the principles that lead us to serve superior food. Thus they will be led to a knowledge of the message for this time.

When thinking men find that our restaurants are closed on the Sabbath, they will make inquiries in regard to the principles that lead us to close our doors on Saturday. In answering their questions we shall have opportunity to acquaint them with the reasons for our faith. We can give them copies of our periodicals and tracts, so that they may be able to understand the difference between "him that serveth God and him that serveth Him not."

Not all our people are as particular as they should be in regard to Sabbath observance. May God help them to reform. It becomes the head of every family to plant his feet firmly on the platform of obedience.

Sabbath Sacredness

Everything that can possibly be done on the six days which God has given to you, should be done. You should not rob God of one hour of holy time. Great blessings are promised to those who place a high estimate upon the Sabbath and realize the obligations resting upon them in regard to its observance.—*Testimonies for the Church,* vol. 2, p. 702 (1871).

Health Foods in All Lands

The Lord has instructed me to say that He has not confined to a few persons all the light there is to be received in regard to the best preparations of health foods. . . .

God is the author of all wisdom, all intelligence, all talent. He will magnify His name by giving to many minds wisdom in the preparation of health foods. And when He does this, the making of these new foods is not to be looked upon as an infringement of the rights of those who are already manufacturing health foods, although in some respects the foods made by the different ones may be similar. God will take ordinary men and will give them skill and understanding in the use of the fruit of the earth. He deals impartially with His workers. Not one is forgotten by Him. He will impress businessmen who are Sabbathkeepers to establish industries that will provide employment for His people. He will teach His servants to prepare less expensive health foods which can be bought by the poor.

In all our plans we should remember that the health-food work is the property of God, and that it is not to be made a financial speculation for personal gain. It is God's gift to His people, and the profits are to be used for the good of suffering humanity everywhere.

Especially in the Southern States of North America many things will be devised and many facilities provided that the poor and needy can sustain themselves by the health-food industries. Under teachers who are laboring for the salvation of their souls, they will be taught how to cultivate and prepare for food those things that grow most readily in their locality.—*Testimonies for the Church*, vol. 7, pp. 128, 129 (1901).

In the Southern States

I have a message to bear in regard to the Southern field. We have a great work to do in this field. Its condition is a condemnation of our professed Christianity. Look at its destitution of ministers, teachers, and medical missionaries. Consider the ignorance, the poverty, the misery, the distress, of many of the people. And yet this field lies close at our doors. How selfish, how inattentive, we have been to our neighbors! We have heartlessly passed them by, doing little to relieve their sufferings. If the gospel commission had been studied and obeyed by our people, the South would have received its proportionate share of ministry. If those who have received the light had walked in the light, they would have realized that upon them rested the responsibility of cultivating this long-neglected portion of the vineyard.

God is calling upon His people to give Him of the means that He has entrusted to them, in order that institutions may be established in the destitute fields that are ripe for the harvest. He calls upon those who have money in the banks to put it into circulation. By giving of our substance to sustain God's work, we show in a practical manner that we love Him supremely and our neighbor as ourselves.

Let schools and sanitariums now be established in many places in the Southern States. Let centers of influence be made in many of the Southern cities by the opening of food stores and vegetarian restaurants. Let there also be facilities for the manufacture of simple, inexpensive health foods. But let not selfish, worldly policy be brought into the work, for God forbids this. Let unselfish

Testimonies for the Church, vol. 7, pp. 56, 57 (1902).

men take hold of this work in the fear of God and with love for their fellow men.

The light given me is that in the Southern field, as elsewhere, the manufacture of health foods should be conducted, not as a speculation for personal gain, but as a business that God has devised whereby a door of hope may be opened for the people. In the South, special consideration should be shown to the poor, who have been terribly neglected. Men of ability and economy are to be chosen to take up the food work; for, in order to make it a success, the greatest wisdom and economy must be exercised. God desires His people to do acceptable service in the preparation of healthful food, not only for their own families, which are their first responsibility, but for the help of the poor everywhere. They are to show Christlike liberality, realizing that they are representing God and that all they have is His endowment.

Brethren, take hold of this work. Give no place to discouragement. Do not criticize those who are trying to do something in right lines, but go to work yourselves.

In connection with the health-food business, various industries may be established that will be a help to the cause in the Southern field. All that men as missionaries for God can do for this field should now be done, for if ever a field needed medical missionary work, it is the South. During the time that has passed into eternity, many should have been in the South, laboring together with God by doing personal work and by giving of their means to sustain themselves and other workers in that field.

As a School Industry

The light given me is that it will not be very long before we shall have to give up using any animal food. Even milk will have to be discarded. Disease is accumulating rapidly. The curse of God is upon the earth, because man has cursed it. The habits and practices of men have brought the earth into such a condition that some other food than animal food must be substituted for the human family. We do not need flesh food at all. God can give us something else.

When we were talking about this land, it was said, "Nothing can be raised here." "Nevertheless," I said, "the Lord can spread a table in the wilderness." Under His direction food will go a long way. When we place ourselves in right relation to Him, He will help us and the food we eat in obedience to Him will satisfy us. We can subsist on very much less than we think we can, if God's blessing is on the food; and if it is for His glory He can multiply it.

We need to understand that God is in the health-reform movement. When we put Christ in it, it is right for us to grasp every probability and possibility.

The health-food business is to be connected with our school, and we should make provision for it. We are erecting buildings for the care of the sick, and food will be required for the patients. Wherever an interest is awakened, the people are to be taught the principles of health reform. If this line of work is brought in, it will be the entering wedge for the work of presenting truth. The health-food business should be established here. It should be one of the industries connected with the school. God has instructed me that parents can find work in this

industry and send their children to school. But everything
that is done should be done with the greatest simplicity.
There is to be no extravagance in anything. Solid work
is to be done, because unless the work is done solidly a
slipshod experience is the result. . . . The work must be
solid. Just as soon as the helpers in this line of work are
controlled by the Holy Spirit, the Lord will give them
tact and intelligence in the manufacturing of foods, just
as He gave the workers on the tabernacle understanding
and ability. He will enable them to do the right kind of
work in building up the tabernacle of the body.

MEDICAL MISSIONARY WORK

The Pioneer Work

Medical missionary work is the pioneer work of the gospel, the door through which the truth for this time is to find entrance to many homes. God's people are to be genuine medical missionaries, for they are to learn to minister to the needs of both soul and body. The purest unselfishness is to be shown by our workers as, with the knowledge and experience gained by practical work, they go out to give treatments to the sick. As they go from house to house they will find access to many hearts. Many will be reached who otherwise never would have heard the gospel message. A demonstration of the principles of health reform will do much toward removing prejudice against our evangelical work. The Great Physician, the originator of medical missionary work, will bless all who thus seek to impart the truth for this time.

Physical healing is bound up with the gospel commission. When Christ sent His disciples out on their first missionary journey, He bade them, "As ye go, preach, saying, The kingdom of heaven is at hand. Heal the sick, cleanse the lepers, raise the dead, cast out devils: freely ye have received, freely give." Matthew 10:7, 8. And when at the close of His earthly ministry He gave them their commission, He said, "These signs shall follow them that believe; In My name shall they cast out devils; they shall speak with new tongues; they shall take up serpents; and if they drink any deadly thing, it shall not hurt them;

Review and Herald, Dec. 17, 1914.

they shall lay hands on the sick, and they shall recover."
Mark 16:17, 18.

The Beloved Physician

Of the disciples after Christ's ascension we read, "They
went forth, and preached everywhere, the Lord working
with them, and confirming the word with signs following." Mark 16:20. Luke is called the "beloved physician." He labored in connection with Paul in Philippi,
and when Paul left that place Luke stayed, doing double
service as a physician and a gospel minister. He was indeed a medical missionary, and his medical skill opened
the way for the gospel to reach many hearts.

The Example of Christ

The divine commission needs no reform. Christ's way
of presenting truth cannot be improved upon. The Saviour gave the disciples practical lessons, teaching them
how to work in such a way as to make souls glad in the
truth. He sympathized with the weary, the heavy-laden,
the oppressed. He fed the hungry and healed the sick.
Constantly He went about doing good. By the good He
accomplished, by His loving words and kindly deeds, He
interpreted the gospel to men.

Brief as was the period of His public ministry, He
accomplished the work He came to do. How impressive
were the truths He taught! How complete His lifework!
What spiritual food He daily imparted as He presented
the bread of life to thousands of hungry souls! His life
was a living ministry of the word. He promised nothing
that He did not perform.

The words of life were presented in such simplicity
that a child could understand them. Men, women, and

children were so impressed with His manner of explaining the Scriptures that they would catch the very intonation of His voice, place the same emphasis on their words, and imitate His gestures. Youth caught His spirit of ministry and sought to pattern after His gracious ways by seeking to assist those whom they saw needing help.

Just as we trace the pathway of a stream of water by the line of living green it produces, so Christ could be seen in the deeds of mercy that marked His pathway at every step. Wherever He went, health sprang up and happiness followed wherever He passed. The blind and deaf rejoiced in His presence. His words to the ignorant opened to them a fountain of life. He dispensed His blessings abundantly and continuously. They were the garnered treasures of eternity, given in Christ, the Lord's rich gift to man.

Christ's work in behalf of man is not finished. It continues today. In like manner His ambassadors are to preach the gospel and to reveal His pitying love for lost and perishing souls. By an unselfish interest in those who need help they are to give a practical demonstration of the truth of the gospel. Much more than mere sermonizing is included in this work. The evangelization of the world is the work God has given to those who go forth in His name. They are to be colaborers with Christ, revealing to those ready to perish His tender, pitying love. God calls for thousands to work for Him, not by preaching to those who know the truth for this time, but by warning those who have never heard the last message of mercy. Work with a heart filled with an earnest longing for souls. Do medical missionary work. Thus you will gain access to the hearts of people, and the way will be prepared for a more decided proclamation of the truth.

Who are laborers together with Christ in this blessed medical missionary work? Who have learned the lessons of the Master and know how to deal skillfully with souls for whom Christ has died? We need, oh, so much! physicians for the soul who have been educated in the school of Christ and who can work in Christ's lines. Our work is to gain a knowledge of Him who is the way, the truth, and the life. We are to interest the people in subjects that concern the health of the body as well as the health of the soul. Believers have a decided message to bear to prepare the way for the kingdom of God.

The great questions of Bible truth are to enter into the very heart of society, to convert and reform men and women, bringing them to see the great need of preparing for the mansions that Christ declared He would prepare for all who love Him. When the Holy Spirit shall do its office work, hearts of stone will become hearts of flesh, and Satan will not work through them to counteract the work that Christ came to earth to do.

Sympathy and Support Needed

Henceforth medical missionary work is to be carried forward with greater earnestness. Medical missions should be opened as pioneer agencies for the proclamation of the third angel's message. How great is the need of means to do this line of work! Gospel medical missions cannot be established without financial aid. Every such enterprise calls for our sympathy and for our means, that facilities may be provided to make the work successful.

A special work is to be done in places where people are constantly coming and going. Christ labored in Capernaum much of the time because this was a place through which travelers were constantly passing and where many often tarried.

Christ sought the people where they were and placed before them the great truths in regard to His kingdom. As He went from place to place, He blessed and comforted the suffering and healed the sick. This is our work. Small companies are to go forth to do the work to which Christ appointed His disciples. While laboring as evangelists they can visit the sick, praying with them and, if need be, treating them, not with medicines but with the remedies provided in nature.

Small Plants in Many Places

There are many places that need gospel medical missionary work, and there small plants should be established. God designs that our sanitariums shall be a means of reaching high and low, rich and poor. They are to be so conducted that by their work attention may be called to the message God has sent to the world.

May the Lord increase our faith and help us to see that He desires us all to become acquainted with His ministry of healing and with the mercy seat. He desires the light of His grace to shine forth from many places. He who understands the necessities of the situation arranges that advantages shall be brought to the workers in various places to enable them more effectually to arouse the attention of the people to the truths that make for deliverance from both physical and spiritual ills.

Compassion and Sympathy to Be Cultivated

The tender sympathies of our Saviour were aroused for fallen and suffering humanity. If you would be His follower, you must cultivate compassion and sympathy.

Indifference to human woes must give place to lively interest in the sufferings of others. The widow, the orphan, the sick and dying, will always need help. Here is an opportunity to proclaim the gospel—to hold up Jesus, the hope and consolation of all men. When the suffering body has been relieved the heart is opened, and you can pour in the heavenly balm. If you are looking to Jesus and drawing from Him knowledge and strength and grace, you can impart His consolation to others, because the Comforter is with you.

You will meet with much prejudice, a great deal of false zeal and miscalled piety; but in both the home and the foreign field you will find more hearts that God has been preparing for the seed of truth than you imagine, and they will hail with joy the divine message when it is presented to them.

Many are suffering from maladies of the soul far more than from diseases of the body, and they will find no relief until they come to Christ, the wellspring of life. The burden of sin, with its unrest and unsatisfied desires, lies at the foundation of a large share of the maladies the sinner suffers. Christ is the Mighty Healer of the sin-sick soul. These poor, afflicted ones need to have a clearer knowledge of Him whom to know aright is life eternal. They need to be patiently and kindly yet earnestly taught how to throw open the windows of the soul and let the sunlight of God's love come in. Complaints of weariness, loneliness, and dissatisfaction will then cease. Satisfying joys will give vigor to the mind and health and vital energy to the body.

Reference for further study: *Christ's Object Lessons,* pages 376-389, "Who Is My Neighbor?"

Medical Evangelism

Melbourne, Australia, September 16, 1892.

I am deeply interested in the subject of medical missionary work and the education of men and women for that work. I could wish that there were one hundred nurses in training where there is one. It ought to be thus. Both men and women can be so much more useful as medical missionaries than as missionaries without the medical education. I am more and more impressed with the fact that a more decided testimony must be borne upon this subject, that more direct efforts must be made to interest the proper persons, setting before them the advantages that every missionary will have in understanding how to treat those who are diseased in body, as well as to minister to sin-sick souls. This double ministration will give the laborer together with God access to homes, and will enable him to reach all classes of society.

An intelligent knowledge of how to treat disease upon hygienic principles will gain the confidence of many who otherwise would not be reached with the truth. In affliction, many are humbled in spirit, and words in favor of the truth spoken to them in tenderness by one who is seeking to alleviate physical sufferings may touch the heart. Prayer—short, weighted with tenderest sympathy, presenting the suffering ones in faith to the Great Physician—will inspire in them a confidence, a rest and trust, that will tend to the health of both soul and body.

I have been surprised at being asked by physicians if I did not think it would be more pleasing to God for them to give up their medical practice and enter the

Medical Missionary, November and December, 1892.

ministry. I am prepared to answer such an inquirer: If you are a Christian and a competent physician, you are qualified to do tenfold more good as a missionary for God than if you were to go forth merely as a preacher of the word. I would advise young men and women to give heed to this matter. Perilous times are before us. The whole world will be involved in perplexity and distress, disease of every kind will be upon the human family, and such ignorance as now prevails concerning the laws of health would result in great suffering and the loss of many lives that might be saved.

While Satan is constantly doing his utmost to take advantage of men's ignorance and to lay the foundation of disease by improper treatment of the body, it is best for those who claim to be sons and daughters of God to avail themselves while they can of the opportunities now presented to gain a knowledge of the human system and how it may be preserved in health. We are to use every faculty of mind which God has given us. The Lord will not work a miracle to preserve anyone in health who will not make an effort to obtain knowledge within his reach concerning this wonderful habitation that God has given. By study of the human organism, we are to learn to correct what may be wrong in our habits and which, if left uncorrected, would bring the sure result, disease and suffering, that make life a burden. The sincerity of our prayers can be proved only by the vigor of our endeavor to obey God's commandments.

Virtue of Character

Evil habits and practices are bringing upon men disease of every kind. Let the understanding be convinced by education as to the sinfulness of abusing and degrading the powers that God has given. Let the mind become intelligent, and the will be placed on the Lord's side, and there will be a wonderful improvement in the physical health. But this can never be accomplished in mere human strength. With strenuous efforts through the grace of Christ to renounce all evil practices and associations and to observe temperance in all things, there must be an abiding persuasion that repentance for the past, as well as forgiveness, is to be sought of God through the atoning sacrifice of Christ. These things must be brought into daily experience; there must be strict watchfulness and unwearied entreaty that Christ will bring every thought into captivity to Himself; His renovating power must be given to the soul, that as accountable beings we may present to God our bodies a living sacrifice, holy and acceptable unto Him, which is our reasonable service.

Will those who claim to believe the solemn, sacred truth for this time arouse their sluggish energies and place themselves in the channel where they can gather to their souls every ray of light that shines upon their pathway? God calls upon all who claim to believe advanced truth to exert every power to the uttermost in gaining knowledge. If we would elevate the moral standard in any country where we may be called to go, we must begin by correcting their physical habits. Virtue of character depends upon the right action of the powers of the mind and body.

Willing Ignorance a Sin

Guilt rests upon us as a people who have had much light, because we have not appreciated or improved the light given upon health reform. Through misunderstanding and perverted ideas many souls are deceived. Those each the truth to others and who should be shepherds of the flock will be held accountable for their willing ignorance and disregard of nature's laws. This is not a matter to be trifled with, to be passed off with a jest. As we approach the close of this earth's history, selfishness and violence and crime prevail as in the days of Noah, when the old world perished in the waters of the Flood. As Bible believers, we need to take our position for righteousness and truth.

As religious aggression subverts the liberties of our nation, those who would stand for freedom of conscience will be placed in unfavorable positions. For their own sake, they should, while they have opportunity, become intelligent in regard to disease, its causes, prevention, and cure. And those who do this will find a field of labor anywhere. There will be suffering ones, plenty of them, who will need help, not only among those of our own faith, but largely among those who know not the truth.

The shortness of time demands an energy that has not been aroused among those who claim to believe the present truth. There is need of personal religion, of repentance, of faith and love. I plead that there be a general awakening among us as a people. In the strength that Christ imparts, we should be able to teach others also how to wrestle with those passions which the light of heaven shows them must be mortified. Let there be constant watchfulness and unwearied prayer for the assistance of the Holy Spirit, and let us avail ourselves of all the help and light that God has given.

Promising Youth to Be Selected

In almost every church there are young men and women who might receive education either as nurses or physicians. They will never have a more favorable opportunity than now. I would urge that this subject be considered prayerfully, that special effort be made to select those youth who give promise of usefulness and moral strength. Let these receive an education . . . to go out as missionaries wherever the Lord may call them to labor. It should ever be kept before them that their work is not only to relieve physical suffering, but to minister to souls that are ready to perish. It is important that everyone who is to act as a medical missionary be skilled in ministering to the soul as well as to the body. He is to be an imitator of Christ, presenting to the sick and suffering the preciousness of pure and undefiled religion. While doing all in his power to relieve physical distress and to preserve this mortal life, he should point to the mercy and the love of Jesus, the Great Physician, who came that "whosoever believeth in Him should not perish, but have everlasting life." John 3:16.

Workers are needed now. As a people, we are not doing one fiftieth of what we might do as active missionaries. If we were only vitalized by the Holy Spirit, there would be a hundred missionaries where there is now one. But where are the missionaries? Has not the truth for this time power to stir the souls of those who claim to believe it? When there is a call to labor, why should there be so many voices to say, "I pray thee, have me excused"? In this country the standard of truth is to be established and exalted. There is great need of workers, and there are many ways in which they can labor. There is work for those in the higher as well as in the more humble positions. . . . Individually all need a heart work. A good work cannot be done by the human agent alone. For the full development and efficiency of the intellectual as well as the spiritual powers, there is, there must be, a vital connection with God, a communion with the highest source of activity. Then with the soul all aglow with zeal for the Master, we can be a blessing to others. Jesus said, "Whosoever drinketh of the water that I shall give him shall never thirst; but the water that I shall give him shall be in him a well of water springing up into everlasting life." John 4:14. Those who become partakers of the grace of Christ will guide others to the living stream.

Is it not a privilege to be thus copartners with Jesus? Is it not an honor to be connected with the grand work of saving souls, acting the part assigned us by our Saviour? And none can impart a blessing to others without receiving benefit himself. "He that watereth shall be watered also himself." Proverbs 11:25.

An Illustration

Christ's work for the paralytic is an illustration of the way we are to work. Through his friends this man had heard of Jesus and requested to be brought into the presence of the Mighty Healer. The Saviour knew that the paralytic had been tortured by the suggestions of the priests, that because of his sins God had cast him off. Therefore His first work was to give him peace of mind. "Son," He said, "thy sins be forgiven thee." This assurance filled his heart with peace and joy. But some who were present began to murmur, saying in their hearts, "Who can forgive sins but God only?" Then that they might know that the Son of man had power to forgive sins, Christ said to the sick man, "Arise, and take up thy bed, and go thy way into thine house." This shows how the Saviour bound together the work of preaching the truth and healing the sick—*Testimonies for the Church,* vol. 6, p. 234 (1900).

The Breadth of the Work

The breadth of gospel medical missionary work is not understood. The medical missionary work now called for is that outlined in the commission which Christ gave to His disciples just before His ascension. "All power is given unto Me in heaven and in earth," He said. "Go ye therefore, and teach all nations, baptizing them in the name of the Father, and of the Son, and of the Holy Ghost: teaching them to observe all things whatsoever I have commanded you: and, lo, I am with you alway, even unto the end of the world." Matthew 28:18-20.

These words point out our field and our work. Our field is the world; our work the proclamation of the truths which Christ came to our world to proclaim. Men and women are to have opportunity to gain a knowledge of present truth, an opportunity to know that Christ is their Saviour, that "God so loved the world, that He gave His only-begotten Son, that whosoever believeth in Him should not perish, but have everlasting life." John 3:16. . . .

Let those who have fitted themselves to engage in medical missionary work in foreign countries go to the places that they expect to make their field of labor, and begin work right among the people, learning the language as they work. Very soon they will find that they can teach the simple truths of God's word.

There is in this country a great, unworked field. The colored race, numbering thousands upon thousands, appeals to the consideration and sympathy of every true, practical believer in Christ. These people do not live in a foreign country, and they do not bow down to idols of wood and stone. They live among us, and again and again, through the testimonies of His Spirit, God has called our attention to them, telling us that here are human beings neglected.

This broad field lies before us unworked, calling for the light that God has given us in trust.

Clear New Ground

Let forces be set at work to clear new ground, to establish new, living interests wherever an opening can be found. Let men learn how to make brief, earnest prayers. Let them learn to speak of the world's Redeemer, to lift up the Man of Calvary higher and still higher. Transplant trees out of your thickly planted nursery. God is not glorified in having such immense advantages centered in one place. We need wise nurserymen who will transplant trees to different localities and give them advantages whereby they may grow. It is a positive duty to go into regions beyond. Rally workers who possess true missionary zeal and let them go forth to diffuse light and knowledge far and near. Let them take the living principles of health reform into communities that to a large degree are ignorant of what they should do. Let men and women teach these principles to classes that cannot have the advantages of the large sanitarium at Battle Creek. It is a fact that the truth of heaven has come to the notice of thousands through the influence of the sanitarium; yet there is a work to be done that has been neglected. We are encouraged as we see the work that is being done in Chicago and in a few other places. But the large responsibility that is now centered in Battle Creek should have been distributed years ago.—*Health, Philanthropic, and Medical Missionary Work*, pages 49, 50 (1895).

Reference for further study: *Testimonies for the Church*, vol. 6, pp. 273-280, "Our Duty to the World."

Christ Our Example

Christ's earthly life, so full of toil and sacrifice, was cheered by the thought that He would not have all His travail for nought. By giving His life for the life of men, He would win the world back to its loyalty. Although the baptism of blood must first be received, although the sins of the world were to weigh upon His innocent soul, yet for the joy that was set before Him He chose to endure the cross and despised the shame.

Study Christ's definition of a true missionary, "Whosoever will come after Me, let him deny himself, and take up his cross, and follow Me." Mark 8:34. Following Christ, as spoken of in these words, is not a pretense, a farce. Jesus expects His disciples to follow closely in His footsteps, enduring what He endured, suffering what He suffered, overcoming as He overcame. He is anxiously waiting to see His professed followers revealing the spirit of self-sacrifice.

Those who receive Christ as a personal Saviour, choosing to be partakers of His suffering, to live His life of self-denial, to endure shame for His sake, will understand what it means to be a genuine medical missionary.

Obedience and Understanding

When all our medical missionaries live the new life in Christ, when they take His word as their guide, they will have a much clearer understanding of what constitutes genuine medical missionary work. This work will have a deeper meaning to them when they render implicit obedience to the law engraven on tables of stone by the finger of God, including the Sabbath commandment, concerning which Christ Himself spoke through Moses to the children of Israel, saying:

Testimonies for the Church, vol. 8, pp. 209, 210 (1903).

"Speak thou also unto the children of Israel, saying, Verily My Sabbaths ye shall keep: for it is a sign between Me and you throughout your generations; that ye may know that I am the Lord that doth sanctify you." "The children of Israel shall keep the Sabbath, to observe the Sabbath throughout their generations, for a perpetual covenant. It is a sign between Me and the children of Israel forever." Exodus 31:13, 16, 17.

Let us diligently study God's word, that we may proclaim with power the message that is to be given in these last days. Many of those upon whom the light of the Saviour's self-sacrificing life is shining refuse to live a life in accordance with His will. They are not willing to live a life of sacrifice for the good of others. They desire to exalt themselves. To such ones truth and righteousness have lost their meaning, and their un-Christlike influence leads many to turn away from the Saviour. God calls for true, steadfast workers, whose lives will counteract the influence of those who are working against Him.

Follow Your Leader

To every medical missionary worker I am instructed to say, Follow your Leader. He is the Way, the Truth, and the Life. He is your example. Upon all medical missionary workers rests the responsibility of keeping in view Christ's life of unselfish service. They are to keep their eyes fixed on Jesus, the Author and Finisher of their faith. He is the source of all light, the fountain of all blessing.

A United Work

Again and again I have been instructed that the medical missionary work is to bear the same relation to the work of the third angel's message that the arm and hand bear to the body. Under the direction of the divine Head they are to work unitedly in preparing the way for the coming of Christ. The right arm of the body of truth is to be constantly active, constantly at work, and God will strengthen it. But it is not to be made the body. At the same time the body is not to say to the arm, "I have no need of thee." The body has need of the arm in order to do active, aggressive work. Both have their appointed work, and each will suffer great loss if worked independently of the other.

The work of preaching the third angel's message has not been regarded by some as God designs it should be. It has been treated as an inferior work, while it should occupy an important place among the human agencies in the salvation of man. The minds of men must be called to the Scriptures as the most effective agency in the salvation of souls, and the ministry of the word is the great educational force to produce this result. Those who disparage the ministry and try to conduct the medical missionary work independently are trying to separate the arm from the body. What would be the result, should they succeed? We should see hands and arms flying about, dispensing means without the direction of the head. The work would become disproportionate and unbalanced. That which God designed should be the hand and arm would take the place of the whole body, and the ministry would be belittled or altogether ignored. This would unsettle minds and bring confusion, and many portions of the Lord's vineyard would be left unworked.

Testimonies for the Church, vol. 6, pp. 288-293 (1904).

The medical missionary work should be a part of the work of every church in our land. Disconnected from the church, it would soon become a strange medley of disorganized atoms. It would consume, but not produce. Instead of acting as God's helping hand to forward His truth, it would sap the life and force from the church and weaken the message. Conducted independently, it would not only consume talent and means needed in other lines, but in the very work of helping the helpless apart from the ministry of the word, it would place men where they would scoff at Bible truth.

Strength in United Effort

The gospel ministry is needed to give permanence and stability to the medical missionary work; and the ministry needs the medical missionary work to demonstrate the practical working of the gospel. Neither part of the work is complete without the other.

The message of the soon coming of the Saviour must be given in all parts of the world, and a solemn dignity should characterize it in every branch. A large vineyard is to be worked, and the wise husbandman will work it so that every part will produce fruit. If in the medical missionary work the living principles of truth are kept pure, uncontaminated by anything that would dim their luster, the Lord will preside over the work. If those who bear the heavy burdens will stand true and steadfast to the principles of truth, the Lord will uphold and sustain them.

The union that should exist between the medical missionary work and the ministry is clearly set forth in the fifty-eighth chapter of Isaiah. There is wisdom and blessing for those who will engage in the work as here presented. This chapter is explicit, and there is in it enough to enlighten anyone who wishes to do the will of God. It presents abundant opportunity to minister to suffering humanity, and at the same time to be an instrument in God's hands of bringing the light of truth before a perishing world. If the work of the third angel's message is carried on in right lines, the ministry will not be given an inferior place, nor will the poor and sick be neglected. In His word God has united these two lines of work, and no man should divorce them.

Weakness in Separation

There may be and there is danger of losing sight of the great principles of truth when doing the work for the poor that it is right to do, but we are ever to bear in mind that in carrying forward this work, the spiritual necessities of the soul are to be kept prominent. In our efforts to relieve temporal necessities, we are in danger of separating from the last gospel message its leading and most urgent features. As it has been carried on in some places, the medical missionary work has absorbed talent and means that belong to other lines of the work, and the effort in lines more directly spiritual has been neglected. Because of the ever-increasing opportunities for ministering to the temporal needs of all classes, there is danger that this work will eclipse the message that God has given us to bear in every city—the proclamation of the soon coming of Christ, the necessity of obedience to the commandments of God and the testimony of Jesus. This message is the burden of our work. It is to be proclaimed with a loud cry and is to go to the whole world. In both home and foreign fields the presentation of health principles must be united with it, but not be independent of it or in any way take its place; neither should this work absorb so much attention as to belittle other branches.

The Lord has instructed us to consider the work in all its bearings, that it may have a proportionate, symmetrical, well-balanced development.

The truth for this time embraces the whole gospel. Rightly presented, it will work in man the very changes that will make evident the power of God's grace upon the heart. It will do a complete work and develop a complete man. Then let no line be drawn between the genuine medical missionary work and the gospel ministry. Let these two blend in giving the invitation, "Come, for all things are now ready." Let them be joined in an inseparable union, even as the arm is joined to the body.

Consider the Cause as a Whole

The Lord has need of all kinds of skillful workmen. "He gave some, apostles; and some, prophets; and some, evangelists; and some, pastors and teachers; for the perfecting of the saints, for the work of the ministry, for the edifying of the body of Christ: till we all come in the unity of the faith, and of the knowledge of the Son of God, unto a perfect man, unto the measure of the stature of the fullness of Christ." Ephesians 4:11-13.

Every child of God should have sanctified judgment to consider the cause as a whole and the relation of each part to every other part, that none may lack. The field is large, and there is a great work of reform to be carried forward, not in one or two lines, but in every line. The medical missionary work is a part of this work of reform, but it should never become the means of separating the workers in the ministry from their field of labor. The education of students in medical missionary lines is not complete unless they are trained to work in connection with the church and the ministry, and the usefulness of those who are preparing for the ministry would be greatly increased if they would become intelligent on the great and important subject of health. The influence of the Holy Spirit is needed that the work may be properly balanced, and that it may move forward solidly in every line.

"Press Together"

The Lord's work is one, and His people are to be one. He has not directed that any one feature of the message should be carried on independently or become all-absorbing. In all His labors He united the medical missionary work with the ministry of the word. He sent out the twelve apostles, and afterward the Seventy, to preach the gospel to the people, and He gave them power also to heal the sick and to cast out devils in His name. Thus should the Lord's messengers enter His work today. Today the message comes to us: "As My Father hath sent Me, even so send I you. And when He had said this, He breathed on them, and saith unto them, Receive ye the Holy Ghost." John 20:21, 22.

Satan will invent every possible scheme to separate those whom God is seeking to make one. But we must not be misled by his devices. If the medical missionary work is carried on as a part of the gospel, worldlings will see the good that is being done; they will be convicted of its genuineness, and will give it their support.

We are nearing the end of this earth's history, and God calls upon all to lift the standard bearing the inscription, "Here are they that keep the commandments of God, and the faith of Jesus." He calls upon His people to work in perfect harmony. He calls upon those engaged in our medical work to unite with the ministry; He calls upon the ministry to co-operate with the medical missionary workers; and He calls upon the church to take up their appointed duty, holding up the standard of true reform in their own territory, leaving the trained and experienced workers to press on into new fields. No word is to be spoken to discourage any, for this grieves the heart of Christ and greatly pleases the adversary. All need to be baptized with the Holy Spirit; all should refrain from censuring and disparaging remarks and draw near to Christ, that they may appreciate the heavy responsibilities which the co-workers with Him are carrying. "Press together; press together," are the words of our divine Instructor. Unity is strength; disunion is weakness and defeat.

Be Guarded

In our work for the poor and unfortunate, we shall need to be guarded, lest we gather responsibilities which we shall not be able to carry. Before adopting plans and methods that require a large outlay of means, we are to consider whether they bear the divine signature. God does not sanction the pushing forward of one line of work without regard to other lines. He designs that the medical missionary work shall prepare the way for the presentation of the saving truth for this time—the proclamation of the third angel's message. If this design is met, the message will not be eclipsed nor its progress hindered.

It is not numerous institutions, large buildings, or great display that God requires, but the harmonious action of a peculiar people, a people chosen by God and precious. Every man is to stand in his lot and place, thinking, speaking, and acting in harmony with the Spirit of God. Then, and not till then, will the work be a complete, symmetrical whole.

Words of Caution to a Leading Physician

Melbourne, Australia, February 3, 1898.

My dear Brother:

Special light has been given me that you are in danger of losing sight of the work for this time. You are erecting barriers to separate your work and those you are educating from the church. This must not be. Those who are receiving instruction in medical missionary lines should be led to realize that their education is to fit them to do better work in connection with the ministers of God. You are to remember, my brother, that the Lord has a people upon the earth whom He respects. But your words, and the way in which they are often spoken, create unbelief in the position that we occupy as a people. You are in danger of failing to hold fast the faith once delivered to the saints, of making shipwreck of your faith. The words were spoken: "A very small leak will sink a ship. One defective link makes a chain worthless."

Educate Medical Missionaries

Remember, my brother, that medical missionary work is not to take men from the ministry, but is to place men in the field, better qualified to minister because of their knowledge of medical missionary work. Young men should receive an education in medical missionary lines and should then go forth to connect with the ministers. They should not be influenced to give themselves exclusively to the work of rescuing the fallen and degraded. That work is found everywhere, and is to be combined with the work of preparing a people to make Bible truth their defense against the sophistries of worldlings and

Testimonies for the Church, vol. 8, pp. 158-162 (1898).

of the fallen church. The third angel is to go forth with great power. Let none ignore this work or treat it as of little importance. The truth is to be proclaimed to the world, that men and women may see the light.

Our Work for Today

What saith the Lord in the fifty-eighth chapter of Isaiah? The whole chapter is of the highest importance. "Is not this the fast that I have chosen?" God asks, "to loose the bands of wickedness, to undo the heavy burdens, and to let the oppressed go free, and that ye break every yoke? Is it not to deal thy bread to the hungry, and that thou bring the poor that are cast out to thy house? when thou seest the naked, that thou cover him; and that thou hide not thyself from thine own flesh? Then shall thy light break forth as the morning, and thine health shall spring forth speedily: and thy righteousness shall go before thee; the glory of the Lord shall be thy rearward. Then shalt thou call, and the Lord shall answer; thou shalt cry, and He shall say, Here I am."

"If thou turn away thy foot from the Sabbath, from doing thy pleasure on My holy day; and call the Sabbath a delight, the holy of the Lord, honorable; and shalt honor Him, not doing thine own ways, nor finding thine own pleasure, nor speaking thine own words: then shalt thou delight thyself in the Lord; and I will cause thee to ride upon the high places of the earth, and feed thee with the heritage of Jacob thy father: for the mouth of the Lord hath spoken it." Isaiah 58:6-9, 13, 14.

This is our work. The light that we have upon the third angel's message is the true light. The mark of the beast is exactly what it has been proclaimed to be. Not all in regard to this matter is yet understood, and will not be understood until the unrolling of the scroll; but a most solemn work is to be accomplished in our world. The Lord's command to His servants is, "Cry aloud, spare not, lift up thy voice like a trumpet, and show My people their transgression, and the house of Jacob their sins." Isaiah 58:1. A message that will arouse the churches is to be proclaimed. Every effort is to be made to give the light, not only to our people, but to the world. I have been instructed that the prophecies of Daniel and the Revelation should be printed in small books, with the necessary explanations, and should be sent all over the world. Our own people need to have the light placed before them in clearer lines.

No Change in God's Cause

There is to be no change in the general features of God's cause. It is to stand out as clear and distinct as prophecy has made it. We are to enter into no confederacy with the world, supposing that by so doing we could accomplish more. My brother, if you stand in the way to hinder the advancement of the work on the lines that God has appointed, you will greatly displease Him. The warning message is to be given, and after you have faithfully accomplished your part of the work, you are not to hinder others of the Lord's servants from going forth to do the work that they should do. Laboring for the degraded and fallen is not to be made the principal and all-important line. This work is to be combined with the work of instructing the churches. Our people are to be taught how to help the needy and the outcast.

No line of our faith that has made us what we are is to be weakened. We have the old landmarks of truth, experience, and duty, and we are to stand firm in defense of our principles, in full view of the world. With hearts filled with interest and solicitude, we are to give the invitation to those in the highways and the byways. Medical missionary work is to be done. But this is only one part of the work that is to be accomplished, and it is not to be made all and in all. It is to be to the work of God as the hand is to the body. There may be unworthy ones connected with the ministry, yet no one can ignore the ministry without ignoring God.

My brother, you are represented to me as in danger of standing apart from our people, feeling that you are a complete whole. But if you bind yourself up with those of your own mind, apart from the church, which is Christ's body, you will make a confederacy that will be broken to pieces, for no union can stand but that which God has framed. Those who are receiving an education in medical lines hear insinuations from time to time that disparage the church and the ministry. These insinuations are seeds that will spring up and bear fruit. The students might better be educated to realize that the church of Christ on earth is to be respected. They need a clear knowledge of the reasons of our faith. This knowledge they must have in order to serve God acceptably. Line upon line, precept upon precept, they must receive the Bible evidence of the truth as it is in Jesus.

Do not, I beg of you, instill into the minds of the students ideas that will cause them to lose confidence in God's appointed ministers. But this you are most certainly doing, whether you are aware of it or not. In His providence the Lord has placed you in a position where you may do a good work for Him in connection with the gospel ministry, bringing the truth before many who otherwise would not become acquainted with it. Temptations will come to you to think that in order to carry forward the medical missionary work you must stand aloof from church organization or church discipline. To stand thus would place you on an unsound footing. The work done for those who come to you for instruction is not complete unless they are educated to work in connection with the church.

The medical missionary work is not to be made all and in all. In this point you are carrying things to extremes. There is a large work to be done. Publications teaching the truth are to be circulated everywhere. Medical students should not be encouraged to circulate only the books treating on health reform. Be careful that you are not found working out your own plans, to the disregard of God's plans.

Rebellion Against Health Reform

There has been a war in the hearts of some ever since the health reform was first introduced. They have felt the same rebellion as did the children of Israel when their appetites were restricted on their journey from Egypt to Canaan. Professed followers of Christ who have all their lives consulted their own pleasure and their own interests, their own ease, and their own appetites are not prepared to change their course of action and live for the glory of God, imitating the self-sacrificing life of their unerring Pattern. A perfect example has been given for Christians to imitate. The words and works of Christ's followers are the channel through which the pure principles of truth and holiness are conveyed to the world. His followers are the salt of the earth, the light of the world.— *Testimonies for the Church*, vol. 2, p. 394 (1870).

Not a Separate Work

In the work of the gospel the Lord uses different instrumentalities, and nothing is to be allowed to separate these instrumentalities. Never should a sanitarium be established as an enterprise independent of the church. Our physicians are to unite with the work of the ministers of the gospel. Through their labors souls are to be saved, that the name of God may be magnified.

Medical missionary work is in no case to be divorced from the gospel ministry. The Lord has specified that the two shall be as closely connected as the arm is with the body. Without this union neither part of the work is complete. The medical missionary work is the gospel in illustration.

But God did not design that the medical missionary work should eclipse the work of the third angel's message. The arm is not to become the body. The third angel's message is the gospel message for these last days, and in no case is it to be overshadowed by other interests and made to appear an unessential consideration. When in our institutions anything is placed above the third angel's message, the gospel is not there the great leading power.

The cross is the center of all religious institutions. These institutions are to be under the control of the Spirit of God; in no institution is any one man to be the sole head. The divine mind has men for every place.

Through the power of the Holy Spirit every work of God's appointment is to be elevated and ennobled and made to witness for the Lord. Man must place himself under the control of the eternal mind, whose dictates he is to obey in every particular.

Testimonies for the Church, vol. 6, pp. 240-242 (1900).

Let us seek to understand our privilege of walking and working with God. The gospel, though it contains God's expressed will, is of no value to men, high or low, rich or poor, unless they place themselves in subjection to God. He who bears to his fellow men the remedy for sin must himself first be moved by the Spirit of God. He must not ply the oars unless he is under divine direction. He cannot work effectually, he cannot carry out the will of God in harmony with the divine mind, unless he finds out, not from human sources, but from infinite wisdom, that God is pleased with his plans.

God's benevolent design embraces every branch of His work. The law of reciprocal dependence and influence is to be recognized and obeyed. "None of us liveth to himself." The enemy has used the chain of dependence to draw men together. They have united to destroy God's image in man, to counterwork the gospel by perverting its principles. They are represented in God's word as being bound in bundles to be burned. Satan is uniting his forces for perdition. The unity of God's chosen people has been terribly shaken. God presents a remedy. This remedy is not one influence among many influences, and on the same level with them; it is an influence above all influences upon the face of the earth, corrective, uplifting, and ennobling. Those who work in the gospel should be elevated and sanctified; for they are dealing with God's great principles. Yoked up with Christ, they are laborers together with God. Thus the Lord desires to bind His followers together, that they may be a power for good, each acting his part, yet all cherishing the sacred principle of dependence on the Head.

The Medical Missionary's Example

In the days of Christ there were no sanitariums in the Holy Land. But wherever the Great Physician went, He carried with Him the healing efficacy that was a cure for every disease, spiritual and physical. This He imparted to those who were under the afflicting power of the enemy. In every city, every town, every village through which He passed, with the solicitude of a loving father He laid His hands upon the afflicted ones, making them whole and speaking words of tenderest sympathy and compassion. How precious to them were His words! From Him flowed a stream of healing power which made the sick whole. He healed men and women with unhesitating willingness and with hearty joyfulness, for He was glad to be able to restore suffering ones to health.

Anxiety of His Family

The Mighty Healer worked so incessantly, so intensely,—and often without food,—that some of His friends feared He could not much longer endure the constant strain. His brothers heard of this, and also of the charge brought by the Pharisees that He cast out devils through the power of Satan. They felt keenly the reproach that came upon them through their relation to Jesus. They decided that He must be persuaded or constrained to cease His manner of labor, and they induced Mary to unite with them, thinking that through His love for her they might prevail upon Him to be more prudent.

Jesus was teaching the people when His disciples brought the message that His mother and His brothers were without and desired to see Him. He knew what

---

Review and Herald, June 9, 1904.

was in their hearts, and "He answered and said unto him that told Him, Who is My mother? and who are My brethren? And He stretched forth His hand toward His disciples, and said, Behold My mother and My brethren! For whosoever shall do the will of My Father which is in heaven, the same is My brother, and sister, and mother." Matthew 12:48-50.

The enmity kindled in the human heart against the gospel was keenly felt by the Son of God, and it was most painful to Him in His home; for His own heart was full of kindness and love, and He appreciated tender regard in the family relation. But with their short measuring line His brothers could not fathom the mission that He came to fulfill and therefore could not sympathize with Him in His trials.

Enmity of the Pharisees

Some of those whom Christ healed He charged to tell no man. He knew that the more the Pharisees and Sadducees and rulers heard of His miracles, the more they would try to hedge up His way. But notwithstanding His precautions, "so much the more went there a fame abroad of Him: and great multitudes came together to hear, and to be healed by Him of their infirmities." Luke 5:15. Again and again He was followed by the priests, who expressed their violent sentiments against Him in order to stir up the enmity of the people. But when He could no longer safely remain in one place He went to another.

In doing medical missionary work we shall meet the same opposition that Christ met. He declares: "Ye shall be hated of all men for My name's sake: but he that endureth to the end shall be saved. But when they persecute you in this city, flee ye into another: for verily I say unto you, Ye shall not have gone over the cities of Israel, till the Son of man be come." Matthew 10:22, 23.

The life of Christ and His ministry to the afflicted are inseparably connected. From the light that has been given me, I know that an intimate relationship should ever exist between the medical missionary work and the gospel ministry. They are bound together in sacred union as one work, and are never to be divorced. The principles of heaven are to be adopted and practiced by those who claim to walk in the Saviour's footsteps. By His example He has shown us that medical missionary work is not to take the place of the preaching of the gospel, but is to be bound up with it. Christ gave a perfect representation of true godliness by combining the work of a physician and a minister, ministering to the needs of both body and soul, healing physical disease, and then speaking words that brought peace to the troubled heart. . . .

Point to Jesus

We should ever remember that the efficiency of the medical missionary work is in pointing sin-sick men and women to the Man of Calvary, who taketh away the sin of the world. By beholding Him they will be changed into His likeness. Our object in establishing sanitariums is to encourage the sick and suffering to look to Jesus and live. Let the workers in our medical institutions keep Christ, the Great Physician, constantly before those to whom disease of body and soul has brought discouragement. Point them to the One who can heal both physical and spiritual diseases. Tell them of the One who is touched with the feeling of their infirmities. Encourage them to place themselves in the care of Him who gave His life to make it possible for them to have life eternal. Keep their minds fixed upon the One altogether lovely, the chiefest among ten thousand. Talk of His love; tell of His power to save.

The Lord desires every worker to do his best. Those who have not had special training in one of our medical institutions may think that they can do very little; but, my dear fellow workers, remember that in the parable of the talents, Christ did not represent all the servants as receiving the same number. To one servant was given five talents; to another, two; and to still another, one. If you have but one talent, use it wisely, increasing it by putting it out to the exchangers. Some cannot do as much as others, but everyone is to do all he can to roll back the wave of disease and distress that is sweeping over our world. Come up to the help of the Lord, against the mighty powers of darkness. God desires every one of His children to have intelligence and knowledge, so that with unmistakable clearness and power His glory shall be revealed in our world. . . .

Christ has empowered His church to do the same work that He did during His ministry. Today He is the same compassionate physician that He was while on this earth. We should let the afflicted understand that in Him there is healing balm for every disease, restoring power for every infirmity.

Reference for further study: *The Ministry of Healing*, pages 17-50, "The True Medical Missionary."

The Gospel in Practice

When health reform was first brought to our notice, about thirty-five years ago, the light presented to me was contained in this scripture: "The Spirit of the Lord God is upon Me; because the Lord hath anointed Me to preach good tidings unto the meek; He hath sent Me to bind up the brokenhearted, to proclaim liberty to the captives, and the opening of the prison to them that are bound; to proclaim the acceptable year of the Lord, and the day of vengeance of our God; to comfort all that mourn; to appoint unto them that mourn in Zion, to give unto them beauty for ashes, the oil of joy for mourning, the garment of praise for the spirit of heaviness; that they might be called trees of righteousness, the planting of the Lord, that He might be glorified. And they shall build the old wastes, they shall raise up the former desolations, and they shall repair the waste cities, the desolations of many generations." Isaiah 61:1-4.

In the light given me so long ago, I was shown that our own people, those who claimed to believe the present truth, should do this work. How were they to do it? In accordance with the directions Christ gave His twelve disciples when He called them together and sent them forth to preach the gospel.

"When He had called unto Him His twelve disciples, He gave them power against unclean spirits, to cast them out, and to heal all manner of sickness and all manner of disease." "These Twelve Jesus sent forth, and commanded them, saying, Go not into the way of the Gentiles, and into any city of the Samaritans enter ye not: but go rather to the lost sheep of the house of Israel. And as ye go, preach, saying, The kingdom of heaven is at

General Conference Bulletin, 1901, pages 202-204 (1901).

(530)

hand. Heal the sick, cleanse the lepers, raise the dead, cast out devils: freely ye have received, freely give." Matthew 10:1, 5-8.

Reforms Called For

In the light given me so long ago, I was shown that intemperance would prevail in the world to an alarming extent and that every one of the people of God must take an elevated stand in regard to reformation in habits and practices. At that time I was eating meat two or three times a day, and I was fainting away two or three times a day. The Lord presented a general plan before me. I was shown that God would give to His commandment-keeping people a reform diet, and that as they received this, their disease and suffering would be greatly lessened. I was shown that this work would progress.

A Sanitarium Needed

Then, in after years, the light was given that we should have a sanitarium, a health institution, which was to be established right among us. This was the means God was to use in bringing His people to a right understanding in regard to health reform. It was also to be the means by which we were to gain access to those not of our faith. We were to have an institution where the sick could be relieved of suffering, and that without drug medication. God declared that He Himself would go before His people in this work.

Well, the work has been steadily increasing. The way was opened for our churches to take hold of it. I proclaimed health reform everywhere I went. At our camp meetings I spoke on Sunday afternoons, and I proclaimed the message of temperance in eating, drinking, and dressing. This was the message I bore for years before I left for Australia.

But there were those who did not come up to the light God had given. There were those in attendance at our camp meetings who ate and drank improperly. Their diet was not in harmony with the light God had given, and it was impossible for them to appreciate the truth in its sacred, holy bearing.

All Classes to Be Benefited

So the light has been gradually coming in. Over and over again instruction was given that our health institutions were to reach all classes of people. The gospel of Jesus Christ includes the work of helping the sick. When I heard that Dr. Kellogg had taken up the medical missionary work, I encouraged him with heart and soul, because I knew that only by this work can the prejudice which exists in the world against our faith be broken down.

In Australia we have tried to do all we could in this line. We located in Cooranbong, and there, where the people have to send twenty-five miles for a doctor, and pay him twenty-five dollars a visit, we helped the sick and suffering all we could. Seeing that we understood something of disease, the people brought their sick to us, and we cared for them. Thus we entirely broke down the prejudice in that place. . . .

Medical missionary work is the pioneer work. It is to be connected with the gospel ministry. It is the gospel in practice, the gospel practically carried out. I have been made so sorry to see that our people have not taken hold of this work as they should. . . .

All heaven is interested in the work of relieving suffering humanity. Satan is exerting all his powers to obtain control over the souls and bodies of men. He is trying to bind them to the wheels of his chariot. My heart is made sad as I look at our churches, which ought to be connected in heart and soul and practice with the medical missionary work....

Ministers to Work on the Gospel Plan

I wish to tell you that soon there will be no work done in ministerial lines but medical missionary work. The work of a minister is to minister. Our ministers are to work on the gospel plan of ministering....

You will never be ministers after the gospel order till you show a decided interest in medical missionary work, the gospel of healing and blessing and strengthening. Come up to the help of the Lord, to the help of the Lord against the mighty powers of darkness, that it be not said of you, "Curse ye Meroz, . . . curse ye bitterly the inhabitants thereof; because they came not to the help of the Lord." Judges 5:23....

It is because of the directions I have received from the Lord that I have the courage to stand among you and speak as I do, notwithstanding the way in which you may look at the medical missionary work. I wish to say that the medical missionary work is God's work. The Lord wants every one of His ministers to come into line. Take hold of the medical missionary work, and it will give you access to the people. Their hearts will be touched as you minister to their necessities. As you relieve their sufferings, you will find opportunity to speak to them of the love of Jesus....

God will help those who love the truth, who give themselves, heart and mind and strength, to Him. God will work mightily with His ministers when their hearts are filled with love for the poor lost sheep of the house of Israel. Hunt up the backsliders, those who once knew what religion was, and give them the message of mercy.

The story of Christ's love will touch a chord in their hearts. Christ draws human beings to Himself with the cord which God has let down from heaven to save the race. The love of Christ can be measured only when this cord is measured. . . .

Medical missionary work, ministering to the sick and suffering, cannot be separated from the gospel. God help those whose attention has been aroused on this subject to have the mind of Christ, the sympathy of Christ. God help you to remember that Christ was a worker, that He went from place to place healing the sick. If we were as closely connected with Christ as were His disciples, God could work through us to heal many who are suffering.

In Faith and Humility

The gospel of Christ is to be lived, practiced in the daily life. The servants of God are to be cleansed from all coldness, all selfishness. Simplicity, meekness, lowliness, are of great value in the work of God. Try to unite the workers in confidence and love. If you cannot do this, be right yourselves, and leave the rest with God. Labor in faith and prayer. Select Christian youth and train them to be, not workers with hearts like iron, but workers who are willing to harmonize.

I pray that the Lord will change the hearts of those who, unless they receive more grace, will enter into temptation. I pray that He will soften and subdue every heart. We need to live in close fellowship with God, that we may love one another as Christ has loved us. It is by this that the world is to know that we are His disciples.— *Testimonies for the Church,* vol. 9, pp. 218, 219 (1909).

Reference for further study: *The Ministry of Healing,* pages 139-160, "Teaching and Healing."

To Gain an Entrance

I am intensely interested in the education of medical students as missionaries. This is the very means of introducing the truth where otherwise it would not find an entrance.

I can see in the Lord's providence that the medical missionary work is to be a great entering wedge, whereby the diseased soul may be reached.

Oh, what a field of usefulness is opened before the medical missionary! Jesus Christ was in every sense of the word a missionary of the highest type, and combined with His missionary work that of the Great Physician, healing all manner of diseases. Many in Christ's day refused to be convinced of their lost condition. When Christ was in their midst as a mighty healer of bodily woe as well as the maladies of the sin-sick soul, some would not come unto Him that they might have life. They refused to be illuminated. So it will be in our day. Some will not be healed of their soul diseases.

Every physician can and ought to be a Christian, and if so, he bears with him a cure for the soul as well as the body. He is doing the work of an apostle as well as of a physician. How much need there is of the preciousness of pure and undefiled religion, that the spiritual teacher may be administering to the soul necessities while relieving the distress of the body! How refreshing it is to the suffering, tempest-tossed soul to hear the words of hope, words from God spoken to the suffering one, to hear the prayers offered in his behalf! How essential that the living missionary should understand the diseases which afflict the human body, to combine the physician, educated to care for diseased bodies, with the faithful,

Medical Missionary Work (1893).

conscientious shepherd of the flock, to give sacredness and double efficiency to the service!

The Lord, in His great goodness and matchless love, has been urging upon His human instrumentalities that missionaries are not really complete in their education unless they have a knowledge of how to treat the sick and suffering. If this had been felt as an important branch of education in the missionary line of labor, many who have lost their lives might have lived. Had they understood how to treat the ailments of the body, and how to study from cause to effect, they could, through their intelligent knowledge of the human body and how to treat its maladies, have reached many darkened minds that otherwise they could not approach.

The Great Physician With Every Worker

The great Physician in Chief is at the side of every true, earnest, God-fearing practitioner who works with his acquired knowledge to relieve the sufferings of the human body. He, the Chief of physicians, is ready to dispense the balm of Gilead. He will hear the prayers offered by the physician and the missionary, if His name will be glorified thereby; and the life of the suffering patient will be prolonged. God is over all. He is the true Head of the missionary of the medical profession, and blessed indeed shall be that physician who has connected himself with the Chief Physician, who has learned from Him not only to treat the suffering bodies, but to watch for souls, to understand how to apply the prescription, and as an undershepherd use the balm of Gilead to heal the bruises that sin has made upon the souls as well as upon the bodies of suffering humanity under the serpent's sting. Oh, how essential that the physician be one divested of selfishness, one who has a correct knowledge of the atonement made by Jesus Christ, so that he can uplift Jesus to the despairing soul, one who holds communion with God! What a treasure he possesses in his knowledge of the treatment of the diseases of the body, and also the knowledge of the plan of salvation. Resting in Jesus as his personal Saviour, he can lead others to hopefulness, to saving faith, to rest and peace, and a new life in Jesus Christ. . . .

The Lord sanctions the efforts of the consecrated worker, the true shepherd. He may have little time to preach discourses, but he can act sermons which will be far more powerful. The truth expressed in living, unselfish deeds is the strongest argument for Christianity. The relieving of the sick, the helping of the distressed, is working in Christ's lines and demonstrates most powerful gospel truths representing Christ's mission and work upon earth. The knowledge of the art of relieving suffering humanity is the opening of doors without number, where the truth can find a lodgment in the heart, and souls be saved unto life—eternal life. Even the most hardhearted and apparently sin-encased souls may be approached in this way and understand something of the mystery of godliness and become so charmed that they will not rest until they have a knowledge of Jesus Christ and His saving grace. . . .

Let there be a company formed somewhat after the order of the Christian Endeavor Society, and see what can be done by each accountable human agent in watching and improving opportunities to do work for the Master. He has a vineyard in which everyone can perform good work. Suffering humanity needs help everywhere.

Medical Missionary Evangelists

Young men who have a practical knowledge of how to treat the sick are now to be sent out to do gospel medical missionary work, in connection with more experienced gospel workers. If these young men will give themselves to the study of the word, they will become successful evangelists. The ministers with whom these young men labor are to give them the same opportunity to learn that Elijah gave Elisha. They are to show them how to teach the truth to others. Where it is possible, these young men should visit the hospitals, and in some cases they may connect with them for a while, laboring disinterestedly.

The purest example of unselfishness is now to be shown by our medical missionary workers. With the knowledge and experience gained by practical work, they are to go out to give treatments to the sick. As they go from house to house, they will find access to many hearts. Many will be reached who otherwise would never have heard the gospel message.

Encouragement to Young Workers

Much good can be done by those who do not hold diplomas as fully accredited physicians. Some are to be prepared to work as competent physicians. Many, working under the direction of such ones, can do acceptable work without spending so long a time in study as it has been thought necessary to spend in the past.

Many will go out to labor for the Master who have not been able to take a regular course of study in school. God will help these workers. They will obtain knowledge from the higher school and will be fitted to take their

Review and Herald, Nov. 19, 1903.

position in the rank and file of workers as nurses. The great Medical Missionary sees every effort that is made to find access to souls by presenting the principles of health reform.

Decided changes are taking place in our world. The Lord has declared that He will turn and overturn. Humble men, who hitherto have been in obscurity, must now be given opportunity to become workers.

To those who go out to do medical missionary work, I would say, Serve the Lord Jesus Christ with sanctified understanding, in connection with the ministers of the gospel and the Great Teacher. He who has given you your commission will give you skill and understanding as you consecrate yourselves to His service, engaging diligently in labor and study, doing your best to bring relief to the sick and suffering.

To those who are tired of a life of sinfulness, but who know not where to turn to obtain relief, present the compassionate Saviour, full of love and tenderness, longing to receive those who come to Him with broken hearts and contrite spirits. Take them by the hand, lift them up, speak to them words of hope and courage. Help them to grasp the hand of Him who has said, "Let him take hold of My strength, that he may make peace with Me; and he shall make peace with Me." Isaiah 27:5.

"Behold," Christ declares, "I come quickly; and My reward is with Me, to give every man according as his work shall be." God calls upon us to voice the words, "Even so, come, Lord Jesus." God will do much more for His people if they will have faith in Him.

18—C.O.H.

Methods and Plans

In all our sanitariums the work done should be of such a character as to win souls to Jesus Christ. We have a wide missionary field in our health institutions, for here people of all countries come to regain their health. The best helpers to have connected with our sanitariums are those men who desire to make the Bible their guide, those who will put forth their mental and moral powers to advance the work in correct ways.

Let the workers in the sanitariums remember that the object of the establishment of these institutions is not alone the relief of suffering and the healing of disease, but also the salvation of souls. Let the spiritual atmosphere of these institutions be such that men and women who are brought to the sanitariums to receive treatment for their bodily ills, shall learn the lesson that their diseased souls need healing.

To preach the gospel means much more than many realize. It is a broad, far-reaching work. Our sanitariums have been presented to me as most efficient means for the promotion of the gospel message.

The work of the true medical missionary is largely a spiritual work. It includes prayer and the laying on of hands; he therefore should be as sacredly set apart for his work as is the minister of the gospel. Those who are selected to act the part of missionary physicians are to be set apart as such. This will strengthen them against the temptations to withdraw from the sanitarium work to engage in private practice. No selfish motives should be allowed to draw the worker from his post of duty. The medical work done in connection with the giving

Medical Missionary Library, No. 5, pp. 14-16 (1906).

of the third angel's message, is to accomplish wonderful results. It is to be a sanctifying, unifying work, corresponding to the work which the great Head of the church sent forth the first disciples to do.

Calling these disciples together, Christ gave them their commission: . . . "And as ye go, preach, saying, The kingdom of heaven is at hand. Heal the sick, cleanse the lepers, raise the dead, cast out devils: freely ye have received, freely give." "Behold, I send you forth as sheep in the midst of wolves: be ye therefore wise as serpents, and harmless as doves." Matthew 10:7, 8, 16.

It is well for us to read this chapter and let its instruction prepare us for our labors. The early disciples were going forth on Christ's errands, under His commission. His spirit was to prepare the way before them. They were to feel that with such a message to give, such blessings to impart, they should receive a welcome in the homes of the people. . . .

Conferences to Employ Medical Missionaries

Through the first disciples a divine gift was proffered to Israel; the faithful evangelist today will do a similar work in every city where our missionaries enter. It is a work which to some extent we have tried to do in connection with some of our sanitariums, but a much wider experience in these lines is to be gained.

Cannot our conference presidents open the way for the students in our schools to engage in this line of labor? Again and again it has been presented to me that "there should be companies organized and educated most thoroughly to work as nurses, as evangelists, as ministers, as canvassers, as gospel students, to perfect a character after the divine similitude." There is a grand work to be done in relieving suffering humanity, and through the labors of students who are receiving an education and training to become efficient medical missionaries the people living in many cities may become acquainted with the truths of the third angel's message. Consecrated leaders and teachers of experience should go out with these young workers at first, giving them instruction how to labor. When favors of food are offered by those who fear and honor God, these favors may be accepted. Thus opportunity will be found for conversation, for explaining the Scriptures, for singing Bible songs and praying with the family. There are many to whom such labor as this would prove a blessing.

And each worker, as he goes forth to this labor, should realize that he is as truly sent of God as were the first disciples. God's eye follows them; His Spirit goes with them. . . .

I am thankful when I think of the advantages enjoyed by the schools that are established near our sanitariums, so that the work of the two educational institutions can blend. The students in these schools, while gaining an education in the knowledge of present truth, can also learn how to be ministers of healing to those whom they go forth to serve.

If ever there was a time when our work should be done under the special direction of the Spirit of God, it is now. Let those who are living at their ease, arouse. Let our sanitariums become what they should be—homes where healing is ministered to sin-sick souls. And this will be done when the workers have a living connection with the Great Healer.

Physicians and Evangelists

Encouraging Words to a Physician

The work you have been doing in the cities is meeting Heaven's approval. What you have done demonstrates that if our physicians and our ministers can work together in the presentation of truth to the people, more can be reached than could be influenced by the minister laboring alone. I trust that your example in this respect may be followed by other physicians.

You need not feel that the Lord has separated you from the sanitarium because you have made more direct efforts to reach the souls in our cities, who need to be converted. You have a burden for this work of presenting the message to the people. Present Christ as the healer of the sin-sick soul. In your work in the field you will gain a broader and more extended influence than if you were confined to an institution.

The acquaintances you make as you attend meetings and present the truth from the physician's standpoint will help to give you an influence, and this line of work will be the means of bringing to our sanitariums a class of people who can be greatly benefited. Arrange your plans so that you can engage in this line of work with freedom, and so that your absence will not hurt the work of the institution.

Present before the people the need of resisting the temptation to indulge appetite. This is where many are failing. Explain how closely body and mind are related and show the need of keeping both in the very best condition. The health talks which you give in the meetings will be one of the best ways of advertising our sanitariums.

A circular letter (1910).

Christ has given us an example. He taught from the Scriptures the gospel truths, and He also healed the afflicted ones who came to Him for relief. He was the greatest physician the world ever knew, and yet He combined with His healing work the imparting of soul-saving truth.

And thus should our physicians labor. They are doing the Lord's work when they labor as evangelists, giving instruction as to how the soul may be healed by the Lord Jesus. Every physician should know how to pray in faith for the sick, as well as to administer the proper treatment. At the same time he should labor as one of God's ministers, to teach repentance and conversion and the salvation of soul and body. Such a combination of labor will broaden his experience and greatly enlarge his influence.

In Touch With the People

One thing I know: the greatest work of our physicians is to get access to the people of the world in the right way. There is a world perishing in sin, and who will take up the work in our cities? The greatest physician is the one who walks in the footsteps of Jesus Christ.

There is a work to be done in all our cities, and those who still work and walk humbly with God, striving daily to be overcomers, will gain precious victories day by day. The work that is done in humility will bear the divine credentials. Let us hide in God. That which I see most clearly is the necessity of men and women's being united in doing the work that needs to be done in our cities. . . . The Lord bears long with men, and He calls earnestly for everyone to repent. Will the ministers, will the physicians, take up this work that has scarcely been touched? May God help us to be faithful and to do the very work that is now most essential.

Now is our time to make decided efforts to awaken the people who have never yet been warned. Much thought and labor is given to the printed page. This is well, but if more efforts were given to sending forth the living missionary to preach the truth, many more souls would be aroused and won to the truth. While Jesus ministers in the true sanctuary above, He is through His Holy Spirit working through His earthly messengers. These agencies will accomplish more than the printed page, if they will go forth in the Spirit and power of Christ. Christ will work through His chosen ministers, filling them with His Spirit, and thus fulfilling to them the assurance, "Lo, I am with you alway, even unto the end of the world." Matthew 28:20.

It is well, in presenting the truth to unbelievers, first to present some subjects upon which they will agree with us. The principles of health and temperance will appeal to their judgment, and we can from these subjects lead them on to understand the binding claims of the fourth commandment. This work our physicians can help in doing. When the people see the value of instruction given regarding healthful living, it gives them confidence to believe that the teachers of these principles have the truth in other lines.

It is the Lord's plan that physicians well versed in Bible truth shall unite with ministers laboring in the cities and aid in giving as a whole the harmonious message of warning that should be given to the world. Some of the very best-qualified men in our institutions should be chosen for this work.

To some it may seem unwise to take men qualified for the position of head physicians and put them to labor in the cities, even though chosen men fill their places in the institutions. But we need to take a broader view of the work and to consider that the Lord is calling for a special line of work to be done in the cities, a work which requires the efforts of men of clear perception, and who, in the power of the Holy Spirit, can present before large congregations the principles of health reform.

The presenting of Bible principles by an intelligent physician will have great weight with many people. There is efficiency and power with one who can combine in his influence the work of a physician and of a gospel minister. His work commends itself to the good judgment of the people.

Practical Hints to Physicians

I am concerned because so many things engage the minds of our physicians which keep them from the work that God would have them do as evangelists. From the light that God has given me, I know that the living preacher who is consecrated and devoted, and knows how to put his trust in God, is greatly needed. We need one hundred workers where now we have one. There is a great work to be done before satanic opposition shall close up the way, and our present opportunities for labor shall be lost. Time is rapidly passing. Our publications are numerous, but the Lord calls for men and women in our churches who have the light to engage in genuine missionary work. Let them in all humility exercise their God-given talents in proclaiming the message that should come to the world at this time.

I hope you will exercise all your capabilities in this work. Present the importance of present truth from the physician's standpoint. The educated physician will find entrance in our cities where other men cannot. Teach the message of health reform. This will have an influence with the people.

The Lord will assuredly guide you if you will seek to do His will, even though it should interfere with some of your desires and plans. As you walk and work in the counsel of God, doors will be opened before you of opportunities for uniting the work of the ministry and that of a physician.

If in the city of Boston and other cities of the East, you and your wife will unite in medical evangelistic work, your usefulness will increase, and there will open before you clear views of duty. In these cities the message of the first angel went with great power in 1842 and 1843, and now the time has come when the message of the third angel is to be proclaimed extensively in the East. There is a grand work before our Eastern sanitariums. The message is to go with power as the work closes up.

Let your words be of a character to exalt the word of God. Live and teach the principles of health reform. Emphasize your belief in the great truths upon which Christian people generally will agree with you. As you advocate the truth of God, you are in every respect to be an example to the believers.

The importance of making our way in the great cities is still kept before me. For many years the Lord has been urging upon us this duty, and yet we see but comparatively little accomplished in our great centers of population. If we do not take up this work in a determined manner, Satan will multiply difficulties which will not be easy to surmount. We are far behind in doing the work that should have been done in these long-neglected cities. The work will now be more difficult than it would have been a few years ago. But if we take up the work in the name of the Lord, barriers will be broken down and decided victories will be ours.

In this work physicians and gospel ministers are needed. We must press our petitions to the Lord and do our best, pressing forward with all the energy possible to make an opening in the large cities. Had we in the past worked after the Lord's plans, many lights would be shining brightly that are going out.

In connection with the presentation of spiritual truths, we should also present what the word of God says upon the questions of health and temperance. In every way possible we must seek to bring souls under the convicting and converting power of God. The believers in our churches need to be aroused to act their part. Let seasons of prayer be appointed, and let us earnestly seek the Lord for an increase of faith and courage. Let ministers and other church members labor for souls as never before. We are not to spend our time merely in repeating over and over the same things to the churches where the truth is well known. Let the church members labor unitedly in their several lines to create an interest. The disciples of Christ are to unite in labor for perishing souls. Let the laborers invite others to unite with them in their efforts, that many may be fired with zeal to work for the Master.

I entreat the church members in every city that they lay hold upon the Lord with determined effort for the baptism of the Holy Spirit. Be assured that Satan is not asleep. Every obstacle possible he will place in the way of those who would advance in this work. Too often these obstacles are regarded as insurmountable. Let everyone now be soundly and truly converted, and then lay hold of the work intelligently and with faith.

Work in the Cities

San Francisco, California, December 12, 1900.

There is a work to be done in California—a work that has been strangely neglected. Let this work be delayed no longer. As doors open for the presentation of truth, let us be ready to enter. Some work has been done in the large city of San Francisco, but as we study the field we see plainly that only a beginning has been made. As soon as possible, well-organized efforts should be put forth in different sections of this city, and also in Oakland. The wickedness of San Francisco is not realized. Our work in this city must broaden and deepen. God sees in it many souls to be saved.

In San Francisco a hygienic restaurant has been opened, also a food store, and treatment rooms. These are doing a good work, but their influence should be greatly extended. Other restaurants similar to the one on Market Street should be opened in San Francisco and in Oakland. Concerning the effort that is now being made in these lines, we can say, Amen and amen. And soon other lines of work that will be a blessing to the people will be established. Medical missionary evangelistic work should be carried forward in a most prudent and thorough manner. The solemn, sacred work of saving souls is to advance in a way that is modest and yet ever elevated.

Where are the working forces? Men and women who are thoroughly converted, men and women of discernment and keen foresight, should act as directors. Good judgment must be exercised in employing persons to do this special work—persons who love God and who walk before Him in all humility, persons who will be effective

Testimonies for the Church, vol. 7, pp. 110-114 (1900).

agencies in God's hand for the accomplishment of the object He has in view—the uplifting and saving of human beings.

Medical missionary evangelists will be able to do excellent pioneer work. The work of the minister should blend fully with that of the medical missionary evangelist. The Christian physician should regard his work as exalted as that of the ministry. He bears a double responsibility, for in him are combined the qualifications of both physician and gospel minister. His is a grand, a sacred, and a very necessary work.

The physician and the minister should realize that they are engaged in the same work. They should labor in perfect harmony. They should counsel together. By their unity they will bear witness that God has sent His only-begotten Son into the world to save all who will believe in Him as their personal Saviour.

Physicians in the Large Cities

Physicians whose professional abilities are above those of the ordinary doctor should engage in the service of God in the large cities. They should seek to reach the higher classes. Something is being done in this line in San Francisco, but much more should be done. Let there be no misconception of the nature and the importance of these enterprises. San Francisco is a large field, and an important portion of the Lord's vineyard.

Medical missionaries who labor in evangelistic lines are doing a work of as high an order as are their ministerial fellow workers. The efforts put forth by these workers are not to be limited to the poorer classes. The higher classes have been strangely neglected. In the higher walks of life will be found many who will respond to the truth, because it is consistent, because it bears the stamp of the high character of the gospel. Not a few of the men of ability thus won to the cause will enter energetically into the Lord's work.

Men of Wealth Will Help

The Lord calls upon those who are in positions of trust, those to whom He has entrusted His precious gifts, to use their talents of intellect and means in His service. Our workers should present before these men a plain statement of our plan of labor, telling them what we need in order to help the poor and needy and to establish this work on a firm basis. Some of these will be impressed by the Holy Spirit to invest the Lord's means in a way that will advance His cause. They will fulfill His purpose by helping to create centers of influence in the large cities. Interested workers will be led to offer themselves for various lines of missionary effort. Hygienic restaurants will be established. But with what carefulness should this work be done!

Every hygienic restaurant should be a school. The workers connected with it should be constantly studying and experimenting, that they may make improvement in the preparation of healthful foods. In the cities this work of instruction may be carried forward on a much larger scale than in smaller places. But in every place where there is a church, instruction should be given in regard to the preparation of simple, healthful foods for the use of those who wish to live in accordance with the principles of health reform. And the church members should impart to the people of their neighborhood the light they receive on this subject.

The students in our schools should be taught how to cook. Let tact and skill be brought into this branch of education. With all deceivableness of unrighteousness,

Satan is working to turn the feet of the youth into paths of temptation that lead to ruin. We must strengthen and help them to withstand the temptations that are to be met on every side regarding the indulgence of appetite. To teach them the science of healthful living is to do missionary work for the Master.

Cooking Schools in Many Places

Cooking schools are to be established in many places. This work may begin in a humble way, but as intelligent cooks do their best to enlighten others the Lord will give them skill and understanding. The word of the Lord is, "Forbid them not, for I will reveal Myself to them as their Instructor." He will work with those who carry out His plans, teaching the people how to bring about a reformation in their diet by the preparation of healthful, inexpensive foods. Thus the poor will be encouraged to adopt the principles of health reform; they will be helped to become industrious and self-reliant.

It has been presented to me that men and women of capability were being taught of God how to prepare wholesome, palatable foods, in an acceptable manner. Many of these were young, and there were also those of mature age. I have been instructed to encourage the conducting of cooking schools in all places where medical missionary work is being done. Every inducement to lead the people to reform must be held out before them. Let as much light as possible shine upon them. Teach them to make every improvement that they can in the preparation of food, and encourage them to impart to others that which they learn.

Shall we not do all in our power to advance the work in all of our large cities? Thousands upon thousands who live near us need help in various ways. Let the ministers of the gospel remember that the Lord Jesus Christ said to His disciples: "Ye are the light of the world. A city that is set on an hill cannot be hid." "Ye are the salt of the earth: but if the salt have lost his savor, wherewith shall it be salted?" Matthew 5:14, 13.

The Lord Working With Them

The Lord Jesus will work miracles for His people. In the sixteenth of Mark we read: "So then after the Lord had spoken unto them, He was received up into heaven, and sat on the right hand of God. And they went forth, and preached everywhere, *the Lord working with them,* and confirmed the word with signs following." Verses 19, 20. Here we are assured that the Lord was qualifying His chosen servants to take up medical missionary work after His ascension.

From the record of the Lord's miracles in providing wine at the wedding feast and in feeding the multitude, we may learn a lesson of the highest importance. The health-food business is one of the Lord's own instrumentalities to supply a necessity. The heavenly Provider of all foods will not leave His people in ignorance in regard to the preparation of the best foods for all times and occasions.

A Means of Overcoming Prejudice

Those who have long known the truth need to seek the Lord most earnestly, that their hearts may be filled with a determination to work for their neighbors. My brethren and sisters, visit those who live near you, and by sympathy and kindness seek to reach their hearts. Be sure to work in a way that will remove prejudice instead of creating it. —*Testimonies for the Church,* vol. 9, p. 34 (1909).

Sanitariums as City Outposts

Like Melrose, one of the chief advantages of the situation at Loma Linda is the pleasing variety of charming scenery. We believe that both places have come into our possession to be used to the very best advantage possible for sanitarium purposes.

But more important than magnificent scenery and beautiful buildings and spacious grounds is the close proximity of these institutions to densely populated districts, and the opportunity thus afforded of communicating to many, many people a knowledge of the third angel's message. We are to have clear spiritual discernment, else we shall fail of understanding the opening providences of God that are preparing the way for us to enlighten the world. The great crisis is just before us. Now is the time for us to sound the warning message, by the agencies that God has given us for this purpose. Let us remember that one most important agency is our medical missionary work. Never are we to lose sight of the great object for which our sanitariums are established—the advancement of God's closing work in the earth.

Loma Linda is in the midst of a very rich district, including three important cities—Redlands, Riverside, and San Bernardino. This field must be worked from Loma Linda, as Boston must be worked from Melrose.

When the New England Sanitarium was removed from South Lancaster to Melrose, the Lord instructed me that this was in the order of His opening providence. The buildings and grounds at Melrose are of a character to recommend our medical missionary work, which is to be carried forward not only in Boston, but in many other

Special Testimonies, Series B, No. 13, pp. 11-13 (1906).

unworked cities in New England. The Melrose property is such that conveniences can be provided that will draw to that sanitarium persons not of our faith. The aristocratic as well as the common people will visit that institution to avail themselves of the advantages offered for restoration of health.

Aggressive Work in Boston

Boston has been pointed out to me repeatedly as a place that must be faithfully worked. The light must shine in the outskirts and in the inmost parts. The Melrose Sanitarium is one of the greatest agencies that can be employed to reach Boston with the truth. The city and its suburbs must hear the last message of mercy to be given to our world. Tent meetings must be held in many places. The workers must put to the very best use the abilities God has given them. The gifts of grace will increase by wide use. But there must be no self-exaltation. No precise lines are to be laid down. Let the Holy Spirit direct the workers. They are to keep looking unto Jesus, the Author and Finisher of their faith. The work for this great city will be signalized by the revelation of the Holy Spirit, if all will walk humbly with God. . . .

We hope that those in charge of the work in New England will co-operate with the Melrose Sanitarium managers in taking aggressive steps to do the work that should be done in Boston. A hundred workers could be laboring to advantage in different portions of the city, in varied lines of service.

Redeeming the Time

The terrible disasters that are befalling great cities ought to arouse us to intense activity in giving the warning message to the people in these congested centers of population while we still have an opportunity. The most favorable time for the presentation of our message in the cities, has passed by. Sin and wickedness are rapidly increasing; and now we shall have to redeem the time by laboring all the more earnestly.

The medical missionary work is a door through which the truth is to find entrance to many homes in the cities. In every city will be found those who will appreciate the truths of the third angel's message. The judgments of God are impending. Why do we not awaken to the peril threatening the men and women living in the great cities of America? Our people do not realize as keenly as they should the responsibility resting upon them to proclaim the truth to the millions dwelling in these unwarned cities.

There are many souls to be saved. Our own souls are to be firmly grounded in a knowledge of the truth, that we may win others from error to the truth. We need now to search the Scriptures diligently, and as we become acquainted with unbelievers, we are to hold up Christ as the anointed, the crucified, the risen Saviour, witnessed to by prophets, testified of by believers, and through whose name we receive the forgiveness of our sins.

We need now a firm belief in the truth. Let us understand what is truth. Time is very short. Whole cities are being swept away. Are we doing our part to give the message that will prepare a people for the coming of their Lord? May God help us to improve the opportunities that are ours.

The Ministry and Medical Work

Both home and foreign missions should be conducted in connection with the ministry of the word. The medical missionary work is not to be carried forward as something apart from the work of the gospel ministry. The Lord's people are to be one. There is to be no separation in His work. Time and means are being absorbed in a work which is carried forward too earnestly in one direction. The Lord has not appointed this. He sent out His twelve apostles and afterward the Seventy to preach the word to the people, and He gave them power to heal the sick and to cast out devils in His name. The two lines of work must not be separated. Satan will invent every possible scheme to separate those whom God is seeking to make one. We must not be misled by his devices. The medical missionary work is to be connected with the third angel's message as the hand is connected with the body; and the education of students in medical missionary lines is not complete unless they are trained to work in connection with the church and the ministry.

There are in the ministry men of faith and experience, men who can say: "That which was from the beginning, which we have heard, which we have seen with our eyes, which we have looked upon, and our hands have handled, of the Word of life; . . . that which we have seen and heard declare we unto you." 1 John 1:1-3. These men are to instruct others. . . .

The medical missionary work is not to take men from the ministry, but to place them in the field. Wherever camp meetings are held, young men who have received an education in medical missionary lines should feel it their duty to act a part. They should be encouraged to

Appeal for the Work in Australia, pages 13-15 (1899).

speak, not only on these special lines, but also upon the points of present truth, giving the reasons why we are Seventh-day Adventists. These young men, given an opportunity to work with older ministers, will receive much help and blessing. . . .

There must be no belittling of the gospel ministry. No enterprise should be so conducted as to cause the ministry of the word to be looked upon as an inferior matter. It is not so. Those who ignore the ministry, are ignoring Christ. The highest of all work is the ministry in its various lines, and it should be kept before the youth that there is no work more blessed of God than that of the gospel minister.

Let not our young men be deterred from entering the ministry. There is danger that through glowing representations some will be drawn out of the path where God bids them walk. Some have been encouraged to take a course of study in medical lines who ought to be preparing themselves to enter the ministry. The Lord calls for more men to labor in His vineyard. The words were spoken, "Strengthen the outposts: have faithful sentinels in every part of the world." God calls for you, young men. He calls for whole armies of young men who are large-hearted and large-minded, and who have a deep love for Christ and the truth. . . .

It is not great and learned men that the ministry needs, it is not eloquent sermonizers. God calls for men who will give themselves to Him to be imbued with His Spirit. The cause of Christ and humanity demands sanctified, self-sacrificing men, those who can go forth without the camp, bearing the reproach. Let them be strong, valiant men, fit for worthy enterprises, and let them make a covenant with God by sacrifice.

ENSAMPLES TO THE FLOCK

The Importance of a Right Example

It is of the greatest importance that ministers and workers set a right example. If they hold and practice lax, loose principles, their example is quoted by those who love to talk rather than to practice, as a full vindication of their course of action. Every mistake that is made grieves the heart of Jesus and does injury to the influence of the truth, which is the power of God for the salvation of souls. The whole synagogue of Satan watches for mistakes in the lives of those who are seeking to represent Christ, and the most is made of every defection.

Take heed lest by your example you place other souls in peril. It is a terrible thing to lose your own soul, but to pursue a course which will cause the loss of other souls is still more terrible. That our influence should result in being a savor of death unto death is a terrible thought, and yet it is possible. With what holy jealousy, then, should we keep guard over our thoughts, our words, our habits, our dispositions, and our characters. God requires more deep, personal holiness on our part. Only by revealing His character can we co-operate with Him in the work of saving souls.

Value of a Consistent Life

The Lord's workers cannot be too careful that their actions do not contradict their words, for a consistent life alone can command respect. If our practice harmonizes

Special Testimonies to Ministers and Workers, No. 7, pp. 36-41 (1896).

with our teaching, our words will have effect; but a piety which is not based upon conscientious principles is as salt without savor. To speak, and do not, is as a sounding brass and a tinkling cymbal. It is of no use for us to strive to inculcate principles which we do not conscientiously practice.

Watch unto prayer. In this way alone can you put your whole being into the Lord's work. Self must be put in the background. Those who make self prominent gain an education that soon becomes second nature to them; and they will soon fail to realize that instead of uplifting Jesus they uplift themselves, that instead of being channels through which the living water can flow to refresh others, they absorb the sympathies and affections of those around them. This is not loyalty to our crucified Lord.

Living Epistles

We are ambassadors for Christ and we are to live, not to save our reputation, but to save perishing souls from perdition. Our daily endeavor should be to show them that they may gain truth and righteousness. Instead of trying to elicit sympathy for ourselves by giving others the impression that we are not appreciated, we are to forget self entirely; and if we fail to do this, through want of spiritual discernment and vital piety, God will require at our hands the souls of those for whom we should have labored. He has made provision that every worker in His service may have grace and wisdom, that he may become a living epistle, known and read of all men.

By watchfulness and prayer we may accomplish just what the Lord designs that we shall. By faithful, painstaking discharge of our duty, by watching for souls as they that must give account, we may remove every stumbling block out of the way of others. By earnest warnings and entreaties, with our own souls drawn out in tender solicitude for those that are ready to perish, we may win souls to Christ.

Grieving the Holy Spirit

I would that all my brethren and sisters would remember that it is a serious thing to grieve the Holy Spirit, and it is grieved when the human agent seeks to work himself and refuses to enter the service of the Lord because the cross is too heavy or the self-denial too great. The Holy Spirit seeks to abide in each soul. If it is welcomed as an honored guest, those who receive it will be made complete in Christ. The good work begun will be finished; the holy thoughts, heavenly affections, and Christlike actions will take the place of impure thoughts, perverse sentiments, and rebellious acts.

The Holy Spirit is a divine teacher. If we heed its lessons we shall become wise unto salvation. But we need to guard well our hearts, for too often we forget the heavenly instruction we have received and seek to act out the natural inclinations of our unconsecrated minds. Each one must fight his own battle against self. Heed the teachings of the Holy Spirit. If this is done, they will be repeated again and again until the impressions are as it were "laid in the rock forever." . . .

Indifference and Opposition

The Lord has given His people a message in regard to health reform. This light has been shining upon their pathway for thirty years, and the Lord cannot sustain His servants in a course which will counteract it. He is displeased when His servants act in opposition to the message upon this point, which He has given them to give to others. Can He be pleased when half the workers laboring in a place teach that the principles of health reform are as closely allied with the third angel's message as the arm is to the body, while their co-workers, by their practice, teach principles that are entirely opposite? This is regarded as a sin in the sight of God. . . .

Nothing brings such discouragement upon the Lord's watchmen as to be connected with those who have mental capacity, and who understand the reasons of our faith, but by precept and example manifest indifference to moral obligations.

The light which God has given upon health reform cannot be trifled with without injury to those who attempt it; and no man can hope to succeed in the work of God while, by precept and example, he acts in opposition to the light which God has sent. The voice of duty is the voice of God,—an inborn, heaven-sent guide,—and the Lord will not be trifled with upon these subjects. He who disregards the light which God has given in regard to the preservation of health, revolts against his own good and refuses to obey the One who is working for his best good.

The Duty of the Christian

It is the duty of every Christian to follow that course of action which the Lord has designated as right for His servants. He is ever to remember that God and eternity are before him, and he should not disregard his spiritual and physical health, even though tempted by wife, children, or relatives to do so. "If the Lord be God, follow Him: but if Baal, then follow him." 1 Kings 18:21.

The Duty to Preserve Health

I am pained at heart as I see so many feeble ministers, so many on beds of sickness, and so many closing the scenes of their earthly history—men who have carried the burden of responsibility in the work of God, whose whole heart was in their work. The conviction that they must cease their labor in the cause they loved was far more painful to them than their sufferings from disease, or even death itself.

Is it not time for us to understand that nature will not long suffer abuse without protesting? Our heavenly Father does not willingly afflict or grieve the children of men. He is not the author of sickness and death. He is the source of life; He would have men live, and He desires them to be obedient to the laws of life and health, that they may live.

Those who accept the present truth and are sanctified through it have an intense desire to represent the truth in their life and character. They have a deep yearning of soul that others may see the light and rejoice in it. As the true watchman goes forth, bearing precious seed, sowing beside all waters, weeping and praying, the burden of labor is very taxing to mind and heart. He cannot keep up the strain continuously, his soul stirred to the very depths, without wearing out prematurely. Strength and efficiency are needed in every discourse. And from time to time fresh supplies of things new and old need to be brought forth from the storehouse of God's word. This will impart life and power to the hearers. God does not want you to become so exhausted that your efforts have no freshness or life.

Those who are engaged in constant mental labor,

Gospel Workers, 1892 edition, pages 172-175 (1892).

whether in study or preaching, need rest and change. The earnest student is constantly taxing the brain, too often while neglecting physical exercise, and as the result the bodily powers are enfeebled and mental effort is restricted. Thus the student fails of accomplishing the very work that he might have done had he labored wisely.

Outdoor Labor a Blessing

If they worked intelligently, giving both mind and body a due share of exercise, ministers would not so readily succumb to disease. If all our workers were so situated that they could spend a few hours each day in outdoor labor, and felt free to do this, it would be a blessing to them; they would be able to discharge more successfully the duties of their calling. If they have not time for complete relaxation, they could be planning and praying while at work with their hands, and could return to their labor refreshed in body and spirit.

Some of our ministers feel that they must every day perform some labor that they can report to the conference, and as the result of trying to do this, their efforts are too often weak and inefficient. They should have periods of rest, of entire freedom from taxing labor. But these cannot take the place of daily physical exercise.

Brethren, when you take time to cultivate your garden, thus gaining the exercise you need to keep the system in good working order, you are just as much doing the work of God as in holding meetings. God is our Father, He loves us, and He does not require any of His servants to abuse their bodies.

Irregular Eating and Indigestion

Another cause both of ill-health and of inefficiency in labor is indigestion. It is impossible for the brain to do its best work when the digestive powers are abused. Many eat hurriedly of various kinds of food, which set up a war in the stomach and thus confuse the brain. The use of unhealthful food, and overeating of even that which is wholesome, should alike be avoided. Many eat at all hours, regardless of the laws of health. Then gloom covers the mind. How can men be honored with divine enlightenment when they are so reckless in their habits, so inattentive to the light which God has given in regard to these things? Brethren, is it not time for you to be converted on these points of selfish indulgence? "Know ye not that they which run in a race run all, but one receiveth the prize? So run, that ye may obtain. And every man that striveth for the mastery is temperate in all things." 1 Corinthians 9:24, 25. Study this solemnly.

Do not, however, feel it your duty to live on an insufficient diet. Learn for yourselves what you should eat, what kinds of food best nourish the body, and then follow the dictates of reason and conscience. At mealtime cast off care and taxing thought. Do not be hurried, but eat slowly and with cheerfulness, your heart filled with gratitude to God for all His blessings. And do not engage in brain labor immediately after a meal. Exercise moderately and give a little time for the stomach to begin its work.

This is not a matter of trifling importance. We must pay attention to it if healthful vigor and a right tone are to be given to the various branches of the work. The character and efficiency of the work depend largely upon the physical condition of the workers. Many committee meetings and other meetings for counsel have taken an unhappy tone from the dyspeptic condition of those assembled. And many a sermon has received a dark shadow from the minister's indigestion.

Health is an inestimable blessing, and one which is more closely related to conscience and religion than many realize. It has a great deal to do with one's capability. Every minister should feel that as he would be a faithful guardian of the flock, he must preserve all his powers in condition for the best possible service.

We are all deficient in practical knowledge concerning this matter. The wonderful mechanism of the human body does not receive half the care that is often given to a mere lifeless machine. Men give years of study in preparation for this ministry, and yet so weaken their powers during this preparatory work that they die prematurely.

Our workers should use their knowledge of the laws of life and health. They should study from cause to effect. Read the best authors on these subjects, and obey religiously that which your reason tells you is truth.

Clear Minds

You need clear, energetic minds, in order to appreciate the exalted character of the truth, to value the atonement, and to place the right estimate upon eternal things. If you pursue a wrong course and indulge in wrong habits of eating, and thereby weaken the intellectual powers, you will not place that high estimate upon salvation and eternal life which will inspire you to conform your life to the life of Christ; you will not make those earnest, self-sacrificing efforts for entire conformity to the will of God which His word requires and which are necessary to give you a moral fitness for the finishing touch of immortality. —*Testimonies for the Church,* vol. 2, p. 66 (1868).

Social Purity

The Lord made a special covenant with ancient Israel: "Now therefore, if ye will obey My voice indeed, and keep My covenant, then ye shall be a peculiar treasure unto Me above all people: for all the earth is Mine: and ye shall be unto Me a kingdom of priests, and an holy nation." Exodus 19:5, 6. He addresses His commandment-keeping people in these last days, "But ye are a chosen generation, a royal priesthood, an holy nation, a peculiar people; that ye should show forth the praises of Him who hath called you out of darkness into His marvelous light." "Dearly beloved, I beseech you as strangers and pilgrims, abstain from fleshly lusts, which war against the soul." 1 Peter 2:9, 11.

Not all who profess to keep the commandments of God possess their bodies in sanctification and honor. The most solemn message ever committed to mortals has been entrusted to this people, and they can have a powerful influence if they will be sanctified by it. They profess to be standing upon the elevated platform of eternal truth, keeping all of God's commandments; therefore, if they indulge in sin, if they commit fornication and adultery, their crime is of tenfold greater magnitude than is that of the classes I have named, who do not acknowledge the law of God as binding upon them. In a peculiar sense do those who profess to keep God's law dishonor Him and reproach the truth by transgressing its precepts.

The Experience of Israel a Warning

It was the prevalence of this very sin, fornication, among ancient Israel, which brought upon them the signal manifestation of God's displeasure. His judgments then followed close upon their heinous sin; thousands fell and their polluted bodies were left in the wilderness. "But with many of them God was not well pleased: for they were overthrown in the wilderness. Now these things were our examples, to the intent we should not lust after evil things, as they also lusted. Neither be ye idolaters, as were some of them; as it is written, The people sat down to eat and drink, and rose up to play. Neither let us commit fornication, as some of them committed, and fell in one day three and twenty thousand. . . . Now all these things happened unto them for ensamples: and they are written for our admonition, upon whom the ends of the world are come. Wherefore let him that thinketh he standeth take heed lest he fall." 1 Corinthians 10:5-12.

Patterns of Piety

Seventh-day Adventists, above all other people in the world, should be patterns of piety, holy in heart and in conversation. . . . Should they who make so high a profession indulge in sin and iniquity, their guilt would be very great. . . . Those who do not control their base passions cannot appreciate the atonement or place a right value upon the soul. Salvation is not experienced or understood by them. The gratification of animal passion is the highest ambition of their lives. God will accept nothing but purity and holiness; one spot, one wrinkle, one defect in the character, will forever debar them from heaven, with all its glories and treasures.

Ample provisions have been made for all who sincerely, earnestly, and thoughtfully set about the work of perfecting holiness in the fear of God. Strength, grace, and glory have been provided through Christ, to be brought by ministering angels to the heirs of salvation. None are so low, so corrupt and vile, that they cannot find in Jesus, who died for them, strength, purity, and righteousness, if they will put away their sins, cease their course of iniquity, and turn with full purpose of heart to the living God. . . .

I was referred to this scripture: "Let not sin therefore reign in your mortal body, that ye should obey it in the lusts thereof. Neither yield ye your members as instruments of unrighteousness unto sin: but yield yourselves unto God, as those that are alive from the dead, and your members as instruments of righteousness unto God." Romans 6:12, 13. Professed Christians, if no further light is given you than that contained in this text, you will be without excuse if you suffer yourselves to be controlled by base passions. . . .

I have long been designing to speak to my sisters and tell them that, from what the Lord has been pleased to show me from time to time, there is a great fault among them. They are not careful to abstain from all appearance of evil. They are not all circumspect in their deportment, as becometh women professing godliness. Their words are not as select and well chosen as those of women who have received the grace of God should be. They are too familiar with their brethren. They linger around them, incline toward them, and seem to choose their society. They are highly gratified with their attention.

From the light which the Lord has given me, our sisters should pursue a very different course. They should be more reserved, manifest less boldness, and encourage in themselves "shamefacedness and sobriety." Both brethren and sisters indulge in too much jovial talk when in each other's society. Women professing godliness indulge in much jesting, joking, and laughing. This is unbecoming and grieves the Spirit of God. These exhibitions reveal a lack of true Christian refinement. They do not strengthen the soul in God, but bring great darkness; they drive away the pure, refined, heavenly angels and bring those who engage in these wrongs down to a low level.

Our sisters should encourage true meekness; they should not be forward, talkative, and bold, but modest and unassuming, slow to speak. They may cherish courteousness. To be kind, tender, pitiful, forgiving, and humble, would be becoming and well-pleasing to God. If they occupy this position, they will not be burdened with undue attention from gentlemen in the church or out. All will feel that there is a sacred circle of purity around these God-fearing women which shields them from any unwarrantable liberties.

With some women professing godliness, there is a careless, coarse freedom of manner which leads to wrong and evil. But those godly women whose minds and hearts are occupied in meditating upon themes which strengthen purity of life, and which elevate the soul to commune with God, will not be easily led astray from the path of rectitude and virtue. Such will be fortified against the sophistry of Satan; they will be prepared to withstand his seductive arts.

Vainglory, the fashion of the world, the desire of the eye, and the lust of the flesh, are connected with the fall of the unfortunate. That which is pleasing to the natural heart and carnal mind is cherished. If the lust of the flesh had been rooted out of their hearts, they would not be so weak. If our sisters would feel the necessity of purifying their thoughts, and never suffer in themselves a carelessness of deportment which leads to improper acts, they need not in the least stain their purity. If they viewed the matter as God has presented it to me, they would have such an abhorrence of impure acts that they would not be found among those who fall through the temptations of Satan, no matter whom he might select as the medium.

A preacher may be dealing in sacred, holy things, and yet not be holy in heart. He may give himself to Satan to work wickedness and to corrupt the souls and bodies of his flock. Yet if the minds of women and youth professing to love and fear God were fortified with His Spirit, if they had trained their minds to purity of thought and educated themselves to avoid all appearance of evil, they would be safe from any improper advances and be secure from the corruption prevailing around them. The apostle Paul wrote concerning himself, "But I keep under my body, and bring it into subjection: lest that by any means, when I have preached to others, I myself should be a castaway." 1 Corinthians 9:27.

If a minister of the gospel does not control his baser passions, if he fails to follow the example of the apostle, and so dishonors his profession and faith as to even name the indulgence of sin, our sisters who profess godliness should not for an instant flatter themselves that sin or crime loses its sinfulness in the least because their minister dares to engage in it. The fact that men who are in responsible places show themselves to be familiar with sin should not lessen the guilt and enormity of the sin in the minds of any. Sin should appear just as sinful, just as abhorrent, as it had been heretofore regarded; and the minds of the pure and elevated should abhor and shun the one who indulges in sin, as they would flee from a serpent whose sting was deadly.

Reference for further study: *Testimonies for the Church,* vol. 5, pp. 591-603, "The Appearance of Evil."

Exercise and Diet

Ministers, teachers, and students do not become as intelligent as they should in regard to the necessity of physical exercise in the open air. They neglect this duty, which is most essential for the preservation of health. They closely apply their minds to books, and eat the allowance of a laboring man. Under such habits, some grow corpulent, because the system is clogged. Others become lean, feeble, and weak, because their vital powers are exhausted in throwing off the excess of food; the liver becomes burdened and unable to throw off the impurities in the blood, and sickness is the result. If physical exercise were combined with mental exertion, the blood would be quickened in its circulation, the action of the heart would be more perfect, impure matter would be thrown off, and new life and vigor would be experienced in every part of the body.

The Nervous System Deranged

When the minds of ministers, schoolteachers, and students are continually excited by study, and the body is allowed to be inactive, the nerves of emotion are taxed, while the nerves of motion are inactive. The wear being all upon the mental organs, they become overworked and enfeebled, while the muscles lose their vigor for want of employment. There is no inclination to exercise the muscles by engaging in physical labor, because exertion seems to be irksome.

Ministers of Christ, professing to be His representatives, should follow His example, and above all others should form habits of strictest temperance. They should keep the life and example of Christ before the people by

Testimonies for the Church, vol. 3, pp. 489-492 (1875).

their own lives of self-denial, self-sacrifice, and active benevolence. Christ overcame appetite in man's behalf; and in His stead they are to set others an example worthy of imitation. Those who do not feel the necessity of engaging in the work of overcoming upon the point of appetite will fail to secure precious victories which they might have gained and will become slaves to appetite and lust, which are filling the cup of iniquity of those who dwell upon the earth.

Self-Denial and Efficiency

Men who are engaged in giving the last message of warning to the world, a message which is to decide the destiny of souls, should make a practical application in their own lives of the truths they preach to others. They should be examples to the people in their eating, in their drinking, and in their chaste conversation and deportment. Gluttony, indulgence of the baser passions, and grievous sins are hidden under the garb of sanctity by many professed representatives of Christ throughout our world. There are men of excellent natural ability whose labor does not accomplish half what it might if they were temperate in all things. Indulgence of appetite and passion beclouds the mind, lessens physical strength, and weakens moral power. Their thoughts are not clear. Their words are not spoken in power, are not vitalized by the Spirit of God so as to reach the hearts of the hearers.

As our first parents lost Eden through the indulgence of appetite, our only hope of regaining Eden is through the firm denial of appetite and passion. Abstemiousness in diet, and control of all the passions, will preserve the intellect and give mental and moral vigor, enabling men to bring all their propensities under the control of the higher powers and to discern between right and wrong, the sacred and the common. All who have a true sense of the sacrifice made by Christ in leaving His home in heaven to come to this world that He might by His own life show man how to resist temptation, will cheerfully deny self and choose to be partakers with Christ of His sufferings.

Which Shall Control?

The fear of the Lord is the beginning of wisdom. Those who overcome as Christ overcame will need to constantly guard themselves against the temptations of Satan. The appetite and passions should be restricted and under the control of enlightened conscience, that the intellect may be unimpaired, the perceptive powers clear, so that the workings of Satan and his snares may not be interpreted to be the providence of God. Many desire the final reward and victory which are to be given to overcomers, but are not willing to endure toil, privation, and denial of self, as did their Redeemer. It is only through obedience and continual effort that we shall overcome as Christ overcame.

The controlling power of appetite will prove the ruin of thousands, when, if they had conquered on this point, they would have had moral power to gain the victory over every other temptation of Satan. But those who are slaves to appetite will fail in perfecting Christian character. The continual transgression of man for six thousand years has brought sickness, pain, and death as its fruits. And as we near the close of time, Satan's temptation to indulge appetite will be more powerful and more difficult to overcome.

A Reform Needed

If Seventh-day Adventists practiced what they profess to believe, if they were sincere health reformers, they would indeed be a spectacle to the world, to angels, and to men. And they would show a far greater zeal for the salvation of those who are ignorant of the truth.

Greater reforms should be seen among the people who claim to be looking for the soon appearing of Christ. Health reform is to do among our people a work which it has not yet done. There are those who ought to be awake to the danger of meat eating, who are still eating the flesh of animals, thus endangering the physical, mental, and spiritual health. Many who are now only half converted on the question of meat eating will go from God's people, to walk no more with them.

In all our work we must obey the laws which God has given, that the physical and spiritual energies may work in harmony. Men may have a form of godliness, they may even preach the gospel, and yet be unpurified and unsanctified. Ministers should be strictly temperate in their eating and drinking, lest they make crooked paths for their feet, turning the lame—those weak in the faith—out of the way. If, while proclaiming the most solemn and important message God has ever given, men war against the truth by indulging wrong habits of eating and drinking, they take all the force from the message they bear.

Evils of Flesh Eating

Those who indulge in meat eating, tea drinking, and gluttony are sowing seeds for a harvest of pain and death.

Review and Herald, May 27, 1902.

The unhealthful food placed in the stomach strengthens the appetites that war against the soul, developing the lower propensities. A diet of flesh meat tends to develop animalism. A development of animalism lessens spirituality, rendering the mind incapable of understanding truth.

The word of God plainly warns us that unless we abstain from fleshly lusts, the physical nature will be brought into conflict with the spiritual nature. Lustful eating wars against health and peace. Thus a warfare is instituted between the higher and the lower attributes of the man. The lower propensities, strong and active, oppress the soul. The highest interests of the being are imperiled by the indulgence of appetites unsanctioned by Heaven.

Great care should be taken to form right habits of eating and drinking. The food eaten should be that which will make the best blood. The delicate organs of digestion should be respected. God requires us, by being temperate in all things, to act our part toward keeping ourselves in health. He cannot enlighten the mind of a man who makes a cesspool of his stomach. He does not hear the prayers of those who are walking in the light of the sparks of their own kindling.

Common Errors in Diet

Intemperance is seen in the quantity as well as in the quality of food eaten. The Lord has instructed me that as a general rule we place too much food in the stomach. Many make themselves uncomfortable by overeating, and sickness is often the result. The Lord did not bring this punishment on them. They brought it on themselves, and God desires them to realize that pain is the result of transgression.

Daily abused, the digestive organs cannot do their work well. A poor quality of blood is made, and thus, through improper eating, the whole machinery is crippled. Give the stomach less to do. It will recover if proper care is shown in regard to the quality and quantity of food eaten.

Many eat too rapidly. Others eat at one meal varieties of food that do not agree. If men and women would only remember how greatly they afflict the soul when they afflict the stomach, and how deeply Christ is dishonored when the stomach is abused, they would deny the appetite and thus give the stomach opportunity to recover its healthy action. While sitting at the table we may do medical missionary work by eating and drinking to the glory of God.

Eating on the Sabbath

To eat on the Sabbath the same amount of food eaten on a working day is entirely out of place. The Sabbath is the day set apart for the worship of God, and on it we are to be specially careful in regard to our diet. A clogged stomach means a clogged brain. Too often so large an amount of food is eaten on the Sabbath that the mind is rendered dull and stupid, incapable of appreciating spiritual things. The habits of eating have much to do with the many dull religious exercises of the Sabbath. The diet for the Sabbath should be selected with reference to the duties of the day on which the purest, holiest service is to be offered to God.

Eating has much to do with religion. The spiritual experience is greatly affected by the way in which the stomach is treated. Eating and drinking in accordance with the laws of health promote virtuous actions. But if the stomach is abused by habits that have no foundation in nature, Satan takes advantage of the wrong that has been done and uses the stomach as an enemy of righteousness, creating a disturbance which affects the entire being. Sacred things are not appreciated. Spiritual zeal diminishes. Peace of mind is lost. There is dissension, strife, and discord. Impatient words are spoken and unkind deeds are done; dishonest practices are followed and anger is manifested—and all because the nerves of the brain are disturbed by the abuse heaped on the stomach.

What a pity it is that often, when the greatest self-denial should be exercised, the stomach is crowded with a mass of unhealthful food, which lies there to decompose. The affliction of the stomach afflicts the brain. The imprudent eater does not realize that he is disqualifying himself for giving wise counsel, disqualifying himself for laying plans for the best advancement of the work of God. But this is so. He cannot discern spiritual things, and in council meetings, when he should say Yea, he says Nay. He makes propositions that are wide of the mark, because the food he has eaten has benumbed his brain power.

Health Reform and Spirituality

The failure to follow sound principles has marred the history of God's people. There has been a continual backsliding in health reform, and as a result God is dishonored by a great lack of spirituality. Barriers have been erected which would never have been seen had God's people walked in the light.

Shall we who have had such great opportunities allow the people of the world to go in advance of us in health reform? Shall we cheapen our minds and abuse our talents by wrong eating? Shall we transgress God's holy law by following selfish practices? Shall our inconsistency become a byword? Shall we live such unchristianlike lives that the Saviour will be ashamed to call us brethren?

Shall we not rather do that medical missionary work which is the gospel in practice, living in such a way that the peace of God can rule in our hearts? Shall we not remove every stumbling block from the feet of unbelievers, ever remembering what is due to a profession of Christianity? Far better give up the name of Christian than make a profession and at the same time indulge appetites which strengthen unholy passions.

A Reformation Called For

God calls upon every church member to dedicate his life unreservedly to the Lord's service. He calls for decided reformation. All creation is groaning under the curse. God's people should place themselves where they will grow in grace, being sanctified, body, soul, and spirit, by the truth. When they break away from all health-destroying indulgences, they will have a clearer perception of what constitutes true godliness. A wonderful change will be seen in the religious experience. . . .

"It is high time to awake out of sleep: for now is our salvation nearer than when we believed. The night is far spent, the day is at hand: let us therefore cast off the works of darkness, and let us put on the armor of light. Let us walk honestly, as in the day; not in rioting and drunkenness, not in chambering and wantonness, not in strife and envying. But put ye on the Lord Jesus Christ, and make not provision for the flesh, to fulfill the lusts thereof." Romans 13:11-14.

A Reformatory Movement

In visions of the night representations passed before me of a great reformatory movement among God's people. Many were praising God. The sick were healed and other miracles were wrought. A spirit of intercession was seen, even as was manifested before the great day of Pentecost. Hundreds and thousands were seen visiting families and opening before them the word of God. Hearts were convicted by the power of the Holy Spirit, and a spirit of genuine conversion was manifest. On every side doors were thrown open to the proclamation of the truth. The world seemed to be lightened with the heavenly influence. Great blessings were received by the true and humble people of God. I heard voices of thanksgiving and praise, and there seemed to be a reformation such as we witnessed in 1844.

Yet some refused to be converted. They were not willing to walk in God's way, and when, in order that the work of God might be advanced, calls were made for freewill offerings, some clung selfishly to their earthly possessions. These covetous ones became separated from the company of believers.—*Testimonies for the Church,* vol. 9, p. 126 (1909).

HOLINESS OF LIFE

Lights Amid Darkness

The Lord has let His light shine upon us in these last days, that the gloom and darkness which have been gathering in past generations because of sinful indulgences, might in some degree be dispelled, and that the train of evils which have resulted because of intemperate eating and drinking might be lessened.

The Lord in wisdom designed to bring His people into a position where they would be separate from the world in spirit and practice, that their children might not so readily be led into idolatry and become tainted with the prevailing corruptions of this age. It is God's design that believing parents and their children should stand forth as living representatives of Christ, candidates for everlasting life. All who are partakers of the divine nature will escape the corruption that is in the world through lust. It is impossible for those who indulge the appetite to attain to Christian perfection. You cannot arouse the moral sensibilities of your children while you are not careful in the selection of their food.—*Testimonies for the Church,* vol. 2, pp. 399, 400 (1870).

This world is a training school for the higher school, this life a preparation for the life to come. Here we are to be prepared for entrance into the heavenly courts. Here we are to receive and believe and practice the truth, until we are made ready for a home with the saints in light.—*Testimonies for the Church,* vol. 8, p. 200 (1904).

A Lesson From Solomon's Fall

The life of Solomon might have been remarkable until its close, if virtue had been preserved. But he surrendered this special grace to lustful passion. In his youth he looked to God for guidance and trusted in Him, and God chose for him and gave him wisdom that astonished the world. His power and wisdom were extolled throughout the land. But his love of women was his sin. This passion he did not control in his manhood, and it proved a snare to him. His wives led him into idolatry, and when he began to descend the declivity of life, the wisdom that God had given him was removed; he lost his firmness of character and became more like the giddy youth, wavering between right and wrong. Yielding his principles, he placed himself in the current of evil, and thus separated himself from God, the foundation and source of his strength. He had moved from principle. Wisdom had been more precious to him than the gold of Ophir. But, alas! lustful passions gained the victory. He was deceived and ruined by women. What a lesson for watchfulness! What a testimony as to the need of strength from God to the very last!

In the battle with inward corruptions and outward temptations, even the wise and powerful Solomon was vanquished. It is not safe to permit the least departure from the strictest integrity. "Abstain from all appearance of evil." 1 Thessalonians 5:22. When a woman relates her family troubles, or complains of her husband, to another man, she violates her marriage vows; she dishonors her husband and breaks down the wall erected to preserve the sanctity of the marriage relation; she throws wide open the door and invites Satan to enter

Testimonies for the Church, vol. 2, pp. 305-307 (1868).

with his insidious temptations. This is just as Satan would have it. If a woman comes to a Christian brother with a tale of her woes, her disappointments and trials, he should ever advise her, if she must confide her troubles to someone, to select sisters for her confidants, and then there will be no appearance of evil, whereby the cause of God may suffer reproach.

Remember Solomon. Among many nations there was no king like him, beloved of his God. But he fell. He was led from God and became corrupt, through the indulgence of lustful passions. This is the prevailing sin of this age, and its progress is fearful. Professed Sabbath-keepers are not clean. There are those who profess to believe the truth who are corrupt at heart. God will prove them, and their folly and sin shall be made manifest. None but the pure and lowly can dwell in His presence. "Who shall ascend into the hill of the Lord? or who shall stand in His holy place? He that hath clean hands, and a pure heart; who hath not lifted up his soul unto vanity, nor sworn deceitfully." Psalm 24:3, 4. "Lord, who shall abide in Thy tabernacle? who shall dwell in Thy holy hill? He that walketh uprightly, and worketh righteousness, and speaketh the truth in his heart. He that backbiteth not with his tongue, nor doeth evil to his neighbor, nor taketh up a reproach against his neighbor. In whose eyes a vile person is contemned; but he honoreth them that fear the Lord. He that sweareth to his own hurt, and changeth not. He that putteth not out his money to usury, nor taketh reward against the innocent. He that doeth these things shall never be moved." Psalm 15.

Counsel to Physicians and Nurses

The Lord has instructed me to present the following scriptures to our physicians: "Furthermore then we beseech you, brethren, and exhort you by the Lord Jesus, that as ye have received of us how ye ought to walk and to please God, so ye would abound more and more. . . . For this is the will of God, even your sanctification." 1 Thessalonians 4:1-3. "As ye have therefore received Christ Jesus the Lord, so walk ye in Him: rooted and built up in Him, and established in the faith, as ye have been taught, abounding therein with thanksgiving. Beware lest any man spoil you through philosophy and vain deceit, after the tradition of men, after the rudiments of the world, and not after Christ." Colossians 2:6-8.

Physicians are placed where peculiar temptations will come to them. If they are not prepared to withstand temptations by the practice of the principles of truth, they will fall when Satan tempts them. There are ministers of the gospel who are too weak to resist temptation. They may have long preached the gospel, and with marked success; they may have won the confidence of the people, but when they think they are strong, they show that they cannot stand alone without being overcome. Unless they govern their habits and passions, unless they keep close to the side of Christ, they will lose eternal life. If ministers are in such danger, physicians are even more so.

The perils of physicians have been opened before me. The physicians in our sanitariums must not allow themselves to think that they are in no danger. They are in positive danger; but they may avoid the perils which surround them if they walk humbly with God, taking heed

---

Special Testimonies, Series B, No. 15, pp. 16-23 (1900).

not to be presumptuous. "Let him that thinketh he stand-eth take heed lest he fall." 1 Corinthians 10:12. A power higher and stronger than human power must hold the fort in our medical institutions.

Experienced Guides and Counselors

Connected with each sanitarium should be a man and his wife of mature age, who are as firm as a rock to the principles of truth, who can act as guides and counselors. The education of men and women in a sanitarium is a most important and delicate work, and unless physicians are constantly prepared for this work by the power of God, they will be tempted to look upon the bodies of ladies with an unsanctified heart and mind.

There should always be connected with our sanitari-ums women of mature age, educated and trained for the work, who are competent to treat lady patients. At what-ever cost, they should be employed; and if they cannot be found, persons having the right dispositions and traits of character should be educated and prepared for this work.

Physicians to Be Circumspect

Physicians must avoid all freedom of manner toward ladies, married or unmarried. They should ever be cir-cumspect in their behavior. It is better that our physi-cians be married men, whose wives can unite with them in the work. Both the doctor and his wife should have a living experience in the things of God. If they are devoted Christians, their work will be as precious as fine gold.

Souls are always in peril. Even married physicians are subject to temptations. Some have fallen in the snares Satan has prepared for them. We are none of us safe from his wily, seductive power. Some are alive to their danger, but realize that Satan is making masterly efforts to overcome them, and by earnest prayer they brace themselves for duty. While in this lower apartment—the world—they are kept by the power of God. By trial they are fitted for the conflict. They are cleansed from sin in the blood of the Lamb.

Trusting in Jesus

No physician is secure who stands in his own strength. Physicians must not enter upon their work with careless, irreverent thoughts. Moment by moment they are to trust in Him who gave His life for fallen humanity and who respects His purchased inheritance. Thus doing, they will rightly regard the purchase of the blood of Christ. They will gird on every piece of the heavenly armor, that they may be protected from the assaults of the enemy. This is a safeguard against sin which the physician must avail himself of if he would be successful in his work.

Our bodies belong to God. He paid the price of redemption for the body as well as the soul. "Ye are not your own; for ye are bought with a price: therefore glorify God in your body, and in your spirit, which are God's." 1 Corinthians 6:19, 20. "The body is not for fornication, but for the Lord; and the Lord for the body." Verse 13. The Creator watches over the human machinery, keeping it in motion. Were it not for His constant care, the pulse would not beat, the action of the heart would cease, the brain would no longer act its part.

The brain is the organ and instrument of the mind and controls the whole body. In order for the other parts of the system to be healthy, the brain must be healthy. And in order for the brain to be healthy, the blood must be pure. If by correct habits of eating and drinking the blood is kept pure, the brain will be properly nourished.

Conditions That Bring Disease

It is the lack of harmonious action in the human organism that brings disease. The imagination may control the other parts of the body to their injury. All parts of the system must work harmoniously. The different parts of the body, especially those remote from the heart, should receive a free circulation of blood. The limbs act an important part and should receive proper attention.

God is the great caretaker of the human machinery. In the care of our bodies we must co-operate with Him. Love for God is essential for life and health. In order to have perfect health our hearts must be filled with hope and love and joy.

The lower passions are to be strictly guarded. The perceptive faculties are abused, terribly abused, when the passions are allowed to run riot. When the passions are indulged, the blood, instead of circulating to all parts of the body, thereby relieving the heart and clearing the mind, is called in undue amount to the internal organs. Disease comes as the result. The man cannot be healthy until the evil is seen and remedied.

"He that is joined unto the Lord"—bound up with Christ in the covenant of grace—"is one spirit. Flee fornication." 1 Corinthians 6:17, 18. Do not stop for one moment to reason. Satan would rejoice to see you overthrown by temptation. Do not stop to argue the case with your weak conscience. Turn away from the first step of transgression.

The Example of Joseph

Would that the example of Joseph might be followed by all who claim to be wise, who feel competent in their own strength to discharge the duties of life. A wise man will not be governed and controlled by his appetites and passions, but will control and govern them. He will draw nigh to God, striving to prepare mind and body to discharge aright the duties of life.

I wish to impress upon the minds of physicians the fact that they cannot do as they please with their thoughts and imaginations and at the same time be safe in their calling. Satan is the destroyer; Christ is the restorer. I desire our physicians to fully comprehend this point. They may save souls from death by a right application of the knowledge they have gained, or they may work against the great Master Builder. They may co-operate with God, or they may counterwork His plans by failing to work harmoniously with Him.

Preservation of Health

All physicians should place themselves under the control of the Great Physician. Under His guidance they will do as they should do. But the Lord will not work a miracle to save physicians who recklessly abuse His building. As far as possible, physicians should observe regularity in their habits of eating. They should take a proper amount of exercise. They should be determined to co-operate with the great Master Builder. God works, and man must come into line and work with Him; for He is the Saviour of the body.

Physicians, above all others, need to realize the relation human beings sustain toward God in regard to the preservation of health and life. They need to study the word of God diligently, lest they disregard the laws of health. There is no need for them to become weak and unbalanced. Under the guidance of the heavenly authority, they may advance in clear, straight lines. But they must give the most earnest heed to the laws of God. They should feel that they are the property of God, that they have been bought with a price, and that therefore they are to glorify Him in all things. By the study of God's word they are to keep the mind awake to the fact that human beings are the Lord's property by creation and by redemption. They are to say, I will do all in my power to save the souls and bodies of those for whom I work. They have been bought with a price, even the blood of Christ, and I must do all I can to help them.

The instruction I have for our physicians is that they must study the word of God with earnestness and diligence. God says, "Come out, . . . and be ye separate, . . . and touch not the unclean." 2 Corinthians 6:17. Obey this word, at whatever cost to social position, worldly honor, or earthly wealth. Trust in the Lord. Walk in all humility of mind before Him. Holding by faith to His word, you may go forward.

Avoid Outward Display

No physician is to trust to outward display, his elegant furniture or stylish equipage, to give him favor and exalt the truth. Physicians who trust to these things are moved by a power from beneath. It is not the grandeur of the house, the elegance of the furniture, the outward display of any kind, that will gain for our sanitariums a true standard. Physicians who are bound up with God will do all in their power to crush out the inclination to vanity and display. . . .

Humility, self-denial, benevolence, and the payment of a faithful tithe, these show that the grace of God is working in the heart. The greatest Teacher, the greatest Physician the world has ever known, gave many lessons on the need of humility. These lessons His followers are to bring into the practical life. They are to live lives of self-denial and self-sacrifice. To many this will be a new experience, but on it their salvation depends. "Whosoever will come after Me," Christ said, "let him deny himself, and take up his cross, and follow Me." Mark 8:34. Following Christ produces the virtues of Christ's character. Humility is a precious grace, peculiarly pleasing to God. Christ says, "Learn of Me; for I am meek and lowly in heart: and ye shall find rest unto your souls." Matthew 11:29. Those who follow Christ will overcome temptation and will receive the glorious reward of eternal life. And to Christ they will render all the praise and glory.

Live Holy Lives

To the young men and young women who are being educated as nurses and physicians I will say, Keep close to Jesus. By beholding Him we become changed into His likeness. Remember that you are not training for courtship or marriage, but for the marriage of Christ. You may have a theoretical knowledge of the truth, but this will not save you. You must know by experience how sinful sin is, and how much you need Jesus as a personal Saviour. Only thus can you become sons and daughters of God. Your only merit is your great need.

Those selected to take the nurses' course in our sanitariums should be wisely chosen. Young girls of a superficial mold of character should not be encouraged to take up this work. Many of the young men who present themselves as being desirous of being educated as physicians have not those traits of character which will enable them to withstand the temptations so common to the work of a physician. Only those should be accepted who give promise of becoming qualified for the great work of imparting the principles of true health reform.

Young ladies connected with our institutions should keep a strict guard over themselves. In word and action, they should be reserved. Never when speaking to a married man should they show the slightest freedom. To my sisters who are connected with our sanitariums, I would say, gird on the armor. When talking to men, be kind and courteous, but never free. Observant eyes are upon you, watching your conduct, judging by it whether you are indeed children of God. Be modest. Abstain from every appearance of evil. Keep on the heavenly armor, or else for Christ's sake sever your connection with the sanitarium, the place where poor shipwrecked souls are to find a haven. Those connected with these institutions are to take heed to themselves. Never, by word or action, are they to give the least occasion for wicked men to speak evil of the truth.

There are two kingdoms in this world, the kingdom of Christ and the kingdom of Satan. To one of these kingdoms each one of us belongs. In His wonderful prayer for His disciples, Christ said, "I pray not that Thou shouldest take them out of the world, but that Thou shouldest keep them from the evil. They are not of the world, even as I am not of the world. Sanctify them through Thy truth: Thy word is truth. As Thou hast sent Me into the world, even so have I also sent them into the world." John 17:15-18.

Exert a Saving Influence

It is not God's will that we should seclude ourselves from the world. But while in the world we should sanctify ourselves to God. We should not pattern after the world. We are to be in the world as a corrective influence, as salt that retains its savor. Among an unholy, impure, idolatrous generation, we are to be pure and holy, showing that the grace of Christ has power to restore in man the divine likeness. We are to exert a saving influence upon the world.

"This is the victory that overcometh the world, even our faith." 1 John 5:4. The world has become a lazar house of sin, a mass of corruption. It knows not the children of God because it knows Him not. We are not to practice its ways or follow its customs. Continually we are to resist its lax principles. Christ said to His followers, "Let your light so shine before men, that they may see your good works, and glorify your Father which is in heaven." Matthew 5:16. It is the duty of physicians and nurses to shine as lights amid the corrupting influences of the world. They are to cherish principles which the world cannot tarnish.

In order for the church to be healthy, it must be composed of healthy Christians. But in our churches and institutions there are many sickly Christians. The light which the Lord has given me is plainly expressed in the third chapter of Philippians. This chapter should be carefully read and studied. The lessons it contains should be practiced.

He who co-operates with the Great Physician will keep nerves, sinews, and muscles in the best condition of health. In order to do its work properly, the human machinery needs careful attention. The harmonious action of the different parts must be preserved.

Be Strong in the Lord

It is so with the soul. The heart is to be carefully kept and guarded. "What shall it profit a man, if he shall gain the whole world, and lose his own soul? Or what shall a man give in exchange for his soul?" Mark 8:36, 37. Christ must abide in the heart by faith. His word is the bread of life and the water of salvation. Trust in its fullness comes to us through constant communion with God. By eating the flesh and drinking the blood of Christ we gain spiritual strength. Christ supplies the lifeblood of the heart, and Christ and the Holy Spirit give nerve power. Begotten again unto a lively hope, imbued with the quickening power of a new nature, the soul is enabled to rise higher and still higher. Paul's prayer to God for the Ephesians was, "That He would grant you, according to the riches of His glory, to be strengthened with might by His Spirit in the inner man; that Christ may dwell in your hearts by faith; that ye, being rooted and grounded in love, may be able to comprehend with all saints what is the breadth, and length, and depth, and height; and to know the love of Christ, which passeth knowledge, that ye might be filled with all the fullness of God." Ephesians 3:16-19.

The blessing of grace is given to men that the heavenly universe and the fallen world may see as they could not otherwise, the perfection of Christ's character. The Great Physician came to our world to show men and women that through His grace they may so live that in the great day of God they can receive the precious testimony, "Ye are complete in Him."

Physicians are to reveal the attributes of Christ, steadfastly persevering in the work God has given them to do. To those who do this work in faithfulness, angels are commissioned to give enlarged views of the character and work of Christ and His power, grace, and love. Thus they become partakers of His image, and day by day grow up to the full stature of men and women in Christ. It is the privilege of the children of God to have a constantly enlarging comprehension of truth, that they may bring love for God and heaven into the work, and draw from others thanksgiving to God because of the richness of His grace.

We have reason for everlasting gratitude to God in that He has left us a perfect example. Every Christian should strive to earnestly follow in the footsteps of the Saviour. We should offer grateful praise and gratitude for giving us such a mighty helper, a safeguard against every temptation, against every species of impropriety in thought, deed, and word.

Our only security against falling into sin is to keep ourselves continually under the molding influence of the Holy Spirit, at the same time engaging actively in the cause of truth and holiness, discharging every God-given duty, but taking no burden which God has not laid upon us. Physicians must stand firmly under the banner of the third angel's message, fighting the good fight of faith perseveringly and successfully, relying on a heavenly armor, the equipment of God's word, never forgetting that they have a leader who never has been and never can be overcome by evil.

Reference for further study: *Testimonies for the Church,* vol. 5, pp. 591-603, "The Appearance of Evil."

The Price of Health

Health may be earned by proper habits of life and may be made to yield interest and compound interest. But this capital, more precious than any bank deposit, may be sacrificed by intemperance in eating and drinking, or by leaving the organs to rust from inaction. Pet indulgences must be given up; laziness must be overcome.

The reason why many of our ministers complain of sickness is, they fail to take sufficient exercise and indulge in overeating. They do not realize that such a course endangers the strongest constitution. Those who . . . are sluggish in temperament should eat very sparingly and not shun physical taxation. Many of our ministers are digging their graves with their teeth. The system, in taking care of the burden placed upon the digestive organs, suffers, and a severe draft is made upon the brain. For every offense committed against the laws of health, the transgressor must pay the penalty in his own body.

When not actively engaged in preaching, the apostle Paul labored at his trade as a tentmaker. This he was obliged to do on account of having accepted unpopular truth. Before he embraced Christianity, he had occupied an elevated position, and was not dependent upon his labor for support. Among the Jews it was customary to teach the children some trade, however high the position they were expected to fill, that a reverse of circumstances might not leave them incapable of sustaining themselves. In accordance with this custom, Paul was a tentmaker; and when his means had been expended to advance the cause of Christ and for his own support, he resorted to his trade in order to gain a livelihood.—*Testimonies for the Church*, vol. 4, pp. 408, 409 (1880).

Simplicity in Dress

As we see our sisters departing from simplicity in dress and cultivating a love for the fashions of the world, we feel troubled. By taking steps in this direction they are separating themselves from God and neglecting the inward adorning. They should not feel at liberty to spend their God-given time in the unnecessary ornamentation of their clothing. How much better might it be employed in searching the Scriptures, thus obtaining a thorough knowledge of the prophecies and of the practical lessons of Christ.

As Christians, we ought not to engage in any employment upon which we cannot conscientiously ask the blessing of the Lord. Do you, my sisters, in the needless work you put upon your garments, feel a clear conscience? Can you, while perplexing the mind over ruffles and bows and ribbons, be uplifting the soul to God in prayer that He will bless your efforts? The time spent in this way might be devoted to doing good to others and to cultivating your own minds.

Many of our sisters are persons of good ability, and if their talents were used to the glory of God, they would be successful in winning many souls to Christ. . . .

Especially should the wives of our ministers be careful not to depart from the plain teachings of the Bible on the point of dress. Many look upon these injunctions as too old-fashioned to be worthy of notice; but He who gave them to His disciples understood the dangers from the love of dress in our time, and sent to us the note of warning. Will we heed the warning and be wise? Extravagance in dress is continually increasing. The end is not yet. Fashion is constantly changing, and our sisters

Testimonies for the Church, vol. 4, pp. 628-647 (1875).

follow in its wake, regardless of time or expense. There is a great amount of means expended upon dress, when it should be returned to God the giver.

Fashionable Dress a Stumbling Block

The plain, neat dress of the poorer class often appears in marked contrast with the attire of their more wealthy sisters, and this difference frequently causes a feeling of embarrassment on the part of the poor. Some try to imitate their more wealthy sisters, and frill and ruffle and trim goods of an inferior quality, so as to approach as nearly as possible to them in dress. Poor girls, receiving but two dollars a week for their work,[1] will expend every cent to dress like others who are not obliged to earn their own living. These youth have nothing to put into the treasury of God. And their time is so thoroughly occupied in making their dress as fashionable as that of their sisters, that they have no time for the improvement of the mind, for the study of God's word, for secret prayer, or for the prayer meeting. The mind is entirely taken up with planning how to appear as well as their sisters. To accomplish this end, physical, mental, and moral health is sacrificed. Happiness and the favor of God are laid upon the altar of fashion.

Many will not attend the service of God upon the Sabbath, because their dress would appear so unlike that of their Christian sisters in style and adornment. Will my sisters consider these things as they are, and will they fully realize the weight of their influence upon others? By walking in a forbidden path themselves, they lead others in the same way of disobedience and backsliding. Christian simplicity is sacrificed to outward display. My sisters,

---

[1] Written in 1875, when money values were much greater than in later years.

how shall we change all this? How shall we recover ourselves from the snare of Satan and break the chains that
have bound us in slavery to fashion? How shall we recover our wasted opportunities? how bring our powers
into healthful, vigorous action? There is only one way,
and that is to make the Bible our rule of life. . . .

Many dress like the world, in order to have an influence over unbelievers; but here they make a sad mistake.
If they would have a true and saving influence, let them
live out their profession, show their faith by their righteous works, and make the distinction plain between the
Christian and the worldling. The words, the dress, the
actions, should tell for God. Then a holy influence will
be shed upon all around them, and even unbelievers will
take knowledge of them that they have been with Jesus.
If any wish to have their influence tell in favor of truth,
let them live out their profession and thus imitate the
humble Pattern.

Pride, ignorance, and folly are constant companions.
The Lord is displeased with the pride manifested among
His professed people. He is dishonored by their conformity to the unhealthful, immodest, and expensive fashions
of this degenerate age. . . .

Dress Reform

To protect the people of God from the corrupting influence of the world, as well as to promote physical and
moral health, the dress reform was introduced among us.
It was not intended to be a yoke of bondage, but a blessing, not to increase labor, but to save labor, not to add to
the expense of dress, but to save expense. It would distinguish God's people from the world and thus serve as
a barrier against its fashions and follies. He who knows

the end from the beginning, who understands our nature and our needs,—our compassionate Redeemer,—saw our dangers and difficulties, and condescended to give us timely warning and instruction concerning our habits of life, even in the proper selection of food and clothing.

Satan is constantly devising some new style of dress that shall prove an injury to physical and moral health; and he exults when he sees professed Christians eagerly accepting the fashions that he has invented. The amount of physical suffering created by unnatural and unhealthful dress cannot be estimated. Many have become lifelong invalids through their compliance with the demands of fashion. . . .

Among these pernicious fashions were the large hoops, which frequently caused indecent exposure of the person. In contrast with this was presented a neat, modest, becoming dress, which would dispense with the hoops and the trailing skirts, and provide for the proper clothing of the limbs. But dress reform comprised more than shortening the dress and clothing the limbs. It included every article of dress upon the person. It lifted the weights from the hips by suspending the skirts from the shoulders. It removed the tight corsets, which compress the lungs, the stomach, and other internal organs, and induce curvature of the spine and an almost countless train of diseases. Dress reform proper provided for the protection and development of every part of the body.[1] . . .

Our Dress a Testimony

Many a soul who was convinced of the truth has been led to decide against it by the pride and love of the world

---

[1] For the reasons why this style of dress is not now advocated, read *Testimonies for the Church*, vol. 4, pp. 635-641.

displayed by our sisters. The doctrine preached seemed clear and harmonious, and the hearers felt that a heavy cross must be lifted by them in taking the truth. When these persons have seen our sisters making so much display in dress, they have said, "This people dress fully as much as we do. They cannot really believe what they profess; and, after all, they must be deceived. If they really thought that Christ was soon coming, and the case of every soul was to be decided for eternal life or death, they could not devote time and money to dress according to the existing fashions." How little did those professedly believing sisters know of the sermon their dress was preaching!

Our words, our actions, and our dress are daily, living preachers, gathering with Christ, or scattering abroad. This is no trivial matter, to be passed off with a jest. The subject of dress demands serious reflection and much prayer. . . .

We would by no means encourage carelessness in dress. Let the attire be appropriate and becoming. Though only a ten-cent calico, it should be kept neat and clean. If there are no ruffles, the wearer can not only save something by making it herself, but she can save quite a little sum by washing and ironing it herself. Families bind heavy burdens upon themselves by dressing their children in accordance with the fashion. What a waste of time! The little ones would look very inviting in a dress without a ruffle or ornament, but kept sweet and clean. It is such a trifle to wash and iron a dress of this style that the labor is not felt to be a burden. . . .

Children Subjected to Fashion

But the greatest evil is the influence upon the children and youth. Almost as soon as they come into the world they are subjected to fashion's demands. Little children hear more of dress than of their salvation. They see their mothers more earnestly consulting the fashion plates than the Bible. More visits are made to the dry-goods dealer and the milliner than to the church. The outward display of dress is made of greater consequence than the adornment of the character. Sharp reprimands are called forth for soiling the fine clothing, and the mind becomes peevish and irritable under continual restraint.

A deformed character does not disturb the mother so much as a soiled dress. The child hears more of dress than of virtue, for the mother is more familiar with fashion than with her Saviour. Her example too often surrounds the young with a poisonous atmosphere. Vice, disguised in fashion's garb, intrudes itself among the children.

Simplicity of dress will make a sensible woman appear to the best advantage. We judge of a person's character by the style of dress worn. Gaudy apparel betrays vanity and weakness. A modest, godly woman will dress modestly. A refined taste, a cultivated mind, will be revealed in the choice of simple and appropriate attire.

The Imperishable Ornament

There is an ornament that will never perish, that will promote the happiness of all around us in this life and will shine with undimmed luster in the immortal future. It is the adorning of a meek and lowly spirit. God has bidden us wear the richest dress upon the soul. By every look into the mirror the worshipers of fashion should be reminded of the neglected soul. Every hour squandered over the toilet should reprove them for leaving the intellect to lie waste. Then there might be a reformation that would elevate and ennoble all the aims and purposes of life. Instead of seeking golden ornaments for the exterior, an earnest effort would be put forth to secure that wisdom which is of more value than fine gold, yea, which is more precious than rubies. . . .

Effect of Dress on Morals

The love of dress endangers the morals and makes woman the opposite of the Christian lady, characterized by modesty and sobriety. Showy, extravagant dress too often encourages lust in the heart of the wearer and awakens base passions in the heart of the beholder. God sees that the ruin of the character is frequently preceded by the indulgence of pride and vanity in dress. He sees that the costly apparel stifles the desire to do good.

The more means persons expend in dress, the less they can have to feed the hungry and clothe the naked; and the streams of beneficence, which should be constantly flowing, are dried up. Every dollar saved by denying one's self of useless ornaments may be given to the needy, or may be placed in the Lord's treasury to sustain the gospel, to send missionaries to foreign countries, to multiply publications to carry rays of light to souls in the darkness of error. Every dollar used unnecessarily deprives the spender of a precious opportunity to do good. . . .

When you place a useless or extravagant article of clothing upon your person, you are withholding from the naked. When you spread your tables with a needless variety of costly food, you are neglecting to feed the hungry. How stands your record, professed Christian? Do not, I beseech you, lay out in foolish and hurtful indulgences that which God requires in His treasury, and the portion which should be given to the poor. Let us not clothe ourselves with costly apparel, but, like women professing godliness, with good works. Let not the cry of the widow and the fatherless go up to Heaven against us. Let not the blood of souls be found on our garments. Let not precious probationary time be squandered in cherishing pride of heart. Are there no poor to be visited? no dim eyes for whom you can read the word of God? no desponding, discouraged ones that need your words of comfort and your prayers? . . .

Do not, my sisters, trifle longer with your own souls and with God. I have been shown that the main cause of your backsliding is your love of dress. This leads to the neglect of grave responsibilities, and you find yourselves with scarcely a spark of the love of God in your hearts. Without delay renounce the cause of your backsliding, because it is sin against your own soul and against God. Be not hardened by the deceitfulness of sin.

As a people, we are looked upon as peculiar. Our position and faith distinguish us from every other denomination. If we are in life and character no better than the world, they will point the finger of scorn at us and say, "These are Seventh-day Adventists." "We have here a sample of the people who keep the seventh day for Sunday." The stigma which should be rightfully attached to such a class is thus placed upon all who are conscientiously keeping the seventh day. Oh, how much better it would be if such a class would not make any pretension to obey the truth!—*Testimonies for the Church,* vol. 5, p. 138 (1882).

Reference for further study: *The Ministry of Healing,* pages 287-294, "Dress."

20—C.O.H.

Extremes in Dress

We as a people do not believe it our duty to go out of the world to be out of the fashion. If we have a neat, plain, modest, and comfortable plan of dress, and world-lings choose to dress as we do, shall we change this mode of dress in order to be different from the world? No, we should not be odd or singular in our dress for the sake of differing from the world, lest they despise us for so doing. Christians are the light of the world, the salt of the earth. Their dress should be neat and modest, their conversation chaste and heavenly, and their deportment blameless.

How shall we dress? If any wore heavy quilts before the introduction of hoops, merely for show and not for comfort, they sinned against themselves by injuring their health, which it is their duty to preserve. If any wear them now merely to look like hoops, they commit sin; for they are seeking to imitate a fashion which is dis-graceful. Corded skirts were worn before hoops were introduced. I have worn a light corded skirt since I was fourteen years of age, not for show but for comfort and decency. Because hoops were introduced I did not lay off my corded skirt for them. Shall I now throw it aside because the fashion of hoops is introduced? No; that would be carrying the matter to an extreme.

I should ever bear in mind that I must be an example and therefore must not run into this or that fashion, but pursue an even and independent course and not be driven to extremes in regard to dress. To throw off my corded skirt that was always modest and comfortable, and put on a thin cotton skirt, and thus appear ridiculous in the other extreme, would be wrong, for then I would not set a right example, but would put an argument into the

Testimonies for the Church, vol. 1, pp. 424-426 (1864).

mouths of hoop wearers. To justify themselves for wearing hoops they would point to me as one who does not wear them, and say that they would not disgrace themselves in that way. By going to such extremes we would destroy all the influence which we might otherwise have had, and lead the wearers of hoops to justify their course. We must dress modestly, without the least regard to the hoop fashion.

There is a medium position in these things. O that we all might wisely find that position and keep it. In this solemn time let us all search our own hearts, repent of our sins, and humble ourselves before God. The work is between God and our own souls. It is an individual work, and all will have enough to do without criticizing the dress, actions, and motives of their brethren and sisters. "Seek ye the Lord, all ye meek of the earth, which have wrought His judgments; seek righteousness, seek meekness: it may be ye shall be hid in the day of the Lord's anger." Zephaniah 2:3. Here is our work. It is not sinners who are here addressed, but all the meek of the earth, who have wrought His judgments, or kept His commandments. There is work for everyone, and if all will obey we shall see sweet union in the ranks of Sabbathkeepers.

Immodest Dresses

We do not think it in accordance with our faith to dress in the American costume, to wear hoops, or to go to an extreme in wearing long dresses which sweep the sidewalks and streets. If women would wear their dresses so as to clear the filth of the streets an inch or two, their dresses would be modest, and they could be kept clean much more easily and would wear longer. Such a dress would be in accordance with our faith.—*Testimonies for the Church,* vol. 1, p. 424 (1864).

Parents as Reformers

The work of temperance must begin in our families, at our tables. Mothers have an important work to do that they may give to the world, through correct discipline and education, children who will be capable of filling almost any position and who can also honor and enjoy the duties of domestic life.

The work of the mother is very important and sacred. She should teach her children from the cradle to practice habits of self-denial and self-control. If her time is mostly occupied with the follies of this degenerate age, if dress and parties engage her precious time, her children fail to receive that education which it is essential they should have in order that they may form correct characters. The anxiety of the Christian mother should not be in regard to the external merely, but that her children may have healthy constitutions and good morals.

Many mothers who deplore the intemperance which exists everywhere do not look deep enough to see the cause. They are daily preparing a variety of dishes and highly seasoned food which tempt the appetite and encourage overeating. The tables of our American people are generally prepared in a manner to make drunkards. Appetite is the ruling principle with a large class. Whoever will indulge appetite in eating too often, and food not of a healthful quality, is weakening his power to resist the clamors of appetite and passion in other respects in proportion as he has strengthened the propensity to incorrect habits of eating. Mothers need to be impressed with their obligation to God and to the world to furnish society with children having well-developed characters.

Testimonies for the Church, vol. 3, pp. 562-568 (1875).

Men and women who come upon the stage of action with firm principles will be fitted to stand unsullied amid the moral pollutions of this corrupt age. It is the duty of mothers to improve their golden opportunities to correctly educate their children for usefulness and duty. . . .

Where Intemperance Begins

We repeat, intemperance commences at our tables. The appetite is indulged until its indulgence becomes second nature. By the use of tea and coffee an appetite is formed for tobacco, and this encourages the appetite for liquors.

Many parents, to avoid the task of patiently educating their children to habits of self-denial, and teaching them how to make a right use of all the blessings of God, indulge them in eating and drinking whenever they please. Appetite and selfish indulgence, unless positively restrained, grow with the growth and strengthen with the strength. When these children commence life for themselves and take their place in society, they are powerless to resist temptation. Moral impurity and gross iniquity abound everywhere. The temptation to indulge taste and to gratify inclination has not lessened with the increase of years, and youth in general are governed by impulse and are slaves to appetite. In the glutton, the tobacco devotee, the winebibber, and the inebriate, we see the evil results of defective education.

When we hear the sad lamentations of Christian men and women over the terrible evils of intemperance, the questions at once arise in the mind: Who have educated the youth and given them their stamp of character? Who have fostered in them the appetites they have acquired? . . .

I saw that Satan, through his temptations, is instituting ever-changing fashions and attractive parties and amusements, that mothers may be led to devote their God-given probationary time to frivolous matters, so that they can have but little opportunity to educate and properly train their children. Our youth want mothers who will teach them from their very cradles to control passion, to deny appetite, and to overcome selfishness. They need line upon line and precept upon precept, here a little and there a little.

Direction was given to the Hebrews how to train their children to avoid the idolatry and wickedness of the heathen nations: "Therefore shall ye lay up these My words in your heart and in your soul, and bind them for a sign upon your hand, that they may be as frontlets between your eyes. And ye shall teach them your children, speaking of them when thou sittest in thine house, and when thou walkest by the way, when thou liest down, and when thou risest up." Deuteronomy 11:18, 19. . . .

The Mother's Responsibility

We address Christian mothers. We entreat that you feel your responsibility as mothers, and that you live not to please yourselves, but to glorify God. . . . Woman is to fill a more sacred and elevated position in the family than the king upon his throne. Her great work is to make her life a living example which she would wish her children to copy. By precept as well as example, she is to store their minds with useful knowledge and lead them to self-sacrificing labor for the good of others. The great stimulus to the toiling, burdened mother should be that every child who is trained aright and who has the inward adorning, the ornament of a meek and quiet spirit, will have a fitness for heaven and will shine in the courts of the Lord. . . .

If children and youth were trained and educated to habits of self-denial and self-control, if they were taught that they eat to live instead of living to eat, there would be less disease and less moral corruption. There would be little necessity for temperance crusades, . . . if in the youth, who form and fashion society, right principles in regard to temperance could be implanted. They would then have moral worth and moral integrity to resist, in the strength of Jesus, the pollutions of these last days.

Temperance in the Home

It is a most difficult matter to unlearn the habits which have been indulged through life and have educated the appetite. The demon of intemperance is not easily conquered. It is of giant strength and hard to overcome. But let parents begin a crusade against intemperance at their own firesides, in their own families, in the principles they teach their children to follow from their very infancy, and they may hope for success. It will pay you, mothers, to use the precious hours which are given you of God in forming, developing, and training the characters of your children, and in teaching them to strictly adhere to the principles of temperance in eating and drinking.

Parents may have transmitted to their children tendencies to appetite and passion, which will make more difficult the work of educating and training these children to be strictly temperate and to have pure and virtuous habits. If the appetite for unhealthy food and for stimulants and narcotics has been transmitted to them as a legacy from their parents, what a fearfully solemn responsibility rests upon the parents to counteract the evil tendencies which they have given to their children! How earnestly and diligently should the parents work to do their duty, in faith and hope, to their unfortunate offspring!

Parents should make it their first business to understand the laws of life and health, that nothing shall be done by them in the preparation of food, or through any other habits, which will develop wrong tendencies in their children. How carefully should mothers study to prepare their tables with the most simple, healthful food, that the digestive organs may not be weakened, the nervous forces unbalanced, and the instruction which they should give their children counteracted, by the food placed before them. This food either weakens or strengthens the organs of the stomach, and has much to do in controlling the physical and moral health of the children. ... Those who indulge the appetite of their children, and do not control their passions, will see the terrible mistake they have made in the tobacco-loving, liquor-drinking slave, whose senses are benumbed and whose lips utter falsehoods and profanity.

When parents and children meet at the final reckoning, what a scene will be presented! Thousands of children who have been slaves to appetite and debasing vice, whose lives are moral wrecks, will stand face to face with the parents who made them what they are. Who but the parents must bear this fearful responsibility?

References for further study: *The Ministry of Healing,* pages 349-406, "The Home;" *Education,* pages 195-201, "Study of Physiology."

Beware of Moral Corruption

If the sisters were elevated and possessed purity of heart, any corrupt advances, even from their minister, would be repulsed with such positiveness as would never need a repetition. Minds must be terribly befogged by Satan, when they can listen to the voice of the seducer because he is a minister, and therefore break God's plain and positive commands and flatter themselves that they commit no sin. Have we not the words of John, "He that saith, I know Him, and keepeth not His commandments, is a liar, and the truth is not in him"? 1 John 2:4. What saith the law? "Thou shalt not commit adultery." Exodus 20:14. When a man professing to keep God's holy law, and ministering in sacred things, takes advantage of the confidence his position gives him and seeks to indulge his base passions, this fact should of itself be sufficient to enable a woman professing godliness to see that, although his profession was as exalted as the heavens, an impure proposal coming from him was from Satan disguised as an angel of light. I cannot believe that the word of God is abiding in the hearts of those who so readily yield up their innocency and virtue upon the altar of lustful passions.

My sisters, avoid even the appearance of evil. In this fast age, reeking with corruption, you are not safe unless you stand guarded. Virtue and modesty are rare. I appeal to you as followers of Christ, making an exalted profession, to cherish the precious, priceless gem of modesty. This will guard virtue. If you have any hope of being finally exalted to join the company of the pure, sinless angels and to live in an atmosphere where there is not

Testimonies for the Church, vol. 2, pp. 457-460 (1868).

the least taint of sin, cherish modesty and virtue. Nothing but purity, sacred purity, will stand the grand review, abide the day of God, and be received into a pure and holy heaven.

Resent Undue Familiarity

The slightest insinuations, from whatever source they may come, inviting you to indulge in sin or to allow the least unwarrantable liberty with your persons, should be resented as the worst of insults to your dignified womanhood. The kiss upon your cheek, at an improper time and place, should lead you to repel the emissary of Satan with disgust. If it is from one in high places, who is dealing in sacred things, the sin is of tenfold greater magnitude and should lead a God-fearing woman or youth to recoil with horror, not only from the sin he would have you commit, but from the hypocrisy and villainy of one whom the people respect and honor as God's servant. He is handling sacred things, yet hiding his baseness of heart under a ministerial cloak. Be afraid of anything like this familiarity. Be sure that the least approach to it is evidence of a lascivious mind and a lustful eye. If the least encouragement is given in this direction, if any of the liberties mentioned are tolerated, no better evidence can be given that your mind is not pure and chaste as it should be, and that sin and crime have charms for you. You lower the standard of your dignified, virtuous womanhood and give unmistakable evidence that a low, brutal, common passion and lust has been suffered to remain alive in your heart and has never been crucified.

As I have been shown the dangers of those who profess better things, and the sins that exist among them, —a class who are not suspected of being in any danger from these polluting sins,—I have been led to inquire,

Who, O Lord, shall stand when Thou appearest? Only those who have clean hands and pure hearts shall abide the day of His coming.

Modesty and Reserve

I feel impelled by the Spirit of the Lord to urge my sisters who profess godliness to cherish modesty of deportment and a becoming reserve, with shamefacedness and sobriety. The liberties taken in this age of corruption should be no criterion for Christ's followers. These fashionable exhibitions of familiarity should not exist among Christians fitting for immortality. If lasciviousness, pollution, adultery, crime, and murder are the order of the day among those who know not the truth and who refuse to be controlled by the principles of God's word, how important that the class professing to be followers of Christ, closely allied to God and angels, should show them a better and nobler way! How important that by their chastity and virtue they stand in marked contrast to that class who are controlled by brute passions!

I have inquired, When will the youthful sisters act with propriety? I know there will be no decided change for the better until parents feel the importance of greater carefulness in educating their children correctly. Teach them to act with reserve and modesty. Educate them for usefulness, to be helps, to minister to others rather than to be waited upon and be ministered to.

Satan controls the minds of the youth in general. Your daughters are not taught self-denial and self-control. They are petted and their pride is fostered. They are allowed to have their own way, until they become headstrong and self-willed, and you are put to your wit's end to know what course to pursue to save them from ruin. Satan is leading them on to be a proverb in the mouth of unbelievers, because of their boldness, their lack of reserve and womanly modesty. The young boys are likewise left to have their own way. They have scarcely entered their teens before they are by the side of little girls of their own age, accompanying them home and making love to them. And the parents are so completely in bondage through their own indulgence and mistaken love for their children that they dare not pursue a decided course to make a change and restrain their too-fast children in this fast age.

With many young ladies the boys are the theme of conversations; with the young men, it is the girls. "Out of the abundance of the heart the mouth speaketh." Matthew 12:34. They talk of those subjects upon which their minds mostly run. The recording angel is writing the words of these professed Christian boys and girls. How will they be confused and ashamed when they meet them again in the day of God! Many children are pious hypocrites. The youth who have not made a profession of religion stumble over these hypocritical ones, and are hardened against any effort that may be made by those interested in their salvation.

The Only Safety

The more responsible the position, the more essential that the influence be right. Every man whom God has chosen to do a special work becomes a target for Satan. Temptations press thick and fast upon him; for our vigilant foe knows that his course of action has a molding influence upon others. . . . The only safety for any of us is in clinging to Jesus and letting nothing separate the soul from the mighty Helper.—*Testimonies for the Church,* vol. 5, pp. 428, 429 (1885).

Servants of Sin

I have been shown that we live amid the perils of the last days. Because iniquity abounds, the love of many waxes cold. The word "many" refers to the professed followers of Christ. They are affected by the prevailing iniquity, and backslide from God; but it is not necessary that they should be thus affected. The cause of this declension is that they do not stand clear from this iniquity. The fact that their love to God is waxing cold because iniquity abounds, shows that they are, in some sense, partakers in this iniquity, or it would not affect their love for God and their zeal and fervor in His cause.

A terrible picture of the condition of the world has been presented before me. Immorality abounds everywhere. Licentiousness is the special sin of this age. Never did vice lift its deformed head with such boldness as now. The people seem to be benumbed, and the lovers of virtue and true goodness are nearly discouraged by its boldness, strength, and prevalence. The iniquity which abounds is not merely confined to the unbeliever and the scoffer. Would that this were the case; but it is not. Many men and women who profess the religion of Christ are guilty. Even some who profess to be looking for His appearing are no more prepared for that event than Satan himself. They are not cleansing themselves from all pollution. They have so long served their lust that it is natural for their thoughts to be impure and their imaginations corrupt. It is as impossible to cause their minds to dwell upon pure and holy things as it would be to turn the course of Niagara and send its waters pouring up the falls.

Testimonies for the Church, vol. 2, pp. 346-353 (1869).

Youth Ensnared

Youth and children of both sexes engage in moral pollution and practice this disgusting, soul-and-body-destroying vice. Many professed Christians are so benumbed by the same practice that their moral sensibilities cannot be aroused to understand that it is sin, and that if continued its sure results will be utter shipwreck of body and mind. Man, the noblest being upon the earth, formed in the image of God, transforms himself into a beast! He makes himself gross and corrupt. Every Christian will have to learn to restrain his passions and be controlled by principle. Unless he does this, he is unworthy of the Christian name.

Some who make a high profession do not understand the sin of self-abuse and its sure results. Long-established habit has blinded their understanding. They do not realize the exceeding sinfulness of this degrading sin, which is enervating the system and destroying their brain nerve power. Moral principle is exceedingly weak when it conflicts with established habit. Solemn messages from Heaven cannot forcibly impress the heart that is not fortified against the indulgence of this degrading vice. The sensitive nerves of the brain have lost their healthy tone by morbid excitation to gratify an unnatural desire for sensual indulgence. The brain nerves which communicate with the entire system are the only medium through which Heaven can communicate to man, and affect his inmost life. Whatever disturbs the circulation of the electric currents in the nervous system, lessens the strength of the vital powers, and the result is a deadening of the sensibilities of the mind. In consideration of these facts, how important that ministers and people who profess godliness should stand forth clear and untainted from this soul-debasing vice!

My soul has been bowed down with anguish as I have been shown the weak condition of God's professed people. Iniquity abounds, and the love of many waxes cold. There are but few professed Christians who regard this matter in the right light and who hold proper government over themselves when public opinion and custom do not condemn them. How few restrain their passions because they feel under moral obligation to do so, and because the fear of God is before their eyes! The higher faculties of man are enslaved by appetite and corrupt passions.

Some will acknowledge the evil of sinful indulgences, yet will excuse themselves by saying that they cannot overcome their passions. This is a terrible admission for any person to make who names Christ. "Let everyone that nameth the name of Christ depart from iniquity." 2 Timothy 2:19. Why is this weakness? It is because the animal propensities have been strengthened by exercise, until they have gained the ascendancy over the higher powers. Men and women lack principle. They are dying spiritually, because they have so long pampered their natural appetites that their power of self-government seems gone. The lower passions of their nature have taken the reins, and that which should be the governing power has become the servant of corrupt passion. The soul is held in lowest bondage. Sensuality has quenched the desire for holiness, and withered spiritual prosperity.

Fruits of Indolence

My soul mourns for the youth who are forming characters in this degenerate age. I tremble for their parents also, for I have been shown that as a general thing they do not understand their obligations to train up their children in the way they should go. Custom and fashion are consulted, and the children soon learn to be swayed by these and are corrupted, while their indulgent parents are themselves benumbed and asleep to their danger. But very few of the youth are free from corrupt habits. They are excused from physical exercise to a great degree for fear they will overwork. The parents bear burdens themselves which their children should bear. Overwork is bad; but the result of indolence is more to be dreaded.

Idleness leads to the indulgence of corrupt habits. Industry does not weary and exhaust one fifth part as much as the pernicious habit of self-abuse. If simple, well-regulated labor exhausts your children, be assured, parents, there is something, aside from their labor, which is enervating their systems and producing a sense of constant weariness. Give your children physical labor which will call into exercise the nerves and muscles. The weariness attending such labor will lessen their inclination to indulge in vicious habits. Idleness is a curse. It produces licentious habits.

Many cases have been presented before me, and as I have had a view of their inner lives, my soul has been sick and disgusted with the rottenheartedness of human beings who profess godliness and talk of translation to heaven. I have frequently asked myself, Whom can I trust? Who is free from iniquity?

An Example of Degradation

My husband and myself once attended a meeting where our sympathies were enlisted for a brother who was a great sufferer with the phthisic. He was pale and emaciated. He requested the prayers of the people of God.

He said that his family were sick, and that he had lost a child. He spoke with feeling of his bereavement. He said that he had been waiting for some time to see Brother and Sister White. He believed that if they would pray for him, he would be healed. After the meeting closed, the brethren called our attention to the case. They said that the church was assisting them; that his wife was sick, and his child had died. The brethren had met at his house, and united in praying for the afflicted family. We were much worn, and had the burden of labor upon us during the meeting, and wished to be excused.

I had resolved not to engage in prayer for anyone, unless the Spirit of the Lord should dictate in the matter. I had been shown that there was so much iniquity abounding, even among professed Sabbathkeepers, that I did not wish to unite in prayer for those of whose history I had no knowledge. I stated my reason. I was assured by the brethren that, as far as they knew, he was a worthy brother. I conversed a few words with the one who had solicited our prayers that he might be healed; but I could not feel free. He wept, and said that he had waited for us to come, and he felt assured that if we would pray for him he would be restored to health. We told him that we were unacquainted with his life; that we would rather those who knew him would pray for him. He importuned us so earnestly that we decided to consider his case, and present it before the Lord that night; and if the way seemed clear, we would comply with his request.

That night we bowed in prayer, and presented his case before the Lord. We entreated that we might know the will of God concerning him. All we desired was that

God might be glorified. Would the Lord have us pray for this afflicted man? We left the burden with the Lord, and retired to rest. In a dream the case of that man was clearly presented. His course from his childhood up was shown, and that if we should pray, the Lord would not hear us; for he regarded iniquity in his heart. The next morning the man came for us to pray for him. We took him aside, and told him we were sorry to be compelled to refuse his request. I related my dream, which he acknowledged was true. He had practiced self-abuse from his boyhood up, and he had continued the practice during his married life, but said he would try to break himself of it.

This man had a long-established habit to overcome. He was in the middle age of life. His moral principles were so weak that when brought in conflict with long-established indulgence they were overcome. The baser passions had gained the ascendancy over the higher nature. I asked him in regard to health reform. He said he could not live it. His wife would throw graham flour out of doors, if it were brought into the house. This family had been helped by the church. Prayer had also been offered in their behalf. Their child had died, the wife was sick, and the husband and father would leave his case upon us, for us to bring before a pure and holy God, that He might work a miracle and make him well. The moral sensibilities of this man were benumbed.

When the young adopt vile practices while the spirit is tender, they will never obtain force to fully and correctly develop physical, intellectual, and moral character. Here was a man debasing himself daily, and yet daring to venture into the presence of God and ask an increase of strength which he had vilely squandered and which, if granted, he would consume upon his lust. What forbearance has God! If He should deal with man according to his corrupt ways, who could live in His sight? What if we had been less cautious and carried the case of this man before God while he was practicing iniquity; would the Lord have heard? Would He have answered? "For Thou art not a God that hath pleasure in wickedness: neither shall evil dwell with Thee. The foolish shall not stand in Thy sight: Thou hatest all workers of iniquity." Psalm 5:4, 5. "If I regard iniquity in my heart, the Lord will not hear me." Psalm 66:18.

This is not a solitary case. Even the marriage relation was not sufficient to preserve this man from the corrupt habits of his youth. I wish I could be convinced that such cases as the one I have presented are rare; but I know they are frequent. Children born to parents who are controlled by corrupt passions are worthless. What can be expected of such children, but that they will sink lower in the scale than their parents? What can be expected of the rising generation? Thousands are devoid of principle. These very ones are transmitting to their offspring their own miserable, corrupt passions. What a legacy! Thousands drag out their unprincipled lives, tainting their associates and perpetuating their debased passions by transmitting them to their children. They take the responsibility of giving to them the stamp of their own characters.

Moral Principle the Only Safeguard

I come again to Christians. If all who profess to obey the law of God were free from iniquity, my soul would be delivered; but they are not. Even some who profess to keep all the commandments of God are guilty of the sin of adultery. What can I say to arouse their benumbed sensibilities? Moral principle, strictly carried out, becomes the only safeguard of the soul. If ever there was a time when the diet should be of the most simple kind, it is now. Meat should not be placed before our children. Its influence is to excite and strengthen the lower passions and has a tendency to deaden the moral powers. Grains and fruits prepared free from grease, and in as natural a condition as possible, should be the food for the tables of all who claim to be preparing for translation to heaven. The less feverish the diet, the more easily can the passions be controlled. Gratification of taste should not be consulted irrespective of physical, intellectual, or moral health.

Indulgence of the baser passions will lead very many to shut their eyes to the light, for they fear that they will see sins which they are unwilling to forsake. All may see if they will. If they choose darkness rather than light, their criminality will be none the less. Why do not men and women read, and become intelligent upon these things, which so decidedly affect their physical, intellectual, and moral strength? God has given you a habitation to care for and preserve in the best condition for His service and glory. Your bodies are not your own. "What? know ye not that your body is the temple of the Holy Ghost which is in you, which ye have of God, and ye are not your own? For ye are bought with a price: therefore glorify God in your body, and in your spirit, which are God's." 1 Corinthians 6:19, 20. "Know ye not that ye are the temple of God, and that the Spirit of God dwelleth in you? If any man defile the temple of God, him shall God destroy; for the temple of God is holy, which temple ye are." 1 Corinthians 3:16, 17.

Blinded by Sin

Satan rejoices to have sinners enter the church as professed Sabbathkeepers, while they allow him to control their minds and affections, using them to deceive and corrupt others.

In this degenerate age many will be found who are so blinded to the sinfulness of sin that they choose a licentious life, because it suits the natural and perverse inclination of the heart. Instead of facing the mirror, the law of God, and bringing their hearts and characters up to God's standard, they allow Satan's agents to erect his standard in their hearts. Corrupt men think it easier to misinterpret the Scriptures to sustain them in their iniquity, than to yield up their corruption and sin and be pure in heart and life.

There are more men of this stamp than many have imagined, and they will multiply as we draw near the end of time. Unless they are rooted and grounded in the truth of the Bible and have a living connection with God, many will be infatuated and deceived. Dangers unseen beset our path. Our only safety is in constant watchfulness and prayer. The nearer we live to Jesus, the more will we partake of His pure and holy character; and the more offensive sin appears to us, the more exalted and desirable will appear the purity and brightness of Christ. . . .

There is always a bewitching power in heresies and in licentiousness. The mind is so deluded that it cannot reason intelligently, and an illusion is continually leading it from purity. The spiritual eyesight becomes blurred, and persons of hitherto untainted morals become confused under the delusive sophistry of those agents of Satan who

Testimonies for the Church, vol. 5, pp. 141-147 (1882).

profess to be messengers of light. It is this delusion which gives these agents power. Should they come out boldly and make their advances openly, they would be repulsed without a moment's hesitation; but they work first to gain sympathy and secure confidence in them as holy, self-sacrificing men of God. As his special messengers, they then begin their artful work of drawing away souls from the path of rectitude, by attempting to make void the law of God.

When ministers thus take advantage of the confidence the people place in them and lead souls to ruin, they make themselves as much more guilty than the common sinner as their profession is higher. In the day of God, when the great Ledger of Heaven is opened, it will be found to contain the names of many ministers who have made pretensions to purity of heart and life and professed to be entrusted with the gospel of Christ, but who have taken advantage of their position to allure souls to transgress the law of God . . . .

If the society of a man of impure mind and licentious habits is chosen in preference to that of the virtuous and pure, it is a sure indication that the tastes and inclinations harmonize, that a low level of morals is reached. This level is called by these deceived, infatuated souls, a high and holy affinity of spirit—a spiritual harmony. But the apostle terms it "spiritual wickedness in high places," against which we are to institute a vigorous warfare.

When the deceiver commences his work of deception, he frequently finds dissimilarity of tastes and habits, but by great pretensions to godliness he gains the confidence, and when this is done, his wily, deceptive power is exercised in his own way, to carry out his devices. By associating with this dangerous element, women become accustomed to breathe the atmosphere of impurity and almost insensibly become permeated with the same spirit. Their identity is lost; they become the shadow of their seducer.

Hypocritical Reformers

Men professing to have new light, claiming to be reformers, will have great influence over a certain class who are convinced of the heresies that exist in the present age and who are not satisfied with the spiritual condition of the churches. With true, honest hearts, these desire to see a change for the better, a coming up to a higher standard. If the faithful servants of Christ would present the truth, pure and unadulterated, to this class, they would accept it and purify themselves by obeying it. But Satan, ever vigilant, sets upon the track of these inquiring souls. Someone making high profession as a reformer comes to them, as Satan came to Christ, disguised as an angel of light, and draws them still farther from the path of right.

The unhappiness and degradation that follow in the train of licentiousness cannot be estimated. The world is defiled under its inhabitants. They have nearly filled up the measure of their iniquity; but that which will bring the heaviest retribution, is the practice of iniquity under the cloak of godliness. The Redeemer of the world never spurned true repentance, however great the guilt; but He hurls burning denunciations against Pharisees and hypocrites. There is more hope for the open sinner than for this class. . . .

As Christ's ambassador, I entreat you who profess present truth to promptly resent any approach to impurity and forsake the society of those who breathe an impure suggestion. Loathe these defiling sins with the most intense hatred. Flee from those who would, even in conversation, let the mind run in such a channel; "for out of the abundance of the heart the mouth speaketh." Matthew 12:34.

As those who practice these defiling sins are steadily increasing in the world and would intrude themselves into our churches, I warn you to give no place to them. Turn from the seducer. Though a professed follower of Christ, he is Satan in the form of man; he has borrowed the livery of heaven that he may the better serve his master. You should not for one moment give place to an impure, covert suggestion; for even this will stain the soul, as impure water defiles the channel through which it passes.

Choose poverty, reproach, separation from friends, or any suffering, rather than to defile the soul with sin. Death before dishonor or the transgression of God's law, should be the motto of every Christian. As a people professing to be reformers, treasuring the most solemn, purifying truths of God's word, we must elevate the standard far higher than it is at the present time. Sin and sinners in the church must be promptly dealt with, that others may not be contaminated. Truth and purity require that we make more thorough work to cleanse the camp from Achans. Let those in responsible positions not suffer sin in a brother. Show him that he must either put away his sins or be separated from the church.

Godliness and Health

The wise man says that wisdom's "ways are ways of pleasantness, and all her paths are peace." Proverbs 3:17. Many cherish the impression that devotion to God is detrimental to health and to cheerful happiness in the social relations of life. But those who walk in the path of wisdom and holiness find that "godliness is profitable unto all things, having promise of the life that now is, and of that which is to come." 1 Timothy 4:8. They are alive to the enjoyment of life's real pleasures, while they are not troubled with vain regrets over misspent hours, nor with gloom or horror of mind, as the worldling too often is when not diverted by some exciting amusement. . . .

Godliness does not conflict with the laws of health, but is in harmony with them. Had men ever been obedient to the law of Ten Commandments, had they carried out in their lives the principles of these ten precepts, the curse of disease that now floods the world would not be. Men may teach that trifling amusements are necessary to keep the mind above despondency. The mind may indeed be thus diverted for the time being; but after the excitement is over, calm reflection comes. Conscience arouses and makes her voice heard, saying, "This is not the way to obtain health or true happiness."

There are many amusements that excite the mind, but depression is sure to follow. Other modes of recreation are innocent and healthful; but useful labor that affords physical exercise will often have a more beneficial influence upon the mind, while at the same time it will strengthen the muscles, improve the circulation, and prove a powerful agent in the recovery of health.

Signs of the Times, Oct. 23, 1884.

"What man is he that desireth life, and loveth many days, that he may see good? Keep thy tongue from evil, and thy lips from speaking guile. Depart from evil, and do good; seek peace, and pursue it. The eyes of the Lord are upon the righteous, and His ears are open unto their cry. The face of the Lord is against them that do evil, to cut off the remembrance of them from the earth. The righteous cry, and the Lord heareth, and delivereth them out of all their troubles." Psalm 34:12-17.

Rightdoing the Best Medicine

The consciousness of rightdoing is the best medicine for diseased bodies and minds. The special blessing of God resting upon the receiver is health and strength. One whose mind is quiet and satisfied in God is on the highway to health. To have the consciousness that the eye of the Lord is upon us, and that His ear is open to our prayers, is a satisfaction indeed. To know that we have a never-failing Friend to whom we can confide all the secrets of the soul, is a happiness which words can never express. Those whose moral faculties are clouded by disease are not the ones to rightly represent the Christian life or the beauties of holiness. They are too often in the fire of fanaticism or the water of cold indifference or stolid gloom.

Those who do not feel that it is a religious duty to discipline the mind to dwell upon cheerful subjects, will usually be found at one of two extremes: they will be elated by a continual round of exciting amusements, indulging in frivolous conversation, laughing and joking, or they will be depressed, having great trials and mental conflicts, which they think but few have ever experienced or can understand. These persons may profess Christianity, but they deceive their own souls. . . .

Idleness and Despondency

Despondent feelings are frequently the result of too much leisure. The hands and mind should be occupied in useful labor, lightening the burdens of others; and those who are thus employed will benefit themselves also. Idleness gives time to brood over imaginary sorrows; and frequently those who do not have real hardships and trials, will borrow them from the future.

There is much deception carried on under the cover of religion. Passion controls the minds of many who have become depraved in thought and feeling in consequence of "pride, fullness of bread, and abundance of idleness." Ezekiel 16:49. These deceived souls flatter themselves that they are spiritually minded and especially consecrated, when their religious experience consists in a sickly sentimentalism rather than in purity, true goodness, and humiliation of self. The mind should be drawn away from self; its powers should be exercised in devising means to make others happier and better. "Pure religion and undefiled before God and the Father is this, To visit the fatherless and widows in their affliction, and to keep himself unspotted from the world." James 1:27.

True Religion Ennobles the Mind

True religion ennobles the mind, refines the taste, sanctifies the judgment, and makes its possessor a partaker of the purity and the holiness of heaven. It brings angels near and separates us more and more from the spirit and influence of the world. It enters into all the acts and relations of life and gives us the "spirit of a sound mind," and the result is happiness and peace.

Said the apostle Paul to his Philippian brethren, "Finally, brethren, whatsoever things are true, whatsoever things are honest, whatsoever things are just, whatsoever things are pure, whatsoever things are lovely, whatsoever things are of good report; if there be any virtue, and if there be any praise, think on these things." Adopt this as the rule of life. "Be careful for nothing; but in everything by prayer and supplication with thanksgiving let your request be made known unto God. And the peace of God, which passeth all understanding, shall keep your hearts and minds through Christ Jesus." Philippians 4:8, 6, 7.

Reference for further study: *Testimonies for the Church,* vol. 4, pp. 552-554, "Health and Religion."

An Advance Step

The work of educating in medical missionary lines is an advance step of great importance in awakening man to his moral responsibilities. Had the ministers taken hold of this work in its various departments in accordance with the light which God has given, there would have been a most decided reformation in eating, drinking, and dressing. But some have stood directly in the way of the advance of health reform. They have held the people back by their indifferent or condemnatory remarks, or by pleasantries and jokes. They themselves and a large number of others have been sufferers unto death, but all have not yet learned wisdom.—*Testimonies for the Church,* vol. 6, p. 377 (1900).

Religion and Contentment

Satan found his way into Eden and made Eve believe that she needed something more than that which God had given for her happiness, that the forbidden fruit would have a special exhilarating influence upon her body and mind and would exalt her even to be equal with God in knowledge. But the knowledge and benefit she thought to gain proved to her a terrible curse.

There are persons with a diseased imagination to whom religion is a tyrant, ruling them as with a rod of iron. Such are constantly mourning over their depravity and groaning over supposed evil. Love does not exist in their hearts; a frown is ever upon their countenances. They are chilled with the innocent laugh from the youth or from anyone. They consider all recreation or amusement a sin and think that the mind must be constantly wrought up to just such a stern, severe pitch. This is one extreme. Others think that the mind must be ever on the stretch to invent new amusements and diversions in order to gain health. They learn to depend on excitement, and are uneasy without it. Such are not true Christians. They go to another extreme. The true principles of Christianity open before all a source of happiness, the height and depth, the length and breadth of which are immeasurable. It is Christ in us a well of water springing up into everlasting life. It is a continual wellspring from which the Christian can drink at will and never exhaust the fountain.

Borrowing Trouble Detrimental

That which brings sickness of body and mind to nearly all, is dissatisfied feelings and discontented repin-

Testimonies for the Church, vol. 1, pp. 565, 566 (1867).

ings. They have not God, they have not the hope which reaches to that within the veil, which is as an anchor to the soul both sure and steadfast. All who possess this hope will purify themselves even as He is pure. Such are free from restless longings, repinings, and discontent; they are not continually looking for evil and brooding over borrowed trouble. But we see many who are having a time of trouble beforehand; anxiety is stamped upon every feature; they seem to find no consolation, but have a continual fearful looking for of some dreadful evil.

Such dishonor God and bring the religion of Christ into disrepute. They have not true love for God, nor for their companions and children. Their affections have become morbid. But vain amusements will never correct the minds of such. They need the transforming influence of the Spirit of God in order to be happy. They need to be benefited by the meditation of Christ, in order to realize consolation, divine and substantial. "For he that will love life, and see good days, let him refrain his tongue from evil, and his lips that they speak no guile: let him eschew evil, and do good; let him speak peace, and ensue it. For the eyes of the Lord are over the righteous, and His ears are open unto their prayers: but the face of the Lord is against them that do evil." 1 Peter 3:10-12. Those who have an experimental knowledge of this scripture are truly happy. They consider the approbation of Heaven of more worth than any earthly amusement; Christ in them the hope of glory will be health to the body and strength to the soul.

The Need of Consecration

Ministers and physicians, in your work you are bearing weighty responsibilities. Let not your thoughts become cheap or common or selfish, for want of the grace of Christ. Our preparation for the home above must be wrought out in this life. The grace of Christ must be woven into every phase of the character.

I am to say to all who claim to be converted, Are your hearts truly changed, and are you watching unto prayer, preserving a thoughtful, consistent course of action, that you may have not a semblance of religion, but the precious, genuine article? Ministers and physicians, when you accepted Christ did you experience a deep sense of spiritual need? How much it means to you who are to be ministers of righteousness, to accept the heavenly gift of light and love and peace and joy in the Holy Spirit. You are to be imbued with such love for Christ that you will yield to Him your whole affections, surrendering your life to Him who gave His life for you. Imbued with the love of Christ, you are to be constrained to perform acts of unselfish service until such acts become your life practice. Daily growth into the life of Christ creates in the soul a heaven of peace; in such a life there is continual fruit bearing.

Brethren and sisters, we need the reformation that all who are redeemed must have, through the cleansing of mind and heart from every taint of sin. In the lives of those who are ransomed by the blood of Christ, self-sacrifice will constantly appear. Goodness and righteousness will be seen. The quiet, inward experience will make the life full of godliness, faith, meekness, patience. This is to be our daily experience. We are to form characters

Review and Herald, May 31, 1906.

free from sin—characters made righteous in and by the grace of Christ. . . . Our hearts are to be cleansed from all impurity in the blood shed to take away sin.

When ministers adorn the doctrine of Christ our Saviour, and when physicians reveal in words and works, and in their influence, the healing grace of Christ, when the Saviour is revealed as the One altogether lovely, a great work will be done in behalf of other souls. God calls for truth in the inner sanctuary of the soul, that the whole being may be a representation of the life of Christ. . . .

I entreat my brethren and sisters who are ministers or physicians, to work out in their lives the precious principles of truth, that others may take knowledge of you that you have been with Jesus and have learned of Him who is pure and holy and undefiled, without rebuke in a sinful and corrupt generation. Then many will be turned to the Lord through the earnest efforts made in their behalf by those who know the truth.

Total Abstinence

When temperance is presented as a part of the gospel, many will see their need of reform. They will see the evil of intoxicating liquors, and that total abstinence is the only platform on which God's people can conscientiously stand. As this instruction is given, the people will become interested in other lines of Bible study.—*Testimonies for the Church,* vol. 7, p. 75 (1902).

Scripture Index

21—C.O.H.

(635)

Index

Appetite—*continued*
  Christ's victory over 122
  conquer, lest temptation to
    indulge increase 574
  control of, learned in childhood
    114
    lesson in, from John the
      Baptist 72-74
  depraved, enshrined as an idol 68
    indulgence of, is sin 21
    of wealthy patients, not to
      cater to 287
  God demands cleansing of 127
  god with many 453
  gratification of, led to destruc-
    tion of Sodom 110
    not chief end of man 116
  indulged at expense of health 122
  indulged at expense of health and
    right principles, example of
    457, 458
  indulgence of, effect of, on spir-
    itual nature 576
    greatest cause of debility 130
    leads to debasing crimes 110
    results of Esau's 110
    results of, to whole life 152
    strengthens animal propen-
      sities 67
    unfits mind for spiritual
      worship 22
    wars against soul 575, 576
  inherited, counteract in childhood
    609, 610
  knowledge of health principles
    aids in battle with 440
  natural provision for gratifica-
    tion of 114
  of children, formed by parents
    125
  overcome through Christ's
    power 125
  power of 122-126
  power of will in control of 125
  principle enabled Daniel to tri-
    umph over 66
  regaining Eden through denial
    of 573, 574
  results of unrestrained indul-
    gence of 24
  results to Adam and Eve, of
    yielding to 108
  ruled antediluvians 109
  slavery to depraved 68
  teach the need of resisting 543
  temptation through, Adam's and
    Eve's 108, 109
  temptation to indulge, measured
    by Christ's temptation 122
  unnatural, indulged, lowers brain
    power 36
  which has no foundation in
    nature 83

  yielding to, broke allegiance
    to God 111
Appetites bequeathed by heredity 49
  See also Indulgence.
Applause not to be sought too
  ardently 384
Appreciation, sense of, gives physician courage 353
Approbation, love of 106
Argue not with weak conscience
  587
Argument for Christianity, deeds of
  unselfishness strongest 537
Ark, illustration of building insti-
  tutions today 278
Arm, right, of third angel's mes-
  sage 331, 434, 513-518
Associates, affected by wrong
  course 45
  character shown by choice of 624
  choice of, determines destiny 416
  importance of right choice of
    414, 415
  See also Youth.
Association, power of, for good or
  evil 414-419
  with worldlings, temptations
    through 423
Athletics, tendency of 189
Attainment, standard of, too low
  259
  See also Students ; Education.
Attainments, possibilities of, before the Christian 107
Australia, health instruction at
  camp meetings in 467
Avondale school, food industry at
  495, 496
  God spread table in wilderness
    at 495

BACKSLIDERS, hunt up 533
Balance, observe proper, in giving
  message 517, 518
Bathing, frequent, benefits of 104
Battle Creek, centralization in 510
  difficulties in establishing insti-
    tutions in 218
  too much centered in 217
Battle Creek Sanitarium, appeal to,
  to help other institutions 310
  donations received by, in early
    days 309
  duty of, to help Rural Health
    Retreat 309
  early experience in 282, 283
  prosperity of 309
Beans, dried, not all can digest 154
Beauty, God the author of all 92
Beer, discard 120
Beginning, humble 226
Behavior, unbecoming, grieves the
  Spirit 570

CAKES, rich 148, 152
Calamities, treat as blessings
    27
  visited upon cities 268
California, work in health lines to
    be done in 549
Call to distant field, wait not for
    425
Calmness, and faith 377
  qualification of nurses 407
Camp meetings, Australian, lec-
    tures on health at 467
  diet at 121
  establishment of health enter-
    prises to follow 468
  labors of medical men at, invited
    433
  preparation for proper diet at
    142
  teaching health reform at 467
  temperance reform urged at 433
  use of literature in work at 465
  See also General meetings.
Cancers largely caused by meat
    eating 133
Canvassers, opportunities of, to
    minister to sick 463
  to teach health principles
    462, 463
  pioneer work of, in medical mis-
    sionary lines 397
  pray for sick 464
Canvassing for health publications
    463
Card playing, Heaven condemns
    195
  tendency of 197
Cause of God, advanced as fruit of
    denial of appetite 131
  consider always as a whole 516
  needs varied talents 516
  neglect no phase of 518
  old landmarks of, to stand
    521, 522
  See also Work of God.
Censure, duty to refrain from 518
  words of, readily spoken against
    God's workers 297
  See also Faultfinding; Criticism.
Centers, for medical missionary
    work, Loma Linda, Mel-
    rose 554-556
  neglect of medical missionary
    work in American 448
  of influence, in all our cities 481
Centralization, contrary to Chris-
    tian principles 217
  counsels regarding 224-227, 275,
    276, 299, 300, 312, 510
Chaplain, qualifications of 289
Character, deformed, mothers
    less concerned with, than
    with dress 601

formed in early youth 112
  given to work, by faithfulness to
    standard 276
  healthy life necessary for perfec-
    tion of 41
  index of future society 112
  perfection of, how attained 384
  power of association to mold 415
  read by associates 363
  ruined through self-indulgence
    14
  shaped by little things of life
    404
  shown by choice of associates
    624
  stability of, how attained 362
  virtuous, useful employment
    an aid to 187
Charity, of institutions, for others
    less favored 308, 309
  of workers, for those in need 308
Charities, organized, work of indi-
    viduals not to be left to 390
Chastity, laws of, transgressed by
    medical men 365
Checkers, Heaven condemns 195
Cheerfulness, aids digestion 53
  essential qualification for nurses
    406
  outdoor life fosters 167
  promotes circulation 54
Cheese, children permitted to
    eat 176
Chess, Heaven condemns 195
Children, care for nervous, regard-
    ing study and exercise 178
  care of clothes to be taught to 103
  confinement of, in school, how
    injurious 176, 177
  cooking to be taught to 486
  diseased, because of appetite of
    parents 78
  "eat to live" 609
  educated in self-indulgence 126
  evil influence of fashion upon
    600, 601
  moral wrecks, parents account-
    able for 610
  neglect to correct habits of,
    brings bitterness 429
  of believers, hypocritical, stum-
    blingblock to others 614
  permitted to eat meat, spices,
    cheese 176
  read to, regarding health 427
  responsibility of parents in
    bringing into world 75
  rules for healthy development
    of 178
  wrong habits of eating take
    heavy toll of 176
Children of God, shining amid dark-
    ness and poverty 14

Christ, attitude of family toward
work of 526
communion of, with nature, reveals secret of power 162
compassion of, for suffering 30,
31, 34
expects disciples to follow closely
in missionary work 511, 512
family of, could not fathom His
mission 527
great Medical Missionary 526-529
Great Physician, today as of old
529
healed all who came 498
healing blind man 30, 31
humble earthly lot of 226
imparting a stream of healing
power 526
interpreted the gospel in His
ministry 498
laying His hands upon afflicted
526
love of, how measured 534
lover of nature 163
medical missionary in every
sense 317, 318
missionary of highest type 535
never was an evangelist like 318
welcomes discouraging conditions
26
work of, hindered by unbelief 31
world's need of 25
Christ's manner of healing 30, 31
Christian Endeavor Society, form
company somewhat like 537
Christian service, organization of
companies for 396, 397
Christians, professed, example of
moral corruption among
618-621
sickly, in our midst 592
Church, duty of, toward reform 517
empowered to do same work
Christ did 529
influence of, increased by faithfulness to health reform 452
reformed in the home 430
reliance of, in power of faith
and obedience 226
responsibility of, toward poor
and suffering 229, 230
throwing burden of sick on
sanitarium 230
too many sick Christians in 592
Church members, all to have part
in building up the work 223
appeal to, for purity of life
623-626
awake to medical missionary
work 425-430
blinded to sin of licentious life
623

duty of, to circulate our literature 464
to engage in medical missionary work 548
to engage in missionary work
546
exhortation to, to labor for souls
548
moral corruption among 583
present-day work of 356
stand as reformers 425
study medical missionary books
for preparation 426
teach health principles 443, 444
See also People of God.
Churches, establishing, all to have
part in 223
popular, resistance to truth by
ministers of 357
Circulation, all parts of body
benefited by 587
cheerfulness beneficial to 54
dependent on exercise 173
perfect health requires perfect
93
poor, effect of 173, 174
quickened by frequent bathing
104
See also Blood.
City missions, intelligent women in
charge of cooking in 449
teaching health principles at
443, 444
treatment rooms needed at 468
See also Medical missionary work.
City surroundings unfavorable to
sanitarium work 267, 273
City work, able physicians in 550
redeem the time in 555, 556
Cities, centers of influence in, men
of wealth will help establish
551
Christ often withdrew from 162
conducting cooking schools in
551, 552
difficulties in working in,
increasing 547
Eastern 547
entreat church members in, to
lay hold upon work 548
hygienic restaurants in 481-491
judgments visited upon 268, 556
labors of Christ in 396, 500
large, conditions in 487
medical missionary work, a door
of entrance to 392, 556
represented in all 393-395
medical missionaries to enter 219
most favorable time for work in,
past 556
physicians and ministers, needed
for 548
to unite in labor for 545, 546

choose practical, if one-sided is necessary 180

cookery a most important branch of 145-153

defective, cause of general intemperance and depravity 607

health not to be sacrificed to obtain 186

in health reform necessary 475-479

in housekeeping, importance of 146, 147

mistaken ideas regarding 182, 186

of medical missionaries, how made complete 516

of workers for gospel service 396

physical labor part of 183

practical, essential 180

riches a curse when they deprive youth of 186

street, acquired through indolence 187

See also Schools.

Educational work must stand as a unit 394, 395

Efficiency, in sanitarium work 260

in workers, health a condition of 193, 194

result of self-denial 573

sanitarium workers to seek 398

Effluvium, poisonous, rising from decaying matter 62

Effort, and prayer, business of life 367

Christ recognizes every, to find access to souls 538, 539

independent, dangers in 514

united, strength in 514-518

Eggs, for small children 136

not to be classed with flesh meats 478

reasons for eventually discarding 478

sometimes beneficial 478

Elect of God, bodies of, made holy 20

to stand untainted 20

Elegance, comfort to be sought before 277

Elements, Satan works through 460

Elijah, message of, to Ahaziah 455

Employees, restaurant, responsibilities of managers toward 483

Employment, for invalids 174

safeguard against evil habits 183, 187

sedentary, sought by many 183

useful, a substitute for unwholesome pleasure 190

Encouragement, speak words of, to workers 243

Endowments, health and spiritual, God has in store for us 139

Energy, exhausted through overwork 98, 99

Entertainments, exciting, effect of, on patients 240

Enthusiasm, need of 35

Epistles, living, workers to be 560

Errors, wrong habits of diet lead to 67

Esau, results to, of indulgence of appetite 110

Europe, establishment of sanitariums in 216, 218, 224

Evangelism, Christ's methods of 34

Evangelists, none like Christ 317, 318

nurses as 395, 396

training of, as medical missionaries 541, 542

See also Medical missionary evangelists.

Eve, temptation and fall of, through appetite 108

Evening, labor not to be prolonged into 99

Evils, neglect of correcting, results in dishonor to parents 429

Example, importance of right 559-562

more powerful than sermons 537

of Christ, to institutional workers 316-318

physicians to be, of principles they teach 547

terrible power of 298

See also Pattern.

Excess, consequences of, be not ignorant of 38

in eating, drinking, and dressing, becomes crime 24

Exercise, aid in regaining health 174

and circulation of blood 173

and diet 572-574

as a restorer 199-201

essential to health 181

healthful, works miracles 171

in garden, pleasing to God 564

lack of, fruitful cause of disease 173

mental and physical, combined 572

mental without physical, effects of 178

not to be neglected 405

outdoor, benefits of, to patients 267

part of regular treatment 171

physical, and labor, benefits of, to patients 200

clothing to be suitable for 52

22—C.O.H.

needs periods of rest 118, 119, 157, 158

overloading, results of 157-160

results of abuse of, on disposition 577, 578

vitality drawn from brain because of abuse of 46

Stomach and brain, sympathy between 134

Stones, rough, fitting for immortality 44

Storybooks and novels, evil results of reading 188

Stove, hovering over 97

Strength, asked from God, then consumed on altar of lust 620, 621

See also Passions.

expending sinfully 43

our source of 593

physical, value of 186

See also Physical.

Students, cooking to be taught to 551

education of, as medical missionaries, for efficient service 557, 558

in principles of healthful living 301

flesh foods not to be served to 130

taught lessons from nature 164

training of, as medical missionaries 419, 541, 542

See also Schools; Education; Teachers; Youth.

Students and teachers, companionship of 191

Study, and exercise to correspond 178

and prayer, value of, for medical workers 361, 362

children injured by too much 176, 177

health books, in home 427

health lost through too much 185

ministers unfitted for pastoral work by constant 193

of nature, health and happiness in 178

relaxation from, a necessity 196

without physical exercise, evils of 179-183

workers to combine exercise with 572, 573

See also Education.

Submission and faith 377-379

Success, danger in 367

God's blessing indispensable to 256

how obtained by sanitarium workers 274

institutional, secret of 263

not gained by expensive dress 292

only through sacrifice 316

proportionate to liberality 309

secret of 255

in sanitariums 205, 256, 278

true, bears heavenly credentials 286

Sufferers, heaven interested in relief of 532

not to be neglected on Sabbath 236

promises of God's word to 213

subjects for tenderest pity and care 385

Suffering, increase of, toward end 506

malady of soul cause of physical 502

regarded as our common lot 19

result of familiarity with, to physicians 326

result of transgression 49

of parents 37

See also Sick; Sickness; Disease.

Sufferings of Christ, our life 332

Sugar, clogs the system 149

evils of free use of 149, 150, 154

substituted for meat 149, 150

See also Diet; Food.

Sugar and milk, harmful combination 149, 150

Suggestions, impure, forsake those who breathe 625, 626

Sunlight, and air, abundant use of 54

in the home 196

true remedy 90

Sunshine, God's means for restoring sick 166

Superintendents, culture and experience needed by 257

Supper, light 156

Surgeon, high wages for 314

Suspicion, words of, against God's workers 297

Sydney Sanitarium, God's design in establishing 221-223

Sympathy, in patients and helpers 350

promotes health and prolongs life 344

to be cultivated 501

See also Compassion.

TABERNACLE, building of, illustration of building institutions 278

Table spread in wilderness, at Avondale 495

See also Avondale.